RHEUMATOLOGY FOR THE HEALTH CARE PROFESSIONAL

HARRY SPIERA, M.D., F.A.C.P.

Dr. Harry Spiera is a physician with broad interests in clinical and investigative rheumatology. He received his M.D. degree from New York University School of Medicine and served his internship and residency at the Mount Sinai Hospital in New York City and at the Veterans Administration Hospital in Brooklyn. He did his rheumatology training at the Columbia University School of Physicians and Surgeons as a Fellow of the Arthritis Foundation. He is current Chief of the Division of Rheumatology at the Mount Sinai School of Medicine and Clinical Professor of Medicine. He is Chairman Emeritus of the Clinical Advisory Board of the SLE Foundation and Chairman of the Medical Advisory Board of the Scleroderma Society. He also serves on the Medical Advisory Board of the Sjogren's Syndrome Foundation. He is a past president of the New York Rheumatism Association.

His research interests are broad. They include the initial description of polymyalgia rheumatica in the United States and subsequent study of its natural history and relationship to giant-cell arteritis. His investigations have also included a study of tryptophane metabolism as it relates to rheumatoid arthritis and other connective tissue diseases. He also has studied rheumatoid factor in rheumatoid arthritis and other chronic disease states in association with Dr. Oreskes. He has described the association of augmentation mammoplasty to scleroderma. His present interests also include the relationship of brain-specific antibodies to central nervous system lupus. He is a Fellow of both the American College of Physicians and the American College of Rheumatology.

IRVIN ORESKES, Ph.D.

Dr. Irwin Oreskes is a scientific researcher, biochemist, and educator in New York City. He received his Ph.D. in Chemistry from the City University of New York. He is currently a member of the Biochemistry graduate faculty of C.U.N.Y., Professor of Medical Laboratory Sciences at Hunter College, and Research Associate Professor at the Mount Sinai School of Medicine. Much of his scientific research has been concerned with the immunology of rheumatoid factor and altered immunoglobulin G in rheumatic diseases. In collaboration with Dr. Spiera he has shown that chronic stimulation of humans with insulin or with heroin can stimulate formation of rheumatoid-factor-like antibodies. He has studied rheumatoid factor model systems in animals and has developed various laboratory tests for clinical chemistry and diagnostic immunology.

Dr. Oreskes is a past dean of Hunter College's School of Health Sciences where he developed an innovative undergraduate program in Medical Laboratory Sciences. He has a continuing interest in the education and networking of different health professionals. He is a member of numerous scienfific organizations including the American Association of Immunologists, the American Association for Clinical Chemistry, and the American College of Rheumatology. He has been a Visiting Professor at The Johns Hopkins University and a Visiting Lecturer at the Welsh National University and other academic institutions.

RHEUMATOLOGY FOR THE HEALTH CARE PROFESSIONAL

Editors

HARRY SPIERA, M.D., F.A.C. P.

Clinical Professor of Medicine; Chief, Division of Rheumatology, The Mount Sinai School of Medicine of C.U.N.Y., New York, N.Y.

IRWIN ORESKES, Ph.D.

Professor of Medical Laboratory Sciences, Hunter College of C.U.N.Y., New York, N.Y.; Director, Rheumatology Laboratory and Research Associate Professor of Medicine Mount Sinai School of Medicine, New York, N.Y.

WARREN H. GREEN, INC.
St. Louis, Missouri, U.S.A.

Published by

WARREN H. GREEN, INC.
8356 Olive Boulevard
St. Louis, Missouri 63132, U.S.A.

ISBN No. 0-87527-464-1

Printed in the United States of America

LIST OF CONTRIBUTORS

LELAND ABBEY, M.D.
Director, Division of Rheumatology
Veterans Administration Hospital
Bronx, New York

JOHN L. ABRUZZO, M.D.
Professor of Medicine
Thomas Jefferson University
Philadelphia, Pennsylvania

BRUCE R. BENDER, M.D.
Fellow, Division of Rheumatology
Jefferson Medical College
Philadelphia, Pennsylvania

BURTON R. BERSON, M.D.
Associate Clinical Professor of Orthopaedic Surgery
The Mount Sinai School of Medicine
New York, New York
Chief of Sports Medicine
Associate Attending Physician
Montefiore Hospital
Bronx, New York

BETTE BLAU, M.A., ADTR
Director of Movement Therapy
Little Village School
Adelphia University
Garden City, New York

SHELDON BLAU, M.D.
Clinical Professor of Medicine
State University of New York at Stoney Brook
Chief of Rheumatology
Nassau County Medical Center
Merrick, New York

MARTIN V. COHEN, Ph.D.
Clinical Psychologist
New York Hospital-Cornell Medical Center
Department of Psychiatry
New York, New York

JAMES M. CORRY, Ph.D.
Department of Health Education
The Mount Sinai Medical Center
New York, New York

ENID W. ENGELHARD, M.S.W./C.S.W.
Director of Social Services
SLE Foundation, Inc.
New York, New York

SANDY B. GANZ, M.S., P.T.
Senior Physical Therapist
Rheumatic Disease Unit
The Hospital for Special Surgery
New York, New York

ELLEN M. GINZLER, M.D., M.P.H.
Associate Professor of Medicine
State University of New York
Health Science Center at Brooklyn
Brooklyn, New York

DOROTHY GOLDSTEIN, M.S.
Director of Medical Affairs
New York Chapter of the
Arthritis Foundation
New York, New York

ROBERT A. GREENWALD, M.D.
Chief of Rheumatology
Long Island Jewish Medical Center
New Hyde Park, New York
Professor of Medicine
State University of New York at
Stoney Brook
Stoney Brook, New York

ALLAN JOSEPHSON, M.D.
Professor of Medicine
State University of New York
Downstate Medical Center
Brooklyn, New York

THOMAS G. KANTOR, M.D.
Professor of Clinical Medicine
New York University School of Medicine
New York, New York

LESLIE KERR, M.D.
Assistant Professor of Medicine
Division of Rheumatology
The Mount Sinai School of Medicine
New York, New York

JUDITH L. KLINGER, O.T.R., M.A.
Senior Occupational Therapist
District Nursing Association
Ridgefield, Connecticut

ROGER N. LEVY, M.D.
Clinical Professor of Orthopaedics
Chief of Arthritis Surgery
The Mount Sinai Medical Center
New York, New York

ESTHER LIPSTEIN, M.D.
Physician-in-Charge
Division of Rheumatology
Queens Hospital Center
Jamaica, New York

MICHAEL D. LOCKSHIN, M.D.
Professor of Medicine
The Hospital for Special Surgery - Cornell Medical Center
New York, New York

RONALD W. MOSKOWITZ, M.D.
Professor of Medicine
Case Western Reserve University
Director, Division of Rheumatic Diseases
University Hospitals of Cleveland
Cleveland, Ohio

IRWIN ORESKES, Ph.D.
Professor of Medical Laboratory Sciences
Hunter College of the C.U.N.Y.
Director, Rheumatology Laboratory and
Research Associate Professor of Medicine
The Mount Sinai School of Medicine of the C.U.N.Y.
New York, New York

K.T. RAJAN, B.Sc., M.B., Ph.D.
Consultant Physician
Department of Rheumatology
East Glamorgan General Hospital
South Wales, Great Britain

ITZHAK A. ROSNER, M.D.
Assistant Professor of Medicine
Division of Rheumatic Diseases
Case Western Reserve University
Cleveland, Ohio

JOYCE Z. SINGER, M.D.
Assistant Professor of Medicine
State University of New York - Health Sciences Center at Brooklyn
Brooklyn, New York

HARRY SPIERA, M.D.
Clinical Professor of Medicine
Chief, Division of Rheumatology
The Mount Sinai School of Medicine
New York, New York

MARY BETTY STEVENS, M.D.
Professor of Medicine
Johns Hopkins University School of Medicine
Baltimore, Maryland

MERYL SUFIAN, Ph.D.
Senior Project Director
Narcotic and Drug Research, Inc.
New York, New York

FREDERICK SWERDLOW, M.D.
Associate Clinical Professor of Medicine
The Mount Sinai School of Medicine
New York, New York

RAMON VALLARINO, M.D.
Director
Rehabilitation Medicine
The Methodist Hospital
Brooklyn, New York

TS'AI-FAN YU, M.D.
Professor of Medicine, Emeritus
The Mount Sinai Medical Center
New York, New York

FOREWORD

Harry Spiera, M.D.
Irwin Oreskes, Ph.D.

Paleontologists tell us that the dinosaur was sometimes a victim of arthritis. Evidence of arthritis have been found in the skeletal remains of prehistoric man. Afflictions involving the musculoskeletal system have been also described by medical writers since antiquity. Gout, one of the more painful and common rheumatic entities was well known to Hippocrates in the fifth century B.C. The later extensive development of baths or spas by the Romans was at least in part an attempt at treatment of rheumatic complaints. By the sixteenth century the word 'rheumatism' was in use to describe certain severe musculoskeletal problems. In the late nineteenth century the entity 'rheumatoid arthritis' had been described. The twentieth century has seen an ever accelerating development of knowledge of the multitude of rheumatic diseases. Since World War II with the more sophisticated application of basic science, clinical science and epidemiology, our understanding of these many diseases has increased exponentially. Today we recognize many rheumatic disease distinguishable from one another by clinical and/or laboratory characteristics.

For all our progress, understanding is still in an early phase and 'new' rheumatic diseases heretofore unrecognized continue to be defined. One example is Lyme arthritis which was first described in 1975. Since then its etiology has been determined and effective treatment made available. The history of how we came to understand this condition exemplifies the successful application of the tools of clinical observation, epidemiology, entomology and microbiology to the solution of a serious medical problem, and illustrates a successful multidisciplinary approach to a medical problem.

Unfortunately the successful resolution of the Lyme disease problem is something of an exception. In the majority of the rheumatic diseases we still do not have a clear-cut knowledge of etiology or cure. Historically this has resulted in the development of a variety of therapeutic approaches, developed by different professions: physician and non-physician, in an attempt to control symptoms, and to retain and restore functional capacity. Unfortunately, this diversity of approach has often been marked by less than ideal inter-disciplinary communication among the concerned health professionals.

Until that happy day when one or more 'magic bullets' are available for specific treatment of the various rheumatic diseases, it may be expected that multi-disciplinary approaches will continue. Even if specific therapies are eventually developed for some of the rheumatic diseases it is likely that the prevalence of certain musculoskeletal problems will increase. This increase is a consequence of the inevitable deterioration of bones, joints and connective tissue that seem to occur with aging. It is clear that longevity is increasing and with it the average age of our population. Thus the need for various health care professionals expert in treating these problems will remain for the foreseeable future.

One of the purposes of this book is to enhance cross-disciplinary understanding among health workers with similar goals in treatment of rheumatic diseases. Adequate educational materials for physicians are available as are increasingly improved material for patients and lay persons. However, material for non-physician health professionals in the rheumatic diseases is inadequate. This book hopes to help fill that need. It is not a textbook of rheumatology and does not attempt to substitute for standard works in the field. What this book does attempt to do is provide concise summaries of the major rheumatic diseases and of therapeutic approaches as developed by different concerned health professionals. Certain social problems are also explored. Chapters are written by known experts who cover major aspects of the rheumatic diseases. They vary in difficulty but all include a bibliography for additional readings.

We hope the book will be of value to:

a) Health professionals primarily concerned with the rheumatic diseases.

b) Other health professionals with peripheral interest.

c) Undergraduate students contemplating careers in one of the health professions.

d) Medical students, residents and physicians with minimal training and experience with rheumatic diseases.

New knowledge about the rheumatic disease is accumulating at an ever increasingly rapid rate. One cannot predict when the 'magic bullets' will be available but one can say with a reasonable degree of certainty that more specific treatments will in time be achieved. When that day comes, health care workers must be prepared to adjust their professional practices in light of new realities. All health professionals need to perfect their understanding to improve their work and to adjust to changing knowledge. Those wedded to particular techniques or diseases may find themselves left behind and cast in the role of obsolete technicians, regardless of their professional credentials and academic degrees. More important, for the patient's benefit, there is need today for better utilization of the information that we do have and better cross-discipline organization and cooperation of the professionals devoted to arthritis health care. It is the editors hope that this book by providing information and by raising some controversial questions will be helpful in achieving these goals.

INTRODUCTION

Irwin Oreskes, Ph.D.
Harry Spiera, M.D.

The array of medical conditions encompassed under the heading "rheumatic" can be bewildering in its extent and variety. More than 100 such diseases are listed in the most recent edition of the *Primer on the Rheumatic Diseases*.* Perusal of this list (see Appendix) will give the reader some idea of the diversity of rheumatic illness. The term "rheuma" used in the writings of Hippocrates have in modern times come to describe that classification of diseases which in one way or another affect the bones, muscles, tendons, cartilage, or other tissues and fluids that make up our joints. In addition to diseases associated with the skeletal system, many rheumatic diseases may also affect the diffuse connective tissue which surrounds cells and organs throughout the body.

The rheumatic diseases represent one of the major public health problems in the U.S. today. It has been suggested that more than 35 million people are affected by one or another of these diseases—a number that approaches 15% of our population. It has been estimated that degenerative joint disease i.e. osteoarthritis (OA) may affect some 16 million, rheumatoid arthritis (RA) 2.5 million; systemic lupus erythematosus (SLE) 500,000; scleroderma and ankylosing spondylitis (AS) 200,000 each and juvenile rheumatoid arthritis (JRA) 100,000 individuals. Added to these numbers are the millions affected with lower back pain or degenerative disc disease. While these conditions are not generally classified as 'rheumatic' they do impinge on the health care system and on arthritis health care workers in a major way.

These figures are admittedly rough estimates. For example, OA is very common in older age. A great majority of those over 55 will show some x-ray signs (but not clinical signs) of this disease. Since the disease is chronic with no presently known cause or cure, it is likely that the number of cases of OA requiring care will continue to increase as the population ages.

Nearly all other rheumatic diseases are also chronic and, here too, we cannot identify their cause or administer their cure. Various epidemiologic studies indicate that the number of *new* cases per year for RA is about 200,000 and for

SLE, about 20,000. Since these diseases are chronic and direct fatal outcomes uncommon, the number of affected individuals continues to increase. This is true even though most of these diseases are not age-linked.

The financial impact of arthritis on the health care system is quite remarkable. It was estimated that in 1982, the total cost ascribed to the rheumatic diseases was about $14 billion, which may be divided roughly into $8 billion for care and $6 billion in lost wages and taxes. Of the care costs, $1.3 billion went to physician providers and $0.3 billion to various non-physician providers. More recent data suggests that the percentage of payments to non-M.D. therapists is increasing.

Nearly $3 billion is currently being spent on drugs and medicines with about 40% of this sum going for non-prescription over-the counter remedies. The very large market for both prescription and non-prescription arthritis drugs has no doubt stimulated development work in the pharmaceutical industry and may be related to the proliferation of NSAID's currently available. Non-proven remedies and "quack" nostrums probably account for an additional $2 billion a year.

It is clear even from these fragmentary data that the cost of care for rheumatic disease patients is considerable. Recognizing that most patients, especially those receiving surgical care are over 65, much of this economic impact is carried by Medicare and Medicaid programs. It is to be expected that with the increasing average age of our population this impact will only increase. Return of inflationary pressures would make the impact worse. In an attempt to moderate these costs the Federal Government has instituted the Diagnosis Related Groups (DRG) system of reimbursement for hospital care, whose primary goal is to limit costs. How this program will impact on both availability and quality of rheumatic disease care is a major health issue today.

It is an article of faith but one amply sustained by past experience that research is the best way to solve the many unanswered questions about etiology, pathogenesis, and treatment of the various rheumatic diseases. In 1986, the Federal Government funded arthritis research and care through the N.I.A.M.S.D. at under $117 million, a sum less than 3% of the total N.I.H. budget. In view of the tremendous social cost of rheumatic diseases, the Arthritis Foundation has argued that the federally funded arthritis research has been and continues to be inadequate. A federal policy which directs medical research funds truly based on societal needs and not on the 'disease of the month' still seems to elude us.

In general, the rheumatic diseases are not characterized by striking increases in mortality. Reliable data are difficult to obtain and individual outcomes often depend on which organ systems are affected. Thus, it is rare to attribute a death to the direct consequences of OA. In RA where systemic involvement is more apparent direct mortality is nevertheless low. However a decrease in life expectancy has been noted. By contrast, scleroderma carries with it significant mortality. The death rate in this condition is about 25% over 10 years. SLE was once thought to be invariably fatal. Now 50% of patients with this condition are alive 15 years after onset. In general, death rates among all rheumatic disease patients have been dropping, this for a number of reasons: 1) Therapeutic improvement, 2) Increase in diagnoses of less severe cases, and 3) Reduced mortality of major non-rheumatic diseases such as coronary disease and stroke.

It is a part of folk-lore that 'arthritis' is a disease of cold and damp places, but modern epidemiologic research does not support this notion. Rheumatoid arthritis has been found wherever it has been looked for, in hot climates as well as in cold. Indeed, the Pima Indians who inhabit the desert Southwest have a higher incidence of RA than the Blackfeet from the cooler Canadian plains. The incidence of RA is the same in Scotland as in Jamaica or the Philippines. Part of the difficulty is one of recognition. It is primarily in advanced Western societies where problems of acute infectious disease have (more or less) been solved that sufficient medical talent is available and concerned to correctly distinguish the various rheumatic diseases. In poor African nations where people have shortened life expectancies and there is limited availability of medical resources, few live long enough to develop OA and those that do are simply ignored by the overburdened existing health care systems. These considerations may give an unwarranted geographic cast to the question of rheumatic disease incidence.

The geographic issue is sometimes confused with the genetic issue. Certain populations have shown distinct predilections to one or another of the rheumatic diseases. The high incidence of RA among the Pimas previously referred to is a case in point. To cite another example, the Maoris of New Zealand have an extraordinarily high incidence (5%) of ankylosing spondylitis.

Gender distribution is a special case of genetic predilection. A number of the rheumatic diseases show increased incidence among females as compared to males, i.e. RA 2.5:1; SLE 5:1, scleroderma 2:1, dermatomyositis 2:1. On the other hand, male predominance is observed in gout, 9:1, and ankylosing spondylitis 3:1. The role of specific sex hormones is suspected but not well understood.

We are beginning to understand the genetic effect in a more insightful way. Extensive studies of tissue transplantation rejection in humans have demonstrated that such reactions are governed by the human leukocyte antigen (HLA) system. For transplants to "take" there must be HLA compatibility between donor and recipient. Since there are over 80 such antigens compatibility is not easily obtained. An unexpected and as yet not well understood phenomena is the finding that the presence of certain HLA-antigen subtypes is associated with an increased incidence of certain of the rheumatic diseases. Thus, individuals who are positive for HLA-B27 are 85 times as likely to develop ankylosing spondylitis as compared to those who are HLA-B27 negative. For Reiter's syndrome this enhanced frequency is 35 times. RA is similarly associated with the DR-4 antigen. Those who are positive for this antigen are 6 times as likely to develop RA compared to those who are negative.

It is of some historical interest that genetic aspects of disease were recognized long before genetics itself was defined as a science. To site just one example, Thomas Belt in 1874 (Belt, T. 'A Naturalist in Nicaragua'. U. Chicago Press 1985, Reprint of 1874 London Edition), noted that "white terriers are more subject than darker-coloured ones to the attack of the fatal distemper." After giving other examples of disease among peaches, chickens, etc., he noted that "immunity from disease is correlated with some slight difference in colour or structure...."

To describe the association between expression of a particular disease and the presence of a particular HLA sub-type is not to explain it. This issue remains as one of the most intriguing questions in medicine today. The mechanisms of these associations remain unknown and it must be emphasized that possession of one of these disease-associated genes does not ensure expression of that particular disease. Thus the vast majority of HLA-B27 positive individuals never develop AS. Unknown environmental factors or physical or psychological stress may serve as precipitating factors in genetically predisposed individuals. One or more fundamental enzyme defects in gout leads to over-production of the end product of purine breakdown uric acid and to formation of urate precipitates in the joints. Hyperuricemic individuals are probably genetically predisposed and in those individuals ingestion of a diet rich in purines may well precipitate or exacerbate gout. Treatment of gouty individuals with low purine diets is often beneficial. The converse does not seem to be true, i.e. purine rich diets do not necessarily trigger gout in non-prone individuals. The question of diet as a stimulant (or therapy!) for many other rheumatic diseases is an area of much discussion and some experimentation. Thus far, other than in gout, convincing relationships have not been established.

Rheumatic disease arising from infections has been recognized for a long time. Arthritis as a consequence of direct joint infection has been described following gonorrhea, tuberculosis, and staphylococcus among others. Lyme arthritis is known to follow certain tick bites and the causative agent is a spirochete. Viral infections, such as rubella are known to cause arthritis.

More interesting from the theoretical viewpoint are those infections that lead to so-called 'reactive' arthritis, i.e., where the organism cannot be demonstrated in the affected joint. This class includes the arthritides following streptococcal (rheumatic fever) or yersinia infection. Reiter's disease is the arthritis which sometimes follows a chlamydia or shigella infection. Many investigators believe this is a more general phenomenon and that RA itself is precipitated by a prior infection by some as yet unidentified organism. All attempts to identify this organism by culturing it from rheumatic synovial fluid have thus far been unavailing.

Most of the rheumatic diseases other than OA are not diseases of old age. RA is seen in children under 2 years of age and pediatric rheumatology is now a recognized subspecialty. SLE is typically seen in young woman from 20 to 40 years of age. However, both of these conditions can and do begin at any age. Therefore, as longevity increases the number of people affected by some rheumatic disease will increase.

OA is perhaps another matter. It is the most widespread of the rheumatic diseases. X-ray and other data has shown evidence of cartilage erosion in some individuals as early as the third decade of life and in 85% of individuals in the 6th decade of life. By age 65 nearly everyone has some sign of the condition. Yet in spite of that no more than 20% of older individuals seem to need medical attention for this condition.

The statistics suggest that some form of cartilage breakdown is an inevitable consequence of aging. What is perhaps not inevitable is that this process must lead to pain or crippling and overt disease. The factors which distinguish, mitigate or prevent overt cartilage disease in old age (in contrast to cartilage erosion) remain unclear.

The rheumatic diseases represent the quintessential chronic disease. Here the realistic goals of therapy are rarely to achieve cures. More often, these goals are to minimize pain, maintain function, slow the progression of the disease and, thereby, improve the quality of life of the patient. Since no cure presently exists for the majority of the rheumatic diseases, a wide variety of therapeutic techniques have been utilized—many useful, some spurious. Evaluation of the merits of any therapy has been difficult and complicating the matter is the pattern of spontaneous remission and exacerbation which characterizes RA and many other rheumatic diseases. It is this pattern that often lends plausibility to assorted anecdotal and unproven therapies when in fact the good results allegedly achieved are due to no more than coincidence.

The multiplicity of legitimate therapies has led to participation in rheumatic health care of a wide variety of health practitioners. In today's pattern of practice, most patients are first seen by primary care or general practice physicians or by internists. Where severity of disease or difficulty of diagnosis makes it appropriate, rheumatologists are called to diagnose, evaluate or prescribe.

Here pathways may diverge. Where the surgical approach seems appropriate then orthopedic surgeons do their thing. If the medical or pharmacologic approach seems best then rheumatologists continue to supervise patient care. All of these physicians may turn to the skills of other non-MD health professionals, e.g. physical and occupational therapists, rehabilitation specialists and orthodists for assorted specialized procedures.

Another branch of medicine, physiatry, has been playing an increasing role in management of some rheumatic patients, especially those whose care requires extensive service by non-MD therapists. Acceptance of the role of physiatrists is varied. They have been striving to define their special place in rheumatic health care.

Insofar as other health care workers play important roles in care of ill patients, so is there a role in rheumatic care for psychiatrists, psychologists, social workers, dieticians, nurses, geriatricians and health educators.

This multiplicity of therapists (and therapies) is at the present time both understandable and useful. Each offers approaches and techniques which in one patient or another may prove to be beneficial. Yet to the patient or for that matter to the general care physician, this array of practitioners can be bewildering. The role of each individual practitioner in the larger picture can likewise be bewildering. Issues of collaboration, cooperation, coordination and organization are serious and pressing if *appropriate* high quality and cost effective care is to be delivered to individual patients.

"Fish Gotta Swim, Birds Gotta Fly." Most therapist (non-MD and MD) are impelled in greater or lesser degree to do what they know best. It sometimes takes more maturity and sophistication to say "no" than to say "yes" to a patient seeking a particular form of therapy. How do we avoid, let alone define, the twin problems of undertreatment vs. overtreatment. In the present state of health care organization, overtreatment tends to be widespread. Some feel that with the development of Federal DRG programs there may be a danger of going the other way. In dealing with these issues one must be mindful that most rheumatic patients at any given time are not very sick and may be reasonably managed with minimal health care. Probably no more than 10% of rheumatic patients require at any given time the full panoply of sophisticated health care. The problem is to make a rational choice between 'more' and 'less.'

It may be argued that there is no such thing as 'more,' that life and well being should not be measured by money and that everything that is technically and scientifically possible should be made available. We have no philosophic quarrel with this view but we must point out that the question put this way is essentially a political one. In practice the politics of health care determine how much society spends on research, on therapy, on rehabilitation. The decision or perhaps better, the compromise is forced on government only after multiple voices contend. These voices represent pragmatic interests more often than idealist theorists. In general the quantity if not the quality of health care is commensurate with the effectiveness and strength of its proponents.

While we believe that greater funds wisely spent are needed for rheumatic disease research and care, we also believe that there can be such a thing as overtreatment—be it excess medication, excess manipulation or excess hospitalization.

How to guard against this tendency? Probably the poorest way is via bureaucratic DRG programs that limit reimbursable hospitalization and therapy to certain experiential averages. While 'policing' may have some value we think that policies which encourage cooperative and comprehensive care may be more effective in lowering health care costs without lowering health care quality.

Additionally we argue for improved education of patients and families so that they better understand their diseases, their therapies and the prospects for improvement. Such education encourages patients to take an active role in their own treatment. Of equal importance is the education of health professionals to better understanding of each other's roles and to develop cooperative approaches in advancing the well being of the patients entrusted to their care.

TABLE OF CONTENTS

III THERAPEUTICS

IV SOCIAL, PSYCHOLOGICAL AND CULTURAL ISSUES

APPENDICES

RHEUMATOLOGY FOR THE HEALTH CARE PROFESSIONAL

I BIOLOGY

"Every country has its particular diseases; the varieties of climate, exposure, soil, situation, trades, arts, manufactures and even the character of a People all pave the way to new complaints, and vary the appearance of those with which we are already acquainted."

A Discourse Upon the Duties of a Physician, C.S. Van Winkle, New York, N.Y., 1819, p. 16.

CHAPTER 1

THE JOINT

Leslie Kerr, M.D.

INTRODUCTION

The joints of the human body endow an otherwise rigid skeleton with the capacity for frictionless motion, stability, and the capacity to withstand compressive forces greater than that of body weight. These attributes in turn allow for the controlled, directed movements necessary for locomotion and coordination. The purpose of this chapter is to describe the structure of joints in order to gain an understanding of how they function.

TYPES OF JOINTS

The joints of the body are classified into three groups: synarthroses, amphiarthroses, and diarthroses.

Synarthroses are immovable joints composed of fibrous tissue, such as sutures between the bones of the skull.

Amphiarthroses contain fibrocartilaginous tissue and are capable of limited motion. Examples of this type of joint are the pubic symphysis and the intervertebral discs.

Diarthrodial joints are those which permit a wide range of motion. Comprising most of the joints in the extremities as well as the intervertebral facet joints, this type of joint is most frequently affected by the pathologic processes to be described in subsequent chapters. These joints are characterized by the presence of a synovial membrane.

STRUCTURE AND FUNCTION OF SYNOVIAL JOINTS — See Figure 1-1

Muscle

The striated muscle surrounding the joint are attached to bone by fibrous tissue bundles known as tendons. Like ligaments, muscles stabilize the joint, via their tendinous insertions to bone, by limiting motion to a single plane and preventing joint rotation. Unlike ligaments, striated muscles contrast voluntarily. This permits ongoing, protective adjustments of joint position and motion.

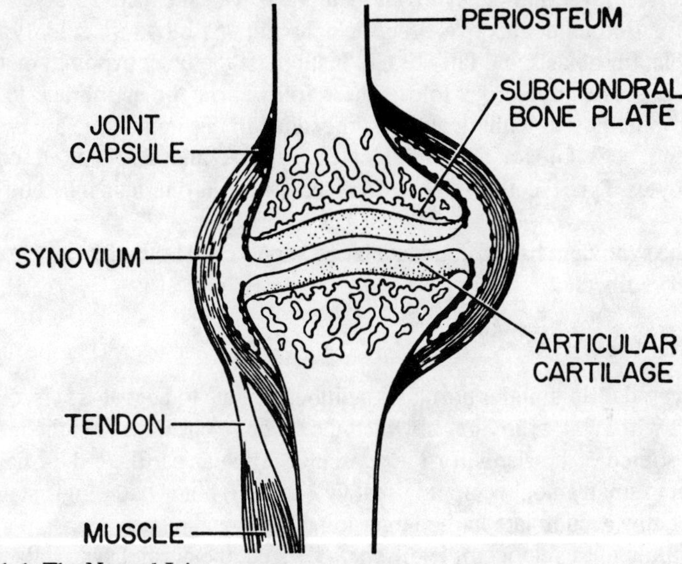

Figure 1-1: The Normal Joint

Fibrous Capsule/Ligaments

The outermost layer of the synovial joint is the fibrous capsule. This capsule consists of dense fibrous tissue which surrounds the entire joint, inserts at the lateral margins of the articular cartilage and merges with the periosteum of the articulating long bones. Within the capsule are localized bands of thickened collagen that connect bone to bone known as ligaments. Both the capsule and ligaments possess an abundant nerve supply which allows perception of joint position (proprioception) and thus protects the joint from inadvertent injury. In addition, both structures stabilize the joint and by limiting motion to certain planes, prevent subluxation and dislocation.

Menisci

These fibrocartilaginous discs are found in the knee, temporomandibular, sternoclavicular, acromioclavicular and distal radioulnar joints. They are attached to the fibrous capsule and maintain the stability of the joint during rotation. Like articular cartilage, menisci lack their own vascular or nerve supply and obtain nutrients from the synovial fluid.

Synovial Tissue

The synovium comprises the inner surface of the fibrous capsule, loosely lining the joint cavity without covering the articular cartilages. It consists of a subsynovial layer and the synovial membrane. The subsynovial layer is composed of fibrous connective tissue which contains blood vessels, lymphatic channels, fibroblasts and fatty tissue. It supports the inner synovial membrane which possesses numerous folds. These folds allow the membrane to stretch during joint motion without tearing. Imbedded in this membrane are two types of lining cells known as synoviocytes Type A and B. Type A cells are phagocytes. Type B cells synthesize and secrete hyaluronic acid into the synovial fluid.

The synovium has an abundant blood supply, and both of its layers contain few nerve fibers.

Synovial Fluid

Synovial fluid under normal conditions is a clear, colorless, viscous fluid located within the synovium in which the articular cartilage is bathed. It is the major source of nutrients for the avascular articular cartilage. Normally it is present in small amounts (approximately 1 to 4 ml) but in pathologic states over 150 ml may accumulate in the larger joints such as the knee.

Although as yet incompletely characterized, the normal synovial endothelial membrane is impermeable to large molecular weight proteins. Thus under normal conditions, large plasma proteins such as fibrinogen are unable to diffuse into synovial fluid. Normal synovial fluid therefore consists only of smaller molecular weight plasma proteins to which hyaluronic acid is added by the synoviocyte. Under pathologic conditions, however, the protein content of synovial fluid may change dramatically. When inflamed, the synovial membrane loses its selective permeability and large molecular weight proteins readily diffuse into synovial fluid. In addition, the inflammatory process itself may stimulate local intra-synovial synthesis of immunoglobulins. An example of local immunoglobulin synthesis is rheumatoid arthritis in which synovial production of rheumatoid factor occur.

Hyaluronic acid is a high molecular weight, viscous polysaccharide consisting of an alternating copolymer of glucosamine and glucuronic acid. Hyaluronic acid can adhere to the surface of articular cartilage and when interposed between the two articulating joint surfaces, functions as a joint lubricant. The extent to which hyaluronic acid serves as the major source of joint lubrication, however, is still unknown. Investigators have described several synovial fluid proteins of smaller molecular weight than hyaluronic acid on the surface of articular cartilage. Thus many substances, as yet uncharacterized, in addition to hyaluronic acid, may play a role in joint lubrication. These substances are collectively referred to as lubricating glycoproteins.

Under normal conditions the synovial fluid cell count is less than 200 MM^3 consisting predominantly of macrophages (>75%) and few, if any, neutrophils. The glucose level is approximately equal to that of serum as are complement levels when corrected for decreasing protein concentration. In pathologic states, however, the characteristics of synovial fluid change dramatically. In the "non-inflammatory" synovial fluids found in conditions such as osteoarthritis, SLE, or trauma, cell counts range between 200 and 9,000MM^3 with less than 25% neutrophils. Synovial fluid glucose and complement levels in these conditions are normal. In the inflammatory arthritides such as rheumatoid arthritis, Reiter's syndrome, psoriatic arthritis, sarcoid, gout, and pseudogout, the synovial fluid cell counts are considerably higher ranging from 3,000 to 100,000MM^3 composed predominantly of neutrophils (>75%). Synovial fluid glucose and complement levels are normal in these conditions, with the exception of rheumatoid arthritis in which the complement levels are decreased. In addition, in acute gout and pseudogout characteristic birefringent crystals can be detected with the aid of a polarizing microscope. The observation of these crystals contained within the synovial fluid neutrophils is diagnostic of crystal-induced synovitis.

In septic arthritis, the synovial fluid is frequently grossly purulent or opaque in appearance due to the extremely high white cell count which ranges from 50,000 to 200,000 MM^3 and is comprised almost exclusively (>90%) of neutrophils. The synovial fluid glucose is almost invariably decreased to less than 50% of the serum glucose value. Synovial fluid complement may be either normal or slightly decreased. Gram stains and/or culture of the fluid frequently reveal bacteria and are diagnostic of a septic process. Thus aspiration and examination of synovial fluid is an extremely important diagnostic test, especially if septic arthritis is suspected clinically.

Articular Cartilage

Articular cartilage is the actual weight bearing surface of the joint which covers the ends of the articulating long bones. It lacks its own blood supply and nerve fibers and it obtains nutrients via diffusion through the synovial membrane and synovial fluid. It is less than 5mm in thickness and consists of water (65–80%), type II collagen fibers and proteoglycans.

Collagen molecules are a heterogenous group of structural support proteins possessing a unique triple helix conformation. This triple helix is composed of three polypeptide chains coiled around each other. Variations in the specific amino acid sequence and content of these polypeptide chains gives rise to several different unique structural types of collagen with varying functions. Type I collagen is the most common form of collagen in the body (>90%) and is found in skin, bone, tendons, synovium, sclera and cornea. Type II collagen is found exclusively in articular cartilage and in the vitreous. Type III collagen provides structural support for blood vessel walls. Type IV collagen is found in basement membranes. Type V collagen is deposited pericellularly and is found in the placenta, skin, and cornea.

Proteoglycans are large, viscous, hydrophobic macromolecules consisting of a protein core to which is attached three types of glycosaminoglycans: Chondroitin-6-sulfate, chondroitin-4-sulfate, and keratan sulfate. These glycosaminoglycan moieties are highly negatively charged. During compressive loads, these negatively charged moieties repel each other, and in so doing, give articular cartilage its property of elasticity.

Articular cartilage has several functions. It synthesizes both the collagen and the proteoglycan of which it is composed. It also provides the contact and weight bearing surface of the joint. In addition, its elastic properties permit reversible deformation during weight bearing which increases surface contact area. By exuding interstitial fluid during weight bearing, it also provides additional joint lubrication. This fluid is reabsorbed when weight bearing ceases. Articular cartilage also binds to its surface lubricating glycoproteins in the synovial fluid which further augment joint lubrication.

Articular cartilage destruction is the end result of any longstanding arthritic process. It can be appreciated from the previous discussion of functional anatomy, how such destruction would compromise joint motion and stability. In septic arthritis, cartilage destruction can be prevented by prompt diagnosis and treatment which terminates the inflammatory process before irreversible damage occurs. In other arthritic conditions such as rheumatoid arthritis and osteoarthritis early preventive measures are usually impossible and at initial patient presentation, articular cartilage loss may have already occurred. In rheumatoid arthritis cartilage is eroded by proliferating, inflammatory synovial tissue (pannus) which releases proteolytic enzymes causing cartilage destruction. In osteoarthritis, chronic trauma in conjunction with poorly defined genetic factors leads to both increased proteoglycan production, but an even more rapid rate of lysosomally mediated collagen degradation with a net less of cartilaginous collagen.

Subchondral Bone

Underneath the articular cartilage is the subchondral bone. It is extremely deformable—a property that decreases local stress by distributing it widely throughout the joint surface.

SUGGESTED READINGS

Hammerman D, Rosenberg LC, Shubert M: Diarthrodial Joints Revisited, J. Bone Surgery, 52A: 725–744, 1970.

Hasselbacher P, ed.: Biology of the Joint, Clinics in Rheumatic Diseases, Vol. 7, No. 1, April 1981, W.B. Saunders & Co.

Kelly, et al, eds.: Textbook of Rheumatology, W.B. Saunders, Philadalphia, 3rd ed., 1989, pp 1–21.

Mankin HJ, Radin E: Structure and Function of Joints, Arthritis and Allied Conditions, 11th ed., D.J. McCarty Jr. ed., Philadelphia, Lea & Febiger, 1989, pp 189–206.

Rodnan GP, Schumacher HR, Zvaiffler NJ eds: Primer of Rheumatic Diseases, 8th ed., Arthritis Foundation, Atlanta, 1983, pp 13–16.

Vernon-Roberts B: Applied Anatomy of Joints; Mason and Currey's Clinical Rheumatology, 3rd ed., H.L.F. Currey ed., Kent, Pitman Medical Ltd., 1980, pp 1–6.

CHAPTER 2

INFLAMMATION

Esther Lipstein, M.D.
Robert A. Greenwald, M.D.

INTRODUCTION

Inflammation is the pathologic process most central to current therapeutic approaches to the rheumatic diseases. Some degree of inflammation is present in virtually every rheumatic disease at one time or another in the natural history of the disease. Even in the disorders generally thought of as "degenerative" such as osteoarthritis, an element or inflammation is usually present. In a disorder such as gout, inflammation is the predominant process, and in rheumatoid arthritis, the severity of the inflammatory process is usually used as a guide to pharmacologic therapy. It is therefore not surprising that a substantial amount of investigative effort has been devoted in the last 15 years to understanding the physiology of inflammation.

The clinical parameters of inflammation were first enumerated by Virchow many years ago: Heat, redness, tenderness, and swelling. The rheumatologist uses these clinical parameters to guide his differential diagnosis as well as his therapy. In some instances, as in rheumatoid arthritis, the inciting agent is unknown. On the other hand, in gout or in a septic process, the stimulus for the inflammatory response is more easily identified. In either case, the response of the host is an interaction of numerous mediators attempting to protect the host from invasion by foreign particles or substances, be it bacteria, viruses, fungi, crystals, or unknown antigens. These mediators affect the blood vessels, the cells, and the surrounding tissues so as to produce the characteristics of inflammation listed above. Interference with the generation of these mediators and/or the host's response(s) is the general goal of anti-inflammatory therapy.

In this chapter, we will review selected aspects of the inflammatory process, concentrating on areas where recent research discoveries have suggested new avenues of approach to therapy. The first part of our review will deal with the chemical aspects of inflammation, and this will be followed by sections on physiologic aspects such as temperature, exercise and motion.

MEDIATORS OF INFLAMMATION

Many substances have been implicated as mediators of inflammation. Most of these mediators are chemical substances released from cells which cause dilatation of blood vessels and edema, the combination of which leads to swelling, heat, erythema and pain. The mediator group includes histamine and serotonin which are vasoactive amines released by tissue cells and/or platelets; anaphylatoxins, fragments of proteins derived primarily from the blood complement system which often serve to escalate inflammation by calling forth additional cells into inflamed areas; kinins, proteins derived from the blood clotting system which increase vascular permeability; prostaglandins derived from polyunsaturated fatty acids, discussed in detail below; and oxygen derived free radicals produced by inflammatory cells.

Prostaglandins

Prostaglandins, and a related group of substances called leukotrienes, are derived from phospholipids in the cell membrane (Figure 2-1). An enzyme called

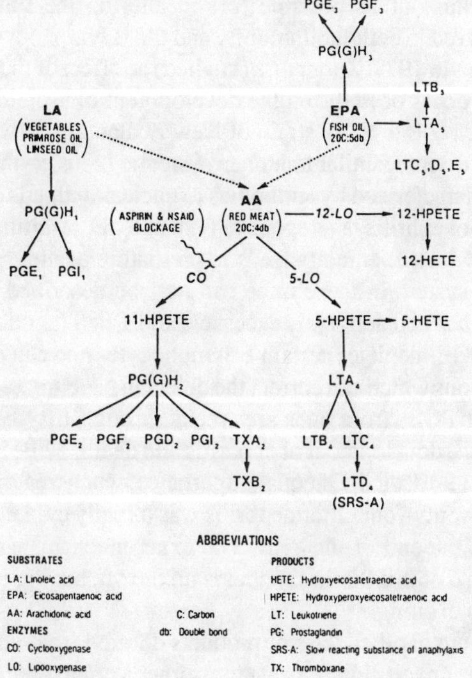

Figure 2-1: Schematic Interrelationship of the Various Mediators of Inflammation

phospholipase acts on these phospholipids to release arachidonic acid from the cell membrane. This substance is a twenty carbon atom fatty acid with four double bonds. Arachidonic acid can also be derived from dietary sources such as red meats and green leafy vegetables.

Several additional enzymes, the most important of which are cyclooxygenase (CO), 5-lipoxygenase (5-LO), and 12-lipoxygenase (12-LO) convert the arachidonic acid into intermediates (PGH_2) and, thence, into active prostaglandins of the two series (PGE_2, PGF_2, PGD_2, and PGI_2), thromboxanes A_2 and B_2, and leukotrienes of the four series (LTB_4, LTD_4, etc.). These derivatives are the ones for which most biologic activity has been demonstrated.

The effects of these prostaglandins vary widely. PGE_2 and PGI_2 are vasodilators, whereas PGF_2 and thromboxane A_2 (produced preferentially by platelets) are vasoconstrictors. PGE_2 has a dual action in that it has been shown to cause inflammation when injected into the skin, where it potentiates the action of agents causing edema, but in other test systems it may be anti-inflammatory by virtue of increasing levels of cyclic-AMP which inhibits the release of histamine and similar mediators.

PGE_1, a prostaglandin derived from linoleic acid, is of particular interest in rheumatology because of its possible role in altering the function of the T lymphocytes involved in cellular immunity and the B lymphocytes which act in antibody formation. In 1977, Zurier *et. al* studied the effect of the administration of pharmacologic doses of PGE_1 on the development of proteinuria, nephritis, and survival in the NZB x NZW strain of New Zealand mice which spontaneously developed a disease similar to human systemic lupus erythematosus. This animal model is characterized by antibodies to nuclear antigens and by immune complex glomerulonephritis, analogous to human SLE, resulting in proteinuria and renal failure, which eventually leads to premature death.

The immune system in these mice can best be described as showing an imbalance in which B cell activity is excessive and T cell function is decreased. Experimentally, PGE_1 depletes certain B lymphocytes and can enhance *in vivo* T cell activity, actions which can correct the defect in NZB mice. Mice receiving daily injections of PGE_1 from ages six weeks through fifty-two weeks were protected against the development of nephritis and death, while in a comparable control group, over 90% died. Of equal importance, when treatment was started on mice at week twenty-four, after nephritis was already evident, all such mice were still alive at the end of the year. The exact mechanism whereby PGE_1 influence the course of this disease model is unknown, but the implications for human disease are exciting.

Leukotrienes are another class of products derived from arachidonic acid. The enzyme 5-LO converts its substrate into either a compound called 5-HETE or into the leukotrienes designated LTB_4 and LTD_4 is a potent chemotactic factor for neutrophils and eosinophils, as are 12-HETE and 5-HETE. LTD_4 causes vasodilation and has been found to be identical to the slow reacting substance of anaphylaxis.

These products of arachidonic acid metabolism may participate in the pathogenesis of rheumatoid arthritis by acting as mediators of inflammation, but they have also been shown to promote bone resorption. Rheumatoid synovium produces large amount of PGE_2 in organ culture, as much as ten fold higher than control tissue. The amount of PGE_2 produced can be correlated well with the bone resorbing activity of the cultures (measured by incubating the synovial tissue with rat skull bones and measuring calcium release), suggesting that PGE_2 may be partly responsible for juxtaarticular bone destruction in RA. When indomethacin is added to the culture, the production of PGE_2 is inhibited because this drug, like most non-steroidal anti-inflammatory agents, inhibits the cyclooxygenase enzyme whose action is required for prostaglandin production. The suppression of PGE_2 synthesis results in loss of the bone resorbing activity as well. PGE_2 also stimulates the secretion of collagenase by macrophages, as well as inhibiting the production of proteoglycans by articular chondrocytes, actions which would worsen the severity of destructive joint disease. However, it must be borne in mind that it is impossible to demonstrate clinically that the drugs which inhibit prostaglandin synthesis also halt the erosive processes of inflammatory arthritis.

Chemotaxis is the process by which certain cells, notably neutrophils (polymorphonuclear leukocytes, PMNs) and macrophages, respond to an inflammatory stimulus by accumulations in the area of the stimulus so as to come to the aid of the host by releasing enzymes and other protective substances. Two products of the lipooxygenase pathway, LTB_4 and 5-HETE, are known to be chemotactic. Substantial elevations of LTB_4 in the synovial fluid of patients with seropositive RA and with seronegative spondyloarthropathy (SSA) has been found, thereby suggesting a mechanism for increased migration of PMNs into inflamed joints. In synovial tissues, 5-HETE was found to be significantly elevated in patients with seropositive RA and with SSA as well, in comparison to the cases with non-inflammatory arthritis. When patients with seropositive RA were given 40 mg of intraarticular methylprednisolone, the concentration of LTB_4 went down substantially, perhaps suggesting a mechanism whereby the use of local steroids may reduce inflammation.

Chemotaxis is a critical component of inflammation, since one of the cardinal pathologic and histologic features of the inflammatory process is an infiltration into the affected tissue by invading cells, usually neutrophils, but also included are monocytes (macrophages) and/or lymphocytes. The mechanisms by which these cells are called forth into the inflamed area are quite complex and many different factors derived from a variety of sources have been identified as being chemotactic. Chemotactic factors have been found that relate to the complement series of proteins, derived from bacterial products, etc., as well as those mentioned above. Chemotaxis is associated with increased neutrophil adhesiveness, margination of neutrophils, and the egress of such cells through vessel walls into inflamed areas.

Many drugs, notably the non-steroidal anti-inflammatory drugs, can be shown to inhibit chemotaxis *in vitro*, but whether or not they work that way in real life is unknown. Colchicine, a remarkably effective agent for treatment of the intense inflammation of gout, seems to work by acting on the neutrophil to inhibit generation of an extremely potent chemotactic factor which the cell produces after contact with a crystal of monosodium urate.

Arachidonic Acid Analogues

Arachidonic acid (AA), as previously noted, is a fatty acid containing twenty carbon atoms and four double bonds. AA analogues are fatty acids of similar structure with differing numbers of carbon atoms and/or double bonds. Eicosapentanoic acid (EPA) contains 20 carbons with five double bonds. It is found in the oil of cold water fish, and may become incorporated into cell membranes in place of AA where it can be acted upon by the same enzymes CO and LO, which convert AA to the mediators previously described.

When EPA is altered in this manner, the three series of prostaglandins (PGE_3, PGF_3), the five series of leukotrienes (LTB_5, LTD_5) and thromboxane A_3 instead of A_2 are formed. Thromboxane A_3 does not have the platelet aggregating properties of thromboxane A_2 and thus generation of the former leads to an anti-thrombotic state. In addition, the enzyme CO found in blood vessel walls can use EPA as a substrate to produce an anti-platelet aggregating agent, probably prostacyclin I_3. Greenland Eskimos have a marine diet containing large amounts of EPA and, as a result, they exhibit poor platelet aggregating properties, and have a prolonged bleeding time. A decreased incidence of myocardial infarctions has been found in this Eskimo population and may relate to this dietary phenomenon.

EPA has been given experimentally to NZB x NZW mice to determine its effect on proteinuria and survival from their lupus-like illness. Five week old mice were fed either beef tallow (low in EPA) or menhadden oil (containing 14.4% EPA). All of the beef tallow animals developed proteinuria and the majority had died by the end of six months. However, none of the mice fed the fish oil diet developed urinary abnormalities and all were alive at six months. Enrichment of the diet with the polyunsaturated fatty acid EPA protected against the development of this disease. The role of similar maneuvers in human disease has not been established.

Psoriasis is an inflammatory skin condition often associated with arthritis.

In psoriatic epidermis, there is heightened activity of the 12-LO and 5-LO enzymatic pathways over that of the cyclooxygenase pathway. The content of 12-HETE, a product of the 12-LO pathway, is 81 times greater in involved skin from psoriatics than from uninvolved, whereas the levels of PGE_2 and PGF_2 (products of the CO pathway) are modestly elevated by only 40% and 86% respectively in involved vs. uninvolved epidermis.

It has been suggested that psoriatic skin may contain an inhibitor of the CO pathway. If such skin is treated with indomethacin, a CO inhibitor, the levels of AA and 12-HETE are increased even further. This causes shunting of the free AA into other metabolic pathways, i.e., 5-LO and 12-LO, resulting in formation of LTB_4 and 12-HETE, both of which are chemoattractants which recruit neutrophils into the inflamed skin sites. The combined effect of indomethacin and endogenous CO inhibitor may cause clinical exacerbation of psoriasis by increasing the diversion of free AA into LTB_4 and 12-HETE.

AA analogues may have a role in the treatment of psoriasis. EPA is transformed into the three series of PGs and thromboxane and into the five series of leukotrienes; substances of lesser inflammatory potency than the four series. Greenland Eskimos rarely have psoriasis, suggesting another possible role of diet (although a strong genetic factor operates in psoriasis as well). Diet can be manipulated by enrichment with vegetable seed oils (linoleic acid) supplemented with evening primrose oil which favors the production of PGE_2 and limits formation of active leukotrienes. One can speculate that joint inflammation in psoriasis may relate to preferential activation of the lipoxygenase pathway with formation of chemoattractants (LTB_4, 12-HETE). Dietary manipulation might play a role in the therapy of this disease, but this has yet to be established.

Oxygen Radicals

In the past five years, a new class of inflammatory mediators derived from oxygen has been intensively studied. These substances are called free radicals, a term which refers to molecules containing unpaired electrons, which are highly reactive. The major free radical of biologic interest is called the superoxide radical, symbolized as [O_2•]. Two related radical species are called hydroxyl radical [OH•] and singlet oxygen. A non-free radical component of the system is hydrogen peroxide [H_2O_2]. These radicals are generated naturally during the course of many biologic processes, foremost among which is the action of various stimuli on the cell membrane of the neutrophil or macrophage. When these inflammatory cells encounter agents, such as bacterial particles, immune complexes or components of the complement system, the cells undergo a metabolic transformation known as respiratory burst characterized by the uptake of oxygen, increased glucose metabolism, and generation of oxygen radicals. The liberation of lysosomal and degradative enzymes often accompanies these other phenomena, and the entire package of events can be viewed as a protective mechanism within the host's defense system.

These oxygen-derived free radicals are capable of having adverse effects on many tissue and molecular substrates. It is not clear which agent, superoxide, hydroxyl, or peroxide, is actually the toxic factor, if any. Trace amounts of iron in tissues probably catalyze the interconversion of one form to another. Suffice it to say that if an oxy radical generating system is used experimentally on various target tissues, one can demonstrate bacterial killing, erythrocyte lysis, neutrophil cell death, liposome lysis, fibroblast or endothelial cell death, increased vascular permeability, brain edema, or disruption of the molecular architecture of hyaluronic acid, DNA, collagen or hemoglobin.

It is probably the generation of superoxide in an inflamed joint which accounts for the decrease of synovial fluid viscosity which is commonly observed clinically. Superoxide generating systems can readily degrade hyaluronic acid, the macromolecular substance in synovial fluid which accounts for the viscosity of joint fluid. It has also been reported that a superoxide system can act on a plasma substrate to create a chemotactic factor which would enhance inflammation. Many other aspects of joint inflammation can be linked by circumstantial evidence to oxygen radicals, although direct evidence of their involvement has not yet been obtained.

Ambitious (and unscrupulous) hucksters have started promoting tablets of superoxide dismutase, also known as Orgotein, for the treatment of arthritis. Superoxide dismutase is an enzyme which scavenges the superoxide radical. Superoxide normally disappears very rapidly *in vivo* anyway, and it is unclear whether an agent that scavenged the radical would be therapeutically useful. The enzyme is, of course, a protein, so presenting it in tablet form is irresponsible and irrational, as it would be readily digested in the intestinal tract. In Europe, it has been used by injection into arthritic joints and good results have been reported, but the studies were not rigorously designed and would not meet American Rheumatism Association or FDA guidelines. It remains to be seen whether or not use of agents that act on free radicals will be of benefit in the treatment of arthritis.

Tissue Degradation

Sustained inflammation in any area of the body eventually results in degradation of the components of the inflamed tissue. The tissues of the joint are particularly susceptible to such damage. There are three major macromolecular species found in joint tissues which may be damaged as a result of the inflammatory process. One is hyaluronic acid, as mentioned above, a long-chain carbohydrate found primarily in synovial fluid. Hyaluronic acid is susceptible to chemical destruction by an enzyme known as hyaluronidase, but this enzyme is not found in neutrophils and levels in joint fluid, even inflamed, are quite low.

If one adds inflamed fluid of low viscosity to normal fluid, the latter is not affected, as it would be if an enzyme were present in the inflamed fluid. The probable mechanism by which hyaluronic acid degradation takes place *in vivo* is by action of oxygen radicals described above.

The second major structural component of joint tissues is collagen. Collagen is a uniquely structured protein composed of three strands of approximately 1,000 amino acids each intertwined in a helical format. Collagen differs from other proteins in that every third amino acid in each strand is glycine and that approximately 20% of the total amino acids are either hydroxylysine or hydroxyproline. The latter amino acids participate in chemical bridging between one collagen molecule and the next, thereby allowing the formation of sheets, ropes and other structures of tightly bound collagen fibrils recognizable as tendons or ligaments. Collagen accounts for the tensile strength of connective tissues, as opposed to providing the resistance to compression, which is the other major physical attribute of connective tissues.

In its native state, i.e., helical and cross-linked, collagen molecules are not subject to enzymatic degradation by normal proteolytic enzymes (enzymes which can degrade other proteins). Native collagen can only be cleaved by specific collagenases. Bacteria can produce such enzymes which can chop the collagen molecules into many small fragments. In septic arthritis, frequent drainage of the inflamed joint to remove such enzymes may, at least theoretically, prevent destruction of tissue. Mammalian collagenases cleave the collagen molecule at a specific point about one-quarter of the way from one end. Once this initial cleavage has occurred, the molecule can denature (unravel) and other enzymes can finish its degradation. White blood cells contain a collagenase capable of doing this, but the pannus, or proliferative synovium of rheumatoid joints, is perhaps the tissue most responsible for secretion of collagenase into the joints, from which not only the cartilage but also the capsule, ligaments and tendons can all be destroyed. The discovery of a collagenase inhibitor safe for long term use might be a major milestone in prevention of tissue destruction in rheumatoid arthritis.

The final component of tissues which may be destroyed by inflammation are the proteoglycans. These are extremely large macromolecules, primarily composed of carbohydrate with a small amount (about 7%) of protein. Their molecular weights range from 2.5 to 70 million. Proteoglycans provide the resiliency (resistance to compression) of cartilage and intervertebral disk. In osteoarthritis, or degenerative joint disease, there is a progressive loss of proteoglycan, the cause and mechanism of which is unknown. In inflammatory conditions, enzymes can cause rapid destruction of these proteoglycans. Neutrophils can secrete the enzyme elastase which is probably the major such enzyme released in inflammation. In addition, proteolytic enzymes can be liberated from cartilage itself, causing its own self destruction.

The degrade macromolecules of the joint may perhaps be "phlogistic" in and of themselves, i.e., they may perpetuate the inflammatory process. Sophisticated immunologic studies of cartilage and ligaments have shown the presence of immunoglobulins reacting with collagen and/or with proteoglycans, suggesting that immune reactivity may play a role in some forms of joint inflammation that appear to be totally non-immunologic.

Inflammation, then, is more than just a painful, disfiguring situation. The release of various substances—collagenase, oxygen radicals, elastase, etc.— will ultimately result in the destruction of the tissue. However, clinical trials have never been able to demonstrate that anti-inflammatory agents, steroidal or non-steroidal, can prevent tissue destruction, or otherwise modify the natural history of the disease for which they are used. We must conclude that either there are other mechanisms by which tissue destruction takes place, currently unknown, or that even maximally tolerated doses of such drugs are insufficient to suppress the inflammatory process. There remains much to be learned about the chemistry of inflammation and the pharmacology of its suppression.

JOINT PHYSIOLOGY

Pressure

Normally, the fluid pressure in a knee joint is less than atmospheric pressure. When synovial fluid volume increases, intra-articular pressures rises accordingly. In the knees of elderly patients with rheumatoid arthritis, there is a disproportionately greater change in pressure with the joint for the same increase in joint fluid volume, indicating increased stiffness of the joint structures. Full flexion of a normal knee can cause a pressure rise of as much as 130 mm Hg with a normal fluid volume. When inflammatory arthritis increases the fluid volume, the effect of full flexion on pressure is accentuated. The combined decrease in synovial fluid volumes and pressure can interfere with synovial blood flow and thereby impair the nutrition of joint tissues. Arthrocentesis of especially large effusions may be useful to alleviate the patient's discomfort.

Oxygen Tension

The mean oxygen tension (partial pressure) in knee joints of three groups of patients; rheumatoid, osteo and traumatic arthritis have been measured. The lowest values were found in the group with rheumatoid arthritis. This lowering of the partial pressure of oxygen can be explained by several factors. There may be a vasculitis of the synovial vessels reducing the oxygen supply, such a vasculitis has been demonstrated angiographically in the rheumatoid hand. The inflamed joint fluid contains many cells which require oxygen for their metabolism, thereby consuming larger quantities than the cells of a normal joint. The combination of decreased delivery of oxygen, due to obliterative endarteritis and increased metabolic demand, causes the oxygen tension in the joint to fall. Such relative anoxia may lead to cell damage or death, including the release of lysosomal enzymes. It has also been shown that exercise itself reduces the oxygen tension in the knee as well (normal or inflamed), perhaps providing a rationale for the clinical experience that immobilization is useful in the treatment of the acutely inflamed joint.

Temperature

Elevated intra-articular temperature has long been recognized as an index of joint inflammation. Studies done as early as 1949 by Horvath and Hollander revealed for example that the mean temperature in rheumatoid joints was 4.2° F higher than normal joints, and 1.5° higher in degenerative disease. The temperature of the adjacent skin was two to three degrees lower than in the joint. Increase joint (but not skin) temperature correlated with disease severity. Surprisingly, application of hot packs increased the skin temperature only, and actually lowered the temperature within the joint. The converse was noted with cool packs. In another study, the same authors showed that exercise, either active or passive, increased the joint temperature as much as 2.5°.

More recently the intra-articular temperature of rabbit joints was measured after injection of monosodium urate crystals, simulating gout, and found to be elevated. Surface temperature correlated poorly with that within the joint. Studies of the effect of exercise on joint temperature elevation showed that passive range of motion amplified urate synovitis, increasing both joint temperature and infiltration of neutrophils into the joint. Isometric exercise, on the other hand, did not increase intra-articular temperature nor did it increase the neutrophil infiltration.

The degradation of collagen is temperature sensitive; the *in vitro* reaction rate increases 300–400% when the temperature is raised from 33° C to 36° C. Although elevated joint temperatures correlate with inflammation, no clinical or radiologic evidence of advancing joint disease could be demonstrated, even after two years of daily heat therapy to the hands of patients with RA.

Exercise

Several studies have been done to assess the effect of exercise on joint inflammation. It has been reported that when canine joints were injected with urate crystals suspended in saline, the severity of the resulting inflammation was increased by exercise. The indices of inflammation evaluated included synovial effusion volume, joint fluid leukocyte count, histology and leakage of carbon (injected intravenously) from synovial vessels. The synovial fluid leukocyte counts were strikingly elevated in the exercised joints. As little as five seconds of exercise resulted in a 30,000 count, while five minutes yielded a count over 100,000; were as little as five seconds of exercise every fifteen minutes for four hours caused a doubling of the leukocyte count in comparison to a rested control knee. More aggressive exercise caused as much as a nine-fold rise in counts. The exercised knees had higher fluid volumes as well. All the injected joints showed histologic evidence of synovitis (PMN infiltration, vascular congestion, etc.), but the changes in the exercised joints were much more severe.

There are several hypotheses which might explain the enhancement of urate inflammation by exercise. Motion may place the crystals in contact with greater areas of synovium and/or increase their contact with neutrophils, thereby resulting in generation of more mediators of inflammation. Joint motion raises intra-articular pressure, which may accelerate cell damage and cause more mediator release. Joint motion could also cause vascular changes with vasodilation accentuating the inflammatory reaction and delivering more inflammatory cells.

Continuous passive motion (CPM) has been advocated for the healing of synovitis. This method of CPM is provided by a mechanical device that slowly and consistently moves the affected joint through a preset range of motion during a specific time period, i.e., a range of 40° to 110° flexion with one cycle every forty seconds. In one study, septic arthritis was induced in rabbits by injecting staphylococcus into the knee joints, applied CPM for ten weeks and compared the exercised joints to immobilized controls. The exercised joints appeared to have been protected against cartilage degradation as assessed by radiologic, histologic and biochemical criteria. It was suggested that CPM prevented synovial adhesions, increased diffusion of nutrients into the cartilage matrix and enhanced the clearance of inflammatory substances from the synovial cavity. Thus, it would appear that carefully controlled exercise can promote the resolution of certain types of inflammation, while in other situations exercise makes the situation worse. Until this conflict is resolved, the applicability of this form of graded exercise for human septic or other arthritis remains to be proven.

CONCLUSION

There remains much to be learned about the pathophysiology of inflammation. Although we now know much more than we did a decade ago about the events which trigger and/or mediate the inflammatory response, many crucial questions remain unanswered. Why does inflammation in some instance, e.g., acute gouty arthritis, usually bring itself to a natural halt (most gout attacks will resolve spontaneously within ten to fourteen days even if untreated), while in other instance, e.g., rheumatoid arthritis, the response becomes self-perpetuating. In what situations are the by-products of inflammation and tissue degradation themselves phlogistic, i.e., when do they cause the inflammation to increase in intensity? If tissue degradation is brought about by release of inflammatory mediators, why don't the so-called "anti-inflammatory" drugs prevent the progression of destructive disease? Until we can answer these and many similar questions, a universally effective treatment for the inflammatory response will not be forthcoming.

SUGGESTED READINGS

Arthritis and Allied Conditions, McCarty, D.J. ed., ch. 1, 2, 10–14. 11th ed., 1989, Lea & Febiger, Philadelphia.

*Biologically Based Immunomodulators in the Therapy of Rheumatic Disease.*Eds. Pincus, S.H., Pisetsky, D.S. and Rosenwasser, L. Elsevier Science Pub. Co., New York 1987.

Inflammation. Ryan, G.B. and Majno, G. The Upjohn Co., Kalamazoo, Michigan 1977.

Primer on the Rheumatic Diseases, 9th edition. Ed. Schumacker, H.R. Chapter 5 "Mediators of Inflammation." The Arthritis Foundation, Atlanta, Georgia 1988.

Synovial Fluid Dynamics, the Regulation of Volume and Pressure. Vol. 2, eds. Holburow, E.S. and Maroundus, A. Pitman Medical Co., London 1983. Levick, S. Jr., "Studies in Joint Diseases."

Textbook of Rheumatology. Eds. Kelly, W.N., Harris, E. Jr., Ruddy, S. and Sledge, C.B. 3rd edition (1989) W.B. Saunders Co., Philadelphia. Chapter 14–23.

Therapeutic Approaches to Inflammatory Diseases. Eds. Lewis, A.J., Ackerman, N.R. and Doherty, N.S. Elsevier Science Publishing Co., New York 1989.

CHAPTER 3

IMMUNOLOGY

Allan Josephson, M.D.
Irwin Oreskes, Ph.D.

INTRODUCTION AND HISTORICAL ASPECTS

All organisms live among other organisms. The interrelations of various life form are extremely complex and are the result of past and continuing evolution. We know that soon after death, the corpse is invaded by an enormous number of bacteria and other organisms. Indeed, biological substances such as milk, blood or tissue, once exposed to the environment are soon nothing more than a rich culture media for ubiquitous fungi and bacteria. All living organisms have developed mechanisms for preventing invasion by other life forms; the more highly evolved the organism, the more complex are the defense systems. These systems sometimes break down, especially when the individual is debilitated or the invader possess a factor which increases its virulence. When this happens we are said to have an infectious disease. The study of those factors which prevent invasions or which permit the infected organism to recover is the science of immunology.

The factors which prevent infections may be quite simple. An intact integument is a good mechanical barrier to the microbes lurking in our environment. Burn patients frequently die of overwhelming sepsis, at least in part resulting from loss of that barrier. Other protective mechanisms are more subtle. Secretions such as tears and mucous wash away particles transporting them back to the environment. Dissolved in our secretions are a variety of substances which may have antibacterial effects. One is lysozyme, an enzyme first described by Alexander Fleming, who also discovered penicillin. Lysozyme has the effect of dissolving the cell walls of many bacteria leading to their death by osmotic rupture.

Other important components of the defense system are cells, some with multilobed nuclei, called polymorphonuclear leukocytes. Others with large nonlobed nuclei are called macrophages. The pioneer immunologist, Ellie Metchnikoff, noted that a foreign body when put in a starfish is soon surrounded by cells similar to human macrophages which ingest and destroy invading bacteria, a process called phagocytosis.

Other early investigators in immunology were intrigued by the fact that humans not only frequently recovered from bacterial and viral infections, but that recovery took between four and seven days with repeated infection by the same organism. Certain bacterial infections such as tuberculous and brucellosis did not follow this pattern, but many did, as did most known viral infections (measles and mumps for example). Indeed, it was noted that while individuals could have had repeated pneumococcal or streptococcal infections, these species really represent families of distinguishable organisms. Repeated infection with the same type of pneumococcus was most unusual. It was also discovered that the serum of a patient who recovered from pneumococcal pneumonia would, when infused into an infected individual cut short the course of the disease or protected an uninfected recipient from infection.

These observations indicated that infection caused the formation in the blood of substances, called antibodies, which assisted in the destruction of the infectious agent and also prevented repeated infections. We now know that antibodies are highly specific. For example, antibodies to Type I pneumococci are of no value in protection against Type III organism. Antibodies are localized in the serum fraction of blood and are heat stable and transferable.

During the pre-antibiotic era, infections were often treated or prevented by manipulations of the immune system. Two techniques were developed. The first was passive immunization in which serum that contained antibodies was transferred to an infected individual; the second was active immunization, in which a non-virulent form of the organism or a chemically extracted portion of an organism, was injected to elicit the production of specific antibodies without an actual infection. This latter technique is in ever widening use.

The description of the serum immune system by one group of scientists and the cellular phagocytic system of polymorphonuclear leukocytes and macrophages by another group, set off a great controversy as to which system was more important. As we shall see, both are important and each depends on the other for effectiveness.

Antibodies

Antibodies are produced in response to infection or injection. The substances inciting their production are called antigens. We can define each in terms of the other. If a substance causes the formation of an antibody, it is an antigen, and that which is formed in response to an antigen is an antibody. Antibodies are very specific for their antigens and will react with them. In many cases putting a solution of a given antigen in contact with a corresponding immune serum will result in the formation of a precipitate composed of the antigen and the antibody complexed together.

Over the years, our knowledge of antibodies has become extraordinarily sophisticated. Antibodies belong to a class of protein known collectively as immunoglobulins and are chemically similar. In general, they consist of amino acids chemically linked together in two long chains, called heavy chains, and two shorter or light chains (Figure 3-1). The basic immunoglobulin monomer unit consists of two heavy and two light polypeptide chains chemically crosslinked by one or more disulfide bonds.

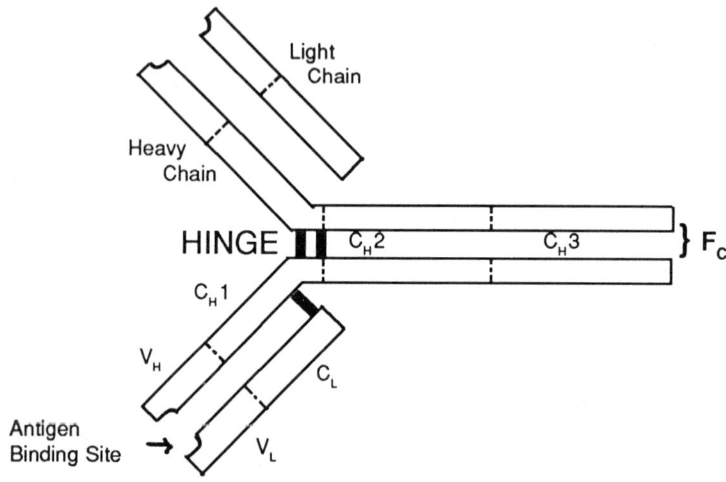

Figure 3-1: Schematic structure of the immunoglobulin G molecule

Detailed chemical investigations have shown that there are two classes of light chains called Kappa (κ) and Lambda (λ) and that any immunoglobulin monomer has either two κ or two λ light chains. There are five classes of heavy chains: μ, γ, α, δ and ε.

If an immunoglobulin has two γ chains, it is called IgG; if two μ chains, IgM; two α chains, IgA; two δ chains, IgD and two ε chains, IgE. The IgM is most often found as a pentamer that is composed of five of the basic four chained monomers linked to each other. IgA A is an antibody found in abundance in secretions as well as in the serum. It is usually a dimer, composed of two basic units when in secretions; although it is most often monomeric in the serum.

The diversity of structure at this level has been associated with different functions of the various antibody classes. IgG can cross the placenta, the others do not. IgA is found in secretions in large amounts, the others in small amounts if at all. IgM is a rapidly produced antibody, but its production provides no immunologic memory; that is, a second infection by the same organism results in an IgM response no faster or greater than the first response.

Production of IgG, on the other hand, is associated with immunologic memory where a second exposure to the same antigen results in a brisk and qualitatively greater IgG antibody response. This is termed the anamnestic response. IgE is particularly adapted to attach to certain cells, the mast cells and basophile, and is responsible for the symptoms of rhinitis and conjunctivitis (hay fever) when certain air-borne antigens, such as pollens, find their way to these antibodies.

The diversity of structure thus far described is only one order of the diversity inherent in this class of proteins. It has been mentioned that antibodies to given organisms will not usually react with organisms of other types. Difference in types of micro-organisms are represented by differences in the chemical composition, sometimes minor differences at that, of the surface components of these organisms. Yet antibodies can distinguish these minor differences. The answer as to what structural characteristics of antibodies define their ability to specifically react with another molecule was somewhat surprising.

The amino acid sequence of half the light chain and approximately one-fourth of the heavy chain is unique for each individual antibody. These are called the variable portions of the heavy (V_H) and light (V_L) chain, and are physically in apposition (Figure 3-1). Thus, the interaction of the variable portions of the heavy and light chains provides a chemical receptor able to combine with the antigen that incites its production. This is a unique phenomenon, as most other proteins, such as hemoglobin, are the same or are only slightly different in amino acid structure among individuals of a given species.

The remainder of the IgG light and heavy chains consist of amino acid domains of relatively constant amino acid sequence. These are termed C_L, C_H1, C_H2 and C_H3. That fragment of the IgG molecule which contain both C_H2 and C_H3 domains is termed Fc.

Antibodies are produced by plasma cells, which are easily recognized by their eccentric nuclei and abundant cytoplasm. They are found in the bone marrow, in lymph nodes and various tissue areas, such as the lamina propria of the gut and bronchi. The plasma cell is a mature form, its precursor being a lymphocyte subclass, known as the B cell. B cells are also found in the circulating blood, where 10 to 15% of circulating lymphocytes are B cells. Their name derives from the observation that in fowl, B cells undergo an obligate maturation process in an organ found in the hindgut, the Bursa of Fabricius. No such organ is found in mammals and the specific site of B cell maturation has never been adequately identified; although the bone marrow is a candidate site.

B cells are readily identified immunohistochemically as they have small amounts of immunoglobulin on their surfaces. If an antigen, such as a component of a bacterium, meets and interacts with a specific receptor on the surface of a B cell, the maturation process begins. The B cell is thereby stimulated and begins to secrete antibodies, maturing to the form we recognize as the plasma cell. The whole group of cells descended from the original B cell is called a clone.

The specific B cell surface receptor is actually preformed antibody. According to the Clonal Selection Theory, we carry enough different preformed antibodies to recognize all possible antigens. Thus, antigen stimulates proliferation of only those B cells with specific complementary surface antibody.

In many cases the antigen is actually captured and phagocytosed by a special type of macrophage and may be in some way "processed" before presentation to the B cell, but it is primarily the inborn and genetically dictated repertoire of antibodies each of us carry that permit us to respond to the many antigens in the environment. Some alteration in the arrangement of this genetic material apparently does occur throughout our lives. This process of somatic mutation serves to increase the diversity of our antibody production.

Antibodies serve to recognize foreign materials and identify them, while the phagocytic cells serve to destroy them. Thus, if a bacterium invades a higher organism, antibodies to surface components of the bacterium are produced, as are antibodies to toxins produced by the bacterium. Although specific antibodies may neutralize the toxins, antibodies which combine with the bacterium will not by themselves kill the pathogen. The destruction of the bacterium is usually accomplished by phagocytosis by polymorphonuclear leukocytes or macrophages. But, while antibodies in the absence of phagocytes are incapable of destroying bacteria, phagocytes, in the absence of antibodies, are only poorly able to engulf the pathogenic organisms. The increase in the ability of cells to phagocytose antibody-coated antigen is called opsonization.

In light of present day knowledge it turns out that the argument between the proponents of phagocytosis on the one hand or interaction with specific antibodies on the other hand as the primary mode of immunologic protection, is a draw.

Complement

Another important link between antibody recognition and phagocytosis is a complex group of proteins collectively called complement. When antibody and antigen interact in the presence of complement, the complement is "fixed." In the process of fixation a component of complement reacts with the antibody-antigen complex and initiates a cascade of protein interaction. A cascade means that an enzyme is activated which acts on the next component, which is in turn activated and so on. At various stages in the cascade, protein inhibitors regulate the process to prevent uncontrolled spontaneous activation. The first complement component, called C_1, is activated by antigen-antibody interactions to become an enzyme, C_1 esterase. After interaction with the next two components,

C_4 and C_2, an enzyme is formed which cleaves C_3, a particularly abundant protein which is found in the plasma in concentrations of approximately 100 mg/dl. When C_3 is cleaved, two fragments are formed, C_3a and C_3b. C_3a is an anaphylatoxin which can cause the release of histamine and other mediators from mast cells. These mediators result in vasodilatation and increases in vascular permeability, producing swelling, redness and heat; the major components of inflammation. The other fragment, C_3b, attaches to the antigen and makes it more readily phagocytosed.

The resulting complex of complement which now includes C_3b, is an enzyme which cleaves C_5 to C_5a and C_5b. C_5a is an active "chemotactic" factor, that attracts polymorphonuclear leukocytes, which in turn find easier access to the antibody-antigen complex by virtue of the previously described increase in vascular permeability.

To recapitulate, the antibody recognizes the antigen as foreign, attaches to the antigen and the resulting complex fixes complement. Factors produced by the complement cascade facilitate the transit of phagocytes, into the local area. The phagocytes, which have receptors for C_3b as well as polymorphonuclear leukocytes, attach to the Fc part of the antibody (Figure 3-1) and engulf the pathogen. The "polymorph" carries a variety of enzymes stored in intra-cellular structures, called oxidants and enzymes, perhaps in sequence, make short work of many bacteria. However, certain bacteria, such as Legionella pneumophilia, not only survive this attack, but actually require intra-cellular residence to replicate. Other defense systems are needed to cope with such obligate intra-cellular pathogens.

The pathway from C_1 esterase activation to C_3 cleavage is termed the classical pathway. Another complement pathway, activated directly by certain bacterial components, such as endotoxin or polysaccharides, utilizes different components to achieve C_3 cleavage, and is termed the alternative pathway.

Examples of congenital defects in many of the steps from antibody production to complement activation have been described. In almost every case, the patient is unable to cope with certain types of infection. These conditions represent one type of immunodeficiency disease.

Humoral Immunity

Because in many cases specific immunity could be transferred from individuals even across species lines by means of serum, the type of immunity just described has been termed humoral immunity. Nevertheless, cells are important at several steps. Humoral antibodies are produced by the B cell. This cell, which comprise 10–15% of all circulating lymphocytes, has on its surface specific antibody molecules. Each immature B cell is thought to express only one of the 10^6–10^8 different antibody combining sites coded for by any individual's DNA.

Should the proper antigen be encountered by such a cell, the interaction of the antigen with the surface antibody stimulates the B cell to proliferate and mature. The mature plasma cell, thus becomes an antibody producing factory.

In the process of proliferation, a whole series of B lymphocytes bearing the same surface antibody is produced, thereby providing a large number of recognition cells for the next encounter, hence the phenomenon of the anamnestic or memory response. The initial recognition antibodies are usually IgM and IgD. As the process continues, the cell that originally produced IgM now switches to IgG, IgA or IgE under certain circumstances. The combining site of all these antibodies, whatever the class, is the same.

Cell Mediated Immunity

The processes of the production of most antibodies is under control of another set of lymphocytes called the T cells. T cells are so named because all members of this group can be shown to have resided for a portion of their history in the thymus. Within the thymus they migrate from the cortical to the medullary zone of that organ and undergo a variety of changes such as alterations in density and acquisition of new surface chemical markers which can be identified.

T cells have long been recognized as being important in the "delayed hypersensitivity" phenomenon. If one injects a small amount of purified extract from the tubercule bacillus into the skin of an individual who has been infected with that organism, even a clinically inapparent infection, an indurated erythematous lesion will appear within forty-eight hours at the site of injection. An individual who had not previously been so infected will not react. One can transfer reactivity to a non-reactor, in the case of lower animals, or with cell extracts in the case of humans. Serum or purified immunoglobulins will not effect the transfer. This reactivity is called cell mediated immunity (CMI). That the positive delayed response does indeed represent a type of immunity, different from, but as important as antibody mediated immunity, has been amply demonstrated. Loss of CMI results in infections from a variety of organisms including the tubercule bacillus, fungi, viruses and other obligate intra-cellular pathogens. Whereas in humoral or antibody mediated immunity, the immunoglobulin circulating in the serum recognizes the chemical configuration of the antigen and reacts with it; in CMI, a surface component of the T lymphocyte bears the recognition apparatus. The chemical nature of this recognition unit has recently been deciphered and while it bears many structural analogies to immunoglobulin, it has in fact, a distinctive structure.

T Cells Subsets

There exist several subsets of T cells, each of which can be characterized by both functional and structural differences. Our ability to recognize these subsets derives from the development of an immunologic method of enormous utility, the monoclonal antibody technique. Two investigators, Kohler and Milstein, developed this method whereby individual clones of antibody forming cells can be kept alive indefinitely. They achieved this clonal immortality by fusing antibody forming cells from mice with cells of a mouse plasma cell tumor known as multiple myeloma. These cell fusions produce monoclonal antibodies that are extremely homogeneous and antigen specific. Among other uses monoclonal antibodies are excellent reagents for detecting T cell surface markers.

Identification of T cell subsets depends on the recognition of cell structures. Thus, all human T cells are positive for the CD2 marker. All mature T cells are CD3 positive. The CD3 surface antigen has been shown to be inherently associated with the combining site or recognition unit on the T cell. Subpopulations of mature T cells, in addition to the CD3 antigen, have on their surface either CD4 or CD8, but not both. (Previous terminology for these T cell markers was T3, T4, T8, respectively.) In general CD4 bearing cells act to promote the immune response and are termed "helper cells." CD8 cells can be further subdivided into "suppressor cells" and "cytotoxic cells."

At this point, it is possible to review the events involved in a cell mediated response. Assume a virus or other intra-cellular pathogen invades a human and infects a variety of cells. A specific type of cell, the dendritic macrophage, phagocytoses some viral particles and processes this antigen which is then presented to a T helper cell. Such cells are activated by interleukin 1 (IL 1), a substance secreted by the macrophage. A series of conditions must be met for the process to proceed. This cell must have a recognition unit on its surface capable of interacting with the viral antigen. It, and the macrophage must also share surface components belonging to the HLA system, which is known by its activity in transplantation rejection. If the macrophage and the T helper cell share the same Class II transplantation antigens, this requirement is met. Activated CD4 cells in turn recruit CD8 cells with another messenger or lymphokine, known as Interleukin 2 (IL2). Cytotoxic CD8 cells bearing the proper recognition unit will then destroy cells which are infected with the virus as these cells will have viral antigen on their surface. For the cytotoxic T cells to so act, however, they must share Class I HLA antigens with the virally infected cells. Other CD8 cells recruited in this process act to suppress the T helper cells and thereby modulate the immune response. Thus, the organism is able to specifically destroy its own cells which are virally infected and in so doing interrupt the viruses' growth phase. Viral material released during the process and other non-intra-cellular antigens are engulfed and destroyed by other types of monocytic macrophages which are both attracted and stimulated by other lymphokines released by the T cells.

The recognition of the antigen by a preprogrammed T cell results in proliferation of that cell accompanied by the release of lymphokines. These lymphokines are non-immunoglobulin glycoproteins which, as a class, act as cell messengers. There are a variety of lymphokines and their properties are now being elucidated. One lymphokine may have more than one activity and they may act synergistically with other lymphokines or other biologically active materials. The ultimate result of the activity of the lymphokine release after antigen recognition is the recruitment of cells, both other lymphocytes and macrophages. The macrophages are large mononuclear cells which are simultaneously attracted to the area of antigenic stimulation and activated. The activation process produces a cell which engulfs not only the specific inciting antigen, but other foreign materials within the same region. The parallel between antibody recognition of antigen, complement activation and mobilization of polymorphs in the humoral response and the recruitment of macrophages in the cell mediated response is striking. Both the polymorphonuclear leukocytes and the macrophage engulf the antigen and activate a series of anatomic and metabolic changes which usually results in the destruction of the microorganism whose surface antigen initiated the process.

From the foregoing, it must not be assumed that T cells have no influence on B cell function. CD4 cells exert helper effects and CD8 cells suppressor effects on antibody production by B cells and together they help regulate antibody production.

The crucial role of the thymus in immune function and regulation is now well recognized. This was not always so. During the late nineteen thirties and beyond, thymuses of young children were irradiated in order to prevent a purely mythical disease, status thymolymphaticus. This concept developed when it was noted that babies dying of sudden infant death syndrome had large thymuses. It is now recognized that a large thymus in early infancy is normal.

Auto-Immunity

The preceding discussion outlines a system which has developed in order to protect an organism from infection by a potential pathogen. Introduction of a microbe which is not easily destroyed or controlled by the body's general defenses will result in infection. The infection will persist unless or until a specific immune response, either antibody or CMI, identifies and targets the invader for destruction by phagocytic cells or other cytotoxic processes. This implies that the immune system must recognize that which is foreign or "non-self." Our tissue cells all have protein and carbohydrate structures on their surfaces. These, too, can act as antigens, that is; signals for the immune system. We know that we can type red blood cells, a technique of identifying surface components. Typing indicates which cells are likely to cause an immune response when injected into a given recipient, by virtue of their having surface antigens which differ from the recipient's red cell antigens. The situation is similar but more complicated when other tissues, such as renal tissue, are transplanted. So many different surface antigens exist that it is almost a certainty than an immune reaction will follow when an individual receives tissue other than blood from a donor who is not his or her identical twin. Only when the immune system is compromised either by a disease process or iatrogenically, is such transplantation feasible.

The problem can be looked at from a different perspective. We should not ask why individuals have such immune responses as it would appear to be a necessary byproduct of a viral defense system. Rather let us ask why each of our immune systems does not respond to our own cells or serum proteins. The many and complicated theories that have been proposed to explain the mechanisms of "self-tolerance" cannot be examined in detail. In general, however, vertebrates do not respond immunologically to potential antigens if they meet them early in development, in prenatal or neonatal life. This means that we do not, or rather, only rarely respond to our own tissues.

Rheumatic Diseases

It was noted many years ago that patients with various rheumatic diseases have altered immune capabilities and can make antibodies to their own antigens. Thus, patients with systemic lupus erythematous (SLE) produce a whole series of autoantibodies. They make antibodies to DNA, the genetic material found in each cell. This is a surprising observation as DNA is a "poor" antigen even when injected from one animal to another of a different species. SLE patients sometimes also make antibodies to their own red cells, platelets, white cells and many other intra-cellular components besides DNA. Such anti-nuclear antibodies (ANA) are sometimes also detected in other disease states or in normals. The prognostic significance of ANA is not clear. Regarding SLE it has been postulated that the disease results from an overall derangement of the immune response, such as diminution of suppressor cell activity. While the cause of this alteration in the immune response is itself unclear, several pathogenetic mechanisms can result from such unbridled antibody production. If a patient makes antibodies against red cells, these cells are more rapidly destroyed and anemia results. Antibodies to white blood cells may diminish the number of phagocytic cells and leave the patient more prone to infection even in the presence of an overactive immune system.

Other damage may be caused indirectly by the unregulated production of autoantibodies. Let us examine the consequences of anti-DNA antibody production. Body cells are normally broken down as part of tissue maintenance. One would assume that this constant breakdown results in a steady supply of DNA.

If lupus patients produce antibodies to DNA, both the antibodies and the antigen will be present together. It has been shown that when large amounts of antibody are mixed with small amounts of antigen a firm precipitate is formed. This precipitate would rapidly be cleared from the blood and tissue fluids by macrophages in tissues. On the other hand, if antibody and antigen are mixed in such proportions that the antigen is in excess, a soluble complex is formed. These complexes can lodge in the filtering mechanisms of the kidney or in blood vessel walls of other organs. When in these areas the complexes may fix complement, and in so doing attract white blood cells. White cells are laden with packets of enzymes, the lysosomes, ordinarily functional in the destruction of engulfed bacteria. The polymorphonuclear leukocytes will attempt to engulf the deposited complexes, but because the deposition is massive, the cells will be unable to internalize the complexes. This "frustrated phagocytosis" as it is called, will result in the extrusion and local spillage of the lysosomal enzymes in the normal tissues. These enzymes can destroy cartilage and other tissue, and in so doing produce what we recognize clinically as an inflammatory reaction. Indeed, the deposition of immune complexes in the kidney has been implicated in the pathogenesis of renal disease in SLE and in other conditions.

Immune complexes have been found in the serum of patients with SLE as noted, and also in the serum of patients with rheumatoid arthritis (RA). In this disease, however, the pattern of tissue destruction is very different. The kidney is rarely, if ever, involved. The joints are the major target organs in rheumatoid arthritis. If it is proposed that immune complexes are the major cause of tissue destruction, (a theory which is far from totally proven), one must be prepared to explain why different clinical syndromes arise through a single pathogenetic process. Differences in size and in other properties of the complex may provide some answers.

Patients with RA only occasionally make anti-nuclear antibodies and then only in small amounts. Anti-DNA antibodies are virtually never seen.

These patients, however, make IgM antibodies called rheumatoid factors (RF). These RF react with sites on the constant region of IgG and have been sometimes termed autoantibodies. The majority of RA patients exhibit RF in the circulation. The stimulus for RF production appears to be either circulating immune complexes, other circulating antibodies that resemble the Fc region of human IgG, or antigens having cross-reactive determinants with human IgG.

Significant numbers of patients with infectious or other diseases also have RF although in lower concentrations (titers). Some normal individuals also have low concentrations of RF. The prevalence of RF in normals is about 1–4% depending on the technique of measurement. With increased age, the prevalence increases. Several studies have indicated that RF arises from different germ line genes in RA as compared to non-RA individuals.

Unfortunately, the role of RF in the pathogenesis of disease has not been established and we may be looking at an epiphenomenon which results from the disease process rather than incites it, i.e., response to a new antigenic determinant formed as a result of inflammatory alteration of IgG. Nevertheless, RF may still play some part in the production of the disease process we see clinically. Complexes are formed by RF with the individual's own IgG and are of higher molecular weight and different composition than those seen in SLE. The varying biological effects of complexes may result from the site of origin of the autoantibodies. RF can be shown to be made by cells in the pannus, or the inflammatory tissue in the joint. If the complexes are formed locally their effects may be noted, at least most intensely, also locally. The local production of these antibodies suggests the concept that some unknown agent be it physical or biological, triggers the disease. There must be some reason that antibodies are produced in one area or another. When RF is produced in the joint, the inflammatory disease process may then be furthered leading to the clinical picture already described.

It is of more than passing interest that much of what we know about the immune system has resulted from investigations of the rheumatic diseases. It has been suspected for many years that some of these diseases, particularly SLE and RA are diseases of autoimmunity, e.g., the turning of the immune system against the host. While those ideas were perhaps naive, they certainly provided hypotheses which are still viable in a more sophisticated form. The ultimate question as to why some individuals have these diseases and others do not, still defies definitive answers. It is true, however, that a search for that answer has contributed to a new era in biological knowledge. Recent research on therapeutic use of natural immunomodulators, such as interferons, interleukins and antibodies with T cell or idiotype specificity suggest new treatment possibilities in RA and SLE.

We trust that this knowledge, when developed, will indeed provide both an answer to the cause and an indication of techniques of prevention and treatment of these maladies.

SUGGESTED READINGS

Cohen, A.S. and Bennett, J.C., editors. *Rheumatology and Immunology*. 2nd edition. Pub. Grune and Stratton, Orlando, FL 1986.

Dixon, F.J. and Fisher, D.W., editors. *The Biology of Immunologic Disease*. Pub. Sinaur Associates, Sunderland, MA 1983.

Golub, E.S. *Immunology, A Synthesis*. Pub. Sinaur Associates, Sunderland, MA 1987.

Haeney, M. *Introduction to Clinical Immunology*. Pub. Butterworth, London 1985.

Male, D. "Immunology, An Illustrated Outline." Pub. C.V. Mosby 1986.

McCarthy, D.J., editor. Arthritis and Allied Conditions, Sec. 11 Scientific Basis for the Study of the Rheumatic Diseases, 11th edition. Lea & Febiger, Philadelphia, 1989.

Morrow, J. and Isenberg, D. "Autoimmune Rheumatic Disease," Pub. Year Book Medical Publishers, Chicago, Ill., 1987.

Roitt, I. "Essential Immunology." Blackwell Scientific Pub. 6th edition, 1988.

Schumacher, H.R., editor. *Primer on the Rheumatic Diseases,* 9th edition. Chapters 6–9. Pub. The Arthritis Foundation, Atlanta, GA 1988.

Tonagawa, S. "The Molecules of the Immune System." **Scientific American,** Vol. 253, pp. 122–131, October 1985.

II SPECIFIC DISEASES

"...all gouty symptoms...are excited by the irritating quality of a certain acrimonious matter circulating in the juices, which matter is supposed either to be generalized from intemperance, or inherited from parents;...and this gouty matter is supposed to discharge itself on some joint, and thus to create a paroxysm of regular, acute, inflamed gout."

The Origin of Gout by John Scot, M.D., 2nd Edition, London, 1783, p. 21.

CHAPTER 4

RHEUMATOID ARTHRITIS

John L. Abruzzo,, M.D.
Bruce R. Bender, M.D.

DESCRIPTION AND CLASSIFICATION

Rheumatoid Arthritis (RA) is a chronic systemic inflammatory disease of unknown cause that primarily affects synovial joints and related structures such as bursae, tendons and ligaments, but can also affect other parts of the body as well, such as the lungs, the heart and blood vessels, the hematologic system, the eyes, subcutaneous tissue, etc. The disease usually affects multiple peripheral joints simultaneously and has a tendency to develop in a bilateral symmetrical manner. Synovial inflammation causes joint stiffness, pain, swelling and warmth. Generalized involvement may be associated with low grade fever, loss of appetite, diminished energy and easy fatigability. Persistence of the disease has debilitating effects on the musculoskeletal system and often leads to frustration, depression and other adverse psychosocial phenomena. Rheumatoid Arthritis affects approximately 1–2% of the general population, but fortunately its course in the majority is relatively benign and non-progressive. The disease is characterized by exacerbations of inflammation and remission. In the severest cases, remissions are only partial and of short duration; but in the more fortunate can be complete and last for many months or even years. There is no specific test for the diagnosis, which usually rests on the recognition of characteristic clinical and laboratory findings and on the exclusion of certain other diseases.

The American Rheumatism Association (ARA) has developed a set of criteria which are useful in the diagnosis and classification of RA (See Table 4-1). As expected, the disease is usually not difficult to diagnose in its most advanced form, but may be impossible to diagnose with certainly early in its course. The ARA criteria lists eleven characteristics of the disease. The disease may be considered "Classical" when seven or more are recognized; "Definite" when five or six are present, and "Probable" if only three or four are evident. The characteristics include: morning stiffness of thirty minutes duration or more; pain on motion or tenderness in at least one joint; soft tissue joint swelling; swelling of at least one other joint; and symmetrical involvement. Additional criteria include the recognition of subcutaneous nodules over bony prominences or on extensor surface or overlying articular regions; typical erosive roentgenographic changes; a positive test for rheumatoid factor in serum; synovial fluid showing a poor mucin precipitate, and characteristic histologic changes in the synovial membrane or subcutaneous nodules.

Another set of criteria, the New York Criteria (See Table 4-2) for the diagnosis of RA may be more helpful in identifying patients whose disease has been more clinically active and progressive, and who are likely to become more disabled and have a greater complexity and severity of problems. Thus, application of both criteria are often helpful for diagnostic purposes, although they are primarily intended as classification criteria they may be most important in studying the disease and its treatment.

At its onset, RA usually follows one of at least three different patterns. The most common pattern is slow and progressive evolution over a period of weeks to months. Complaints may include fatigue, malaise, or diffuse aches and pains *not* initially localized by the patient to joints. Sooner or later morning stiffness and bilateral symmetrical joints involvement especially at the hands, wrists, feet and knees becomes evident in most cases. Morning stiffness may occasionally be the first complaint even before the onset of joint pain, and can be thought of as a discomfort throughout a restricted range of joint motion when the patient initiates easy movements after arising from sleep; following a period of sustained joint immobility and relaxation. Muscular weakness is also common, and may be described as difficulty with activities of daily living such as climbing the stairs, opening jars, opening doors, etc. Other systemic symptoms may also occur and include low grade fever, weight loss, loss of appetite, sleep disturbance and depression.

A second pattern of onset is marked by more sudden development and predominance of fatigue, fever, malaise and morning stiffness. Joint pain and muscular weakness are less prominent among the initial symptoms. The least common pattern of onset is the sudden development of severe pain in multiple joints usually associated with diffuse muscle aches as well.

The course of RA is every bit as variable as its mode of onset. RA is generally regarded as a chronic disease that is characterized by remissions and exacerbations that eventually may cause joint deformities, impairment of motion and functional loss. Nevertheless, the great majority of patients with RA experience at least one or more remissions. Remissions occur most frequently during the first few years of the disease and may last anywhere from a month or two or a number of years. Remissions are sometimes complete and are characterized by complete disappearance of symptoms and all signs of joint inflammation. More often, however, remissions are incomplete and, as the disease progresses, incomplete remissions are more common. After the initial episode, a small percentage of patients experience a complete remission lasting for many years and a small percentage experience *no* remissions at all. Instead, the disease is progressive and destructive resulting in crippling deformities in one to two years. The great majority of patients, however, follow a course somewhere between these extremes. Many have a relatively benign and non-progressive course with a favorable outcome resulting in relatively insignificant permanent functional loss, although temporary functional deficiencies lasting anywhere from a few days to a few months may occur periodically.

Approximately 20% of patients with RA will eventually develop permanent impairments with significant loss of function and disability. A disease characterized by an unpredictable course and a broad range of functional outcomes presents innumerable therapeutic challenges. Fortunately, most patients respond favorably to medical management that includes the appropriate selection and use of anti-inflammatory drugs or other disease suppressing agents. Health professionals including physical and occupation therapists, nurses, vocational counselors, social workers and community agencies all may be needed for the individual with RA.

RA may present atypical forms as well. One such form is its confinement to a relatively few joints and rarely even a single joint. Another is the presence of a palindromic pattern. In this form, acute painful swelling usually develops in one or a few joints over several hours and subsides completely within a few hours, or it may last up to two or three weeks. In this form, the disease resembles acute gout. On rare occasions rheumatoid disease exists predominantly and even solely as multiple painless subcutaneous nodules referred to as rheumatoid nodulosis. Joint involvement may be minimal or absent. Finally, description of other more systemic and complex forms of the disease is beyond the scope of this chapter, i.e., rheumatoid vasculitis, Felty's syndrome and Sjögren's syndrome.

Clinical management in general requires periodic assessment of the status of the disease. This is usually accomplished by physical examination and appropriate laboratory and radiologic examinations. The extent and severity of joint inflammation may be assessed by grading the amount of heat, pain and tenderness, and swelling of individual joints; by the duration and severity of morning stiffness; the severity of fatigue, and the presence or absence of fever. Periodic assessment of the functional status is just as important as assessing the severity of inflammation. Determination of the erythrocyte sedimentation rate (ESR) is frequently helpful as the ESR generally correlates with the severity and extent of inflammation. Progression of the disease to more advanced anatomical stages, i.e., degrees of degradation of the anatomical integrity of the articular cartilage and subchondral bone, ligament, tendons and other capsular tissues that are associated with clinically significant permanent joint deformities, can also be assessed by a careful periodic physical examination and by occasional radiologic examination. Functional status is usually related to the severity, extent and location of the joint inflammation, and also to the degree of permanent deformity and structural changes in tendons, ligaments, and other periarticular structures. One method of clinical assessment was described by Steinbrocker in 1949 (Table 4-3) and has been used effectively for many years. The method defines the progression of the disease by physical and radiological means and divides patients into four stages; early, moderate, severe and terminal. It then defines the functional capacity as four classes ranging from complete functional capability with the retained ability to carry on all usual duties without handicaps (Class I), to largely or wholly incapacitated, at which point the patient is either bedridden or confined to a wheelchair, and capable of little or no self-care (Class 4).

It is implicit in this method of assessment that a patient classified as Stage I, Class 3 or 4, would most likely have acute generalized joint inflammation causing severe but potentially completely reversible disability. On the other hand, a patient classified as Stage IV Class 4 most likely has long-standing disease that has resulted in many non-reversible anatomical changes. Such a patient may still additionally have active joint inflammation contributing to the severe level of disability. Careful clinical evaluation would thus be needed before proper therapeutic interventions should be undertaken. These would include the need for more potent and probably more toxic drugs, physical and occupational modalities and surgery.

Periodic assessment is also important because it is basically not possible to predict the outcome of the disease from its early presenting features, even though certain characteristics, such as the development of subcutaneous rheumatoid nodules and high serum titers of rheumatoid factor correlate with more destructive, disabling disease. These features usually occur as the disease progresses rather than in the first few months after onset. Thus, their predictive value is reduced.

A better appreciation of the relationships between the joint inflammation of rheumatoid arthritis, the limitation of joint motion, the results of synovial tissue proliferation, resulting deformities and poor function, may be gained with the help of the diagram on page 5 of a normal diarthrodial joint. Diarthrodial joints possess a true tissue cavity that allows for relatively free mobility. The opposing surfaces of the articulating bones are separated by articular cartilage that covers each of the surfaces and by a small amount of fluid within the cavity of the joint. The joints are enclosed by a capsule consisting of connective tissue richly supplied with blood vessels and nerve endings. Its inner-most surface is made of synovial cells. The synovial cells essentially form a membrane which extends from the edge of one articular cartilage to the edge of the opposing articular cartilage by proceeding around the inner-most part of the joint capsule. Synovial tissue does not cover the surface of the articular cartilage. The inner surface of the joint capsule is formed of redundant folds and pouches of synovial tissue that help allow freedom of joint motion. The fibrous joint capsule, ligaments and the periarticular muscles provide stability and strength to the joints. Compressive forces normally applied to joints such as the knee joint may range from 2–10 times that of the body weight. Motion of weight bearing diarthrodial joints such as the knees, hips and ankles is characterized by rapid acceleration and deceleration. This type of motion causes particularly high stress to the major load bearing regions of the joints. In RA, inflammation of the synovium causes the symptoms associated with disease. It causes the synovial tissue to swell and fluid to accumulate within the joint cavity. Increased fluid in a body cavity is termed an effusion. Fortunately, this process is potentially reversible especially with the application of rest, splints, and the use of anti-inflammatory medications. The functional deficiencies resulting directly from this process are thus also reversible. Later in the course of the disease, however, the functional deficiencies become progressively less reversible as the development of chronic essentially non-reversible destructive changes take place within and around the joints.

SPECIFIC JOINTS

The Hand and Wrist

Of the many clinical features of rheumatoid arthritis, the chronic deformities found in the hands and wrist are probably most characteristic of the disease. In general, joint deformities occur as a result of several factors operating together over a period of time. Most important is destruction of articular tissues as a result of sustained inflammation, the remodeling of some of the structures especially articular cartilage and bone, and the biomechanical forces of various muscles during use and possibly even at rest. Progressive weakening of the extensor carpiulnaris is associated with volar subluxation of the ulnar side of the wrist. The precise mechanisms for the frequent development of this deformity are complex and incompletely understood. Weakening of the radial collateral ligaments and joint capsules occur simultaneously with the inflammation and muscle imbalance. Synovial cystic swelling is usually observed and is usually more pronounced on the dorsal side of the wrist. It is the result of synovial proliferation and increased intra-articular pressure.

The metacarpophalangeal joints show proliferative swelling mainly on the extensor surface. Weakening of the collateral ligaments and strong flexor forces pull the base of the proximal phalanges to produce volar subluxation. Ulnar deviation at the metacarpophalangeal joint is most common and probably occurs because of failures of the radial collateral ligaments associated with intrinsic muscle decompositions. Ulnar deviation is more likely to occur than radial deviation because of the natural design of the joints of the hand. When the disease is far advanced, the extensor tendons slide laterally into the groove on the ulnar side of the joints producing a fixed deformity. Similar factors operating at the proximal interphalangeal joints result in either hyperextension deformities or flexion deformities with the reverse occurring at the distal interphalangeal joints. The first type is often referred to as a swan-neck deformity; the second, a boutonniere deformity. In conjunction with deformities range of motion is usually restricted but sometimes joint range is actually increased as a result of the destructive and stretching process. The degree of disability resulting from the various deformities differs greatly from individual to individual but loss of flexion in the fingers generally produces much greater disability than an equivalent loss of extension. This is especially significant when the ring and little fingers are affected. Deformities of the thumb may be classified into opposition, adduction, and abduction and result in loss of the appropriate movement. This is very important because normal opposition, adduction and abduction are needed for so many activities of daily living such as gripping a door knob, a pan or utensil. The intrinsic muscles of the hand may develop fixed flexion contractures that may be preventable by a supervised exercise program.

Flexor tenosynovitis is another common feature of rheumatoid arthritis as is painless "attrition" extensor tendon rupture. The third, second, fourth, fifth and first flexor tendons are involved in the order listed. These lesions cause "trigger" fingers that are usually effectively treated by splinting and injection therapy. Indications for hand surgery include intractable pain at the metacarpophalangeal joints due to subluxation, tendon ruptures, and defective thumb or finger function and fixed deformities.

The Elbow

Inflammation of the tendon sheaths and synovial membranes, accompanied by swelling of surrounding soft tissue structures (synovitis) usually involves both the radiohumeral and ulnohumeral joints. Acute involvement is usually associated with a joint effusion and may be effectively treated by aspiration and corticosteroid injection. Acute synovitis at the elbow usually causes bulging, tenderness and thickening along either side of the olecranon process that may be distinguished from olecranon bursitis where the tenderness, thickening and bulging is found directly over the olecranon process.

Chronic synovitis of the elbow usually causes some loss of both extension and flexion that unless severe, may be unnoticed by the patient as the elbow is essentially an interconnecting hinge joint between the hand and the upper thorax.

Motion at the shoulder and wrist can usually offset loss of motion at the elbow so that function is relatively unimpaired.

The Shoulder

The acromioclavicular joint is the most frequently involved portion of the shoulder. Synovitis here may be signaled by pain when the patient turns and places his or her weight on the side as during sleep. Involvement of the rotator cuff is potentially more significant in that with weakening of the rotator cuff tendons by chronic synovitis the rotator cuff tendons are vulnerable to tear and significant loss of shoulder abduction. Conservative treatment with rest, physical modalities and repeated intra-articular steroid injections help control pain and return range of motion for more normal function.

The Cervical Spine

The cervical spine is involved in up to two thirds of patients. The most common complaint is painful restriction of neck motion. Chronic erosive synovitis involving the atlanto-axial joint can lead to subluxation and potentially dangerous complications, including cervical cord damage and brain stem involvement. The most common symptom of significant atlanto-axial involvement is pain radiating from the back of the neck to the top of the head. A sensation of burning and/or numbness may be elicited when the patient turns her head. Symptoms such as difficulty speaking or swallowing, difficulty with bladder control, unilateral weakness, sudden onset of ataxia and/or "drop" attacks are causes for alarm and immediate attention. In general, patients with significant atlanto-axial disease should be cautioned about potential whiplash injuries and airway intubation for general anesthesia. The patient should be given careful instructions on the use of a cervical collar and a proper head rest when riding in motor vehicles. They should be strongly advised to avoid situations of sudden acceleration or deceleration that might precipitate spinal cord compression.

The Hip

Hip involvement is fortunately relatively uncommon but when it occurs it is especially serious because synovitis of this large weight-bearing joint is often severely disabling and its persistence leads to anatomical changes that cause permanent disability. Furthermore, the deep location of the hips make their examination more difficult. Signs of inflammation such as increased warmth and joint effusions are almost impossible to detect by physical examination. Painful restriction of range of motion is the most dependable sign of hip synovitis and is usually referred to the inguinal and groin regions. Pain localized to the lateral aspect of the hip is frequently a symptom of trochanteric bursitis. The distinction is important to make because an injection of a steroid medication into the trochanteric bursa is usually highly effective treatment for trochanteric bursitis. External rotation is usually the first motion of the hip joints to become restricted. Radiographic images include joint space narrowing, slight subchondral sclerosis and diffuse osteopenia. With disease progression, acetabular resorption is association with a medial and cephalad migration of the femoral head that may culminate in the protrusion of the head into the pelvis. This condition is referred to as acetabulum protrusii and occurs in less than 5% of patients. More commonly the femoral head undergoes cystic changes with resorption, partial collapse and remodeling as in other weight-bearing joints. Advanced deformities of the hips are usually associated with severe pain and disability. Orthopedic reconstructive surgery is an effective form of treatment that is frequently indicated.

The Knees

The knees are commonly involved in rheumatoid arthritis and in contrast to the hip, synovial inflammation is readily apparent by examination. Joint effusions are easily aspirated and can be subjected to laboratory examination as well. Synovitis results in quadriceps muscle atrophy very rapidly and an inability to fully extend the knee. Flexion contractures also occur commonly and interfere with ambulation. Persistence of disease can cause laxity of the collateral ligaments, joint instability and difficulty with walking or bending. Forceful flexion of the knees as with bending and stair climbing cause very high intra-articular pressures that may lead to rupture of the joint capsule at points of weakness and more commonly synovial out-pouchings. These usually occur posteriorly and are termed Baker's or popliteal cysts. It has been shown by use of contrast dyes that essentially one way valvular actions allow joint fluid to pass from the knee cavity into the popliteal cyst, but not to return. Popliteal cysts may compress superficial veins or may themselves rupture with the dissection of fluid into the calf using swelling of the calf and a clinical syndrome that mimics deep vein thrombophlebitis.

The Ankles and Feet

The articulations of the feet are involved frequently and early in the disease. The changes that take place in many ways resemble those found in the hands. The metatarsophalangeal joints are almost always involved, and are usually the first joints to show bone erosions. Synovitis at these joints is especially painful and disabling with respect to walking because the normal stride places great pressure on these inflamed joints during the push-off phase. Progressive involvement is associated with metatarsal head subluxation, lateral toe deformity, and dorsal tendon contractures producing "cock-up" toes. In addition, ligament laxity results in a spreading of the forefoot. Numerous increased points of friction and pressure with the interior surfaces of shoes can lead to corns and calluses or ulcerations of the skin and infections.

The ankles are less commonly involved than the knees. Chronic disease with resultant ligamentous laxity usually results in instability and a permanently everted foot deformity.

EPIDEMIOLOGY

Rheumatoid arthritis affects about one percent of the adult U.S. population. In general, the prevalence of definite, chronic rheumatoid arthritis is about the same world wide when the age of the particular population is taken into account. The increased prevalence in certain populations of Yakima and Chippewa Indians, Jamaicans and urban South African Blacks suggest potentially important environmental or genetic factors affecting these groups. Disease prevalence increases with advancing age to the seventh decade. Generally, disease that begins in the elderly is thought to be milder than that beginning at an early age. Although rheumatoid arthritis is seldom a fatal disease, mortality appears to be increasing. Individuals having severe generalized disease early in its course appear to be at increased risks and death is most often caused by cardiovascular, renal and infectious complications.

ETIOLOGY AND PATHOGENESIS

Infectious agents have long been considered as possible etiologic agents, but none have been definitely identified. Investigations in the fields of bacteriology, virology and immunology have helped us to understand the mechanisms of joint inflammation and autoimmune responses. Accumulated evidence suggests that the disease may be initiated by one or more environmental agents acting on a genetically vulnerable and possibly immunologically deficient host to cause a sustained and possibly abnormal immune response by the host. This may result in the development of chronic inflammatory synovitis.

Nutritional and metabolic factors appear to be of incidental importance in etiology. Viral factors have been searched for intensively, but to date no intact replicating viruses have been consistently recovered from synovial tissue. However, since patients with rheumatoid arthritis have an increased frequently of antibodies to a nuclear antigen found in the Epstein-Barr virus, it is possible that this virus has an etiologic role. Virus-induced new antigens could develop on synovial cell membranes or on virus infected lymphocyte or macrophage membranes to stimulate normal defense mechanism that include an immunological response against host (auto) antigens. The Epstein-Barr virus is a ubiquitous organism containing double-strained DNA that infects almost all people before thirty years of age. The viruses are selectively found in B lymphocytes, which are thus activated to proliferate and produce antibodies. It has been suggested that rheumatoid patients have genetically determined deficiencies that alter their ability to handle the virus in the same way that non-rheumatoid persons would. The responsible genetic factors are not known, but it is thought that they involve the short arm of the sixth chromosome where the major histocompatibility genes (HLA) are located. Genes located on the D locus of this chromosome help govern the function of the immune system, and HLA-DR4, a specific D locus antigen can be found on B lymphocyte surface membranes about twice as frequently in rheumatoid arthritis as in the general population. Further research may clarity the way in which the immune system interacts with microbes and/or their components and could lead to the development of the chronic synovitis of rheumatoid arthritis. At present, it appears that both humoral and cell-mediated function of the immune system participates in this process as a result of significant interactions between antigen processing macrophages and T and B lymphocytes that occur within affected synovium.

In the presence of stimulating antigens, T lymphocytes release soluble chemical factors (lymphokines) locally that signal and regulate further immune functions as enhancement or suppression of B lymphocyte activity or that can cause damage to joint tissues directly. When B lymphocytes are stimulated, they proliferate and differentiate into plasma cells that synthesize specific immunoglobulins (antibodies). This latter process is referred to as the humoral part of the immune system because antibodies are stable proteins that are carried in the blood and are thus capable of acting at distant as well as local sites. Antibodies may interact with antigens to form immune complexes, or they may interact with one another (self-association) to form IgG-anti-IgG immune complexes. Immune complexes activate the complement system and the products of these complex interactions contribute to the pathologic process of inflammation. Humoral immune processes appear to play a major role in the initiation and perpetuation of rheumatoid inflammation.

RF (rheumatoid factors) are antibodies that are capable of reacting with other immunoglobulins to form immune complexes. Some, having a molecular weight of about 160,000 and a sedimentation constant of 7S on analytic ultracentrifugation, are classified as IgG. Others, (classical RF) are IgM antibodies that have a molecular weight of about one million and 19S sedimentation constant. The latter is found in about 80% of patients with RA and can be detected by agglutination procedures such as the latex fixation test. This is a useful, though not specific test for the disease. The primary stimulus for the continuing production of RF in patients with RA is not known.

The joint tissue destruction associated with these immune processes appears to result from the elaboration of factors such as enzymes including lysosomal proteases released from leukocytes, collagenases, etc. Rheumatoid synovitis can be simply thought of as two types of inflammation occurring at the same time, i.e., an acute exudative component and a chronic inflammatory component. The exudative component is represented in the synovial membrane and joint effusion. Polymorphonuclear leukocytes and immune complexes may be identified at these sites and complement activity and consumption are increased. The chronic inflammatory component of RA is predominantly confined to the tissues beneath the synovial membrane and is represented by a mononuclear infiltration that is sometimes prominent around blood vessels. These inflammatory processes result in the elaboration of chemical mediators that cause cartilage degeneration, bone erosions and the other clinical signs of rheumatoid joint destruction.

In summary, the synovitis of RA consists of a chronic inflammatory phase in which RF are synthesized and released into synovial fluid to form immune complexes which in turn are responsible for triggering the second phase, acute inflammation. The stimulus for the chronic cellular infiltrative phase of the disease affects the so-called transitional areas of the synovial membrane where T and B lymphocytes undergo blastic transformation. The agent initiating these events may be a virus. Alternatively, there may be a genetically related defect causing an error of immunoregulation by suppressor T lymphocytes. Suffice it to say that the exact mechanisms of the error of immunoregulation is an area of intense interest and continued study.

TREATMENT

Proper management of the individual patient requires the recognition that RA is a systemic disorder with variable modes of onset, course and outcome. A large number of medicines, procedures and rehabilitative modalities are available and, if utilized appropriately, can help minimize deformity and maintain a relatively pain-controlled, if not pain-free, productive life. Drug therapy generally proceeds in a stepwise fashion as the disease persists or progresses. (See Table 4-4). However, a comprehensive management program includes drug therapy, patient education, psychosocial support as well as counseling and a carefully planned program of physical therapy. Each of these four primary components of the care plan must be tailored to the individual patient, adjusted on the basis on periodic assessment in accordance with the following three factors: (1) Intensity, extent and location of inflammation; (2) The anatomical stage of the disease and rate of its progression and (3) Functional considerations.

In general, the primary objective in early disease is to suppress synovial inflammation in an effort to control symptoms and prevent deformities. However, when the patient is in a later phase of disease ("end-stage"), it may be too late to effectively limit progression of the disease by suppressing inflammation. In this case, surgery and rehabilitation assumes more primary roles.

DRUG THERAPY

Drug therapy is prescribed during any stage of the disease and is aimed at suppressing rheumatoid inflammation when clinically evident. Salicylates or other non-steroidal anti-inflammatory agents are emphasized early in the course of the disease, but may be used at any stage along with the occasional intra-articular use of steroids for individually acute or disabling joint involvement. The anti-malarial drugs and/or pulse intravenous, or oral steroids may be added for patients with acute generalized and disabling disease who have not responded adequately to non-steroidal anti-inflammatory drugs. These drugs, in particular the corticosteroids, must only be used after careful deliberation and with great caution because of the complications associated with long-term use even at low doses.

Once erosions of bone and deterioration of articular cartilage have developed (Stage 2 or beyond), the further likelihood of destructive synovitis and a disabling disease justifies attempts at control with drugs having potential for controlling the rheumatoid process, but also for causing potentially fatal adverse reactions. Thus, intra-muscular gold or D-penicillamine should be prescribed after careful consideration and discussion with the patient. These drugs may also be used concurrent with a non-steroidal anti-inflammatory agent. Azathioprine or methotrexate, immunosuppressive agents may be used in place of gold and D-penicillamine for the still refractory patient. Other immunosuppressive agents, lymphoplasmapheresis, and total nodal irradiation may be considered under experimental protocols.

The physical therapy program utilizes fundamentals including heat, therapeutic exercise, patient and family education, and local or total body rest. Napping may be encouraged as needed. The concept of rest should include attention to reactive depression associated with the attendant loss of normal function. The patient must be helped in learning to cope with all the associated problems of RA. Rest periods should be incorporated into the daily routine as needed.

The patient should be made aware of social services, and referred to physical and occupational therapists as indicated. The nutritional state must be reviewed periodically, family counseling for sexual and marital difficulties must be offered as necessary, and corrective orthopedic surgery must be considered as needed. For a more detailed review of the individual modalities of the comprehensive care plan, the reader is referred to other chapters in this book.

SUGGESTED READINGS

Abruzzo, J.L. Mortality and rheumatoid arthritis. **Arth and Rheum.** 25:8, 1020–1023, 1982.

Bennett, P.H. and Burch, T.A. New York Symposium on population studies in the rheumatic diseases: New diagnostic criteria. **Bull Rheum Dis.** 17:453, 1967.

Brewerton, D.A. Hand deformities in rheumatoid disease. **Ann Rheum Dis.** 16:183–197, 1957.

Deppter, J.M. and Zvaifler, N.J. Epstein-Barr Virus: In relationship to the pathogenesis of rheumatoid arthritis. **Arth and Rheum.** 24:6, 75761, 1981.

Kelly, M.N., Harris, E.D., Jr., Ruddy, S., and Sledge, C.B. (eds.) Textbook of Rheumatology. WB Saunders, Philadelphia, 3rd edition, 1989. Sec. 7 Rheumatoid Arthritis.

Luukainen, R., Isomaki, H. and Kajander, A. Prognostic value of the type of onset of rheumatoid arthritis. **Ann Rheum Dis.** 42:274–275, 1983.

McCarthy, D.J. (ed.) Arthritis and Allied Conditions. Lea & Febiger, Philadelphia, 11th edition, 1989. Sec. 4 Rheumatoid Arthritis.

Ropes, M.W., Bennett, G.A., Cobb, S., Jacox, R., and Jessar, R.A. 1958 Revision of diagnostic criteria for rheumatoid arthritis. **Bull Rheum Dis.** 9:175–176, 1958.

Steinbrocker, O., Traeger, C.H., and Batterman, R.C. Therapeutic criteria in rheumatoid arthritis. **JAMA** 140:659–662, 1949.

TABLE 4-1 [1,2,3]
CRITERIA FOR THE CLASSIFICATION OF RHEUMATOID ARTHRITIS

A. Classic Rheumatoid Arthritis
This diagnosis requires 7 of the following criteria. In criteria 1 through 5 the joint signs or symptoms must be continuous for at least 6 weeks. Any one of the features listed under Exclusions will exclude a patient from this and all other categories.

1. Morning stiffness
2. Pain on motion or tenderness in at least 1 joint (observed by a physician)
3. Swelling (soft tissue thickening or fluid, not bony overgrowth alone) in a least 1 joint (observed by a physician)
4. Swelling (observed by a physician) of at least 1 other joint (any interval free of joint symptoms between the 2 joint involvements may not be more than 3 months)
5. Symmetric joint swelling (observed by a physician) with simultaneous involvement of the same joint on both sides of the body (bilateral involvement of proximal interphalangeal, metacarpophalangeal, or metatarsophalangeal joints is acceptable without absolute symmetry). Terminal phalangeal joint involvement will not satisfy this criterion
6. Subcutaneous nodules (observed by a physician) over bony prominences, on extensor surfaces, or in juxtaarticular regions
7. Roentgenographic changes typical of rheumatoid arthritis (which must include at least bony decalcification localized to or most marked adjacent to the involved joints and not just degenerative changes). Degenerative changes do not exclude patients from any group classified as having rheumatoid arthritis.
8. Positive agglutination test — demonstration of the "rheumatoid factor" by any method which, in 2 laboratories, has been positive in not over 5% of normal controls, or positive streptococcal agglutination test. [The latter is now obsolete.]
9. Poor mucin precipitate from synovial fluid (with shreds and cloudy solution). (An inflammatory synovial effusion with 2,000 or more white cells/mm³, without crystals can be substituted for this criterion.)
10. Characteristic histologic changes in synovium with 3 or more of the following: marked villous hypertrophy; proliferation of superficial synovial cells often with palisading; marked infiltration of chronic inflammatory cells (lymphocytes or plasma cells predominating) with tendency to form "lymphoid nodules"; deposition of compact fibrin either on surface or interstitially; foci of necrosis.
11. Characteristic histologic changes in nodules showing granulomatous foci with central zones of cell necrosis, surrounded by a palisade of proliferated mononuclear and peripheral fibrosis and chronic inflammatory cell infiltration.

B. Definite Rheumatoid Arthritis
This diagnosis requires 5 of the above criteria. In criteria 1 through 5 the joint signs or symptoms must be continuous for at least 6 weeks.

— Continued to page 49 —

C. Probable Rheumatoid Arthritis
This diagnosis requires 3 of the above criteria. In at least one of criteria 1 through 5 the joint signs or symptoms must be continuous for at least 6 weeks.

D. Possible Rheumatoid Arthritis
This diagnosis requires 2 of the following criteria and total duration of joint symptoms must be at least 3 months.

1. Morning stiffness.
2. Tenderness or pain on motion (observed by a physician) with history of recurrence or persistence for 3 weeks.
3. History or observation of joint swelling.
4. Subcutaneous nodules (observed by a physician).
5. Elevated sedimentation rate or C-reactive protein.
6. Iritis [of dubious value as a criterion except in juvenile arthritis].

E. Exclusions

1. The typical rash of systemic lupus erythematosus (with butterfly distribution, follicle plugging, and areas of atrophy)
2. High concentration of lupus erythematosus cells (4 or more in 2 smears prepared from heparinized blood incubated not over 2 hours) [or other clearcut evidence of systemic lupus erythematosus.]
3. Histologic evidence of periarteritis nodosa with segmental necrosis of arteries associated with nodular leukocytic infiltration extending perivascularly and tending to include many eosinophils.
4. Weakness of neck, trunk, and pharyngeal muscles or persistent muscle swelling or dermatomyositis.
5. Definite scleroderma (not limited to the fingers). [This is an arguable point.]
6. A clinical picture characteristic of rheumatic fever with migratory joint involvement and evidence of endocarditis, especially if accompanied by subcutaneous nodules or erythema marginatum or chorea. (An elevated antistreptolysin titer will not rule out the diagnosis of rheumatoid arthritis.)
7. A clinical picture characteristic of gouty arthritis with acute attacks of swelling, redness, and pain in one or more joints, especially if relieved by colchicine or accompanied by urate crystals.
8. Tophi
9. A clinical picture characteristic of acute infectious arthritis of bacterial or viral origin with: an acute focus of infection or in close association with a disease of known infectious origin; chills; fever; and an acute joint involvement, usually migratory initially (especially if there are organisms in the joint fluid or response to antibiotic therapy)
10. Tubercle bacilli in the joints or histologic evidence of joint tuberculosis.
11. A clinical picture characteristic of Reiter's syndrome with urethritis and conjunctivitis associated with acute joint involvement, usually migratory initially.
12. A clinical picture characteristic of the shoulder - hand syndrome with unilateral involvement of shoulder and hand, with diffuse swelling of the hand followed by atrophy and contractures.
13. A clinical picture characteristic of hypertrophic osteoarthropathy with clubbing of fingers and/or hypertrophic periostitis along the shafts of the long bones especially if an intrapulmonary lesion (or other appropriate underlying disorder) is present.
14. A clinical picture characteristic of neuroarthropathy with condensation and destruction of bones of involved joints and with associated neurologic findings.
15. Homogentisic acid in the urine, detectable grossly with alkalinization.
16. Histologic evidence of sarcoid or positive Kveim test.
17. Multiple myeloma as evidenced by marked increase in plasma cells in the bone marrow, or Bence-Jones protein in the urine.
18. Characteristic skin lesions of erythema nodosum.
19. Leukemia or lymphoma with characteristic cells in peripheral blood, bone marrow, or tissues.
20. Agammaglobulinemia

It should be noted that these criteria were developed before the new classification of rheumatic diseases adopted by the American Rheumatism Association in 1963, in which ankylosing spondylitis, psoriatic arthritis, and arthritis associated with ulcerative colitis and regional enteritis are listed as distinct from rheumatoid arthritis. Also, many additional distinct rheumatic diseases have been recognized since this time. Two or more diseases can coexist so exclusions are not absolute.

Proposed 1987 Revised American Rheumatism Association Criteria for Rheumatoid Arthritis [2, 3]

Four or more criteria must be present to diagnose rheumatoid arthritis:

1. Morning stiffness for at least one hour and present for at least six weeks.
2. Swelling of three or more joints for at least six weeks.
3. Swelling of wrist, metacarpophalangeal or proximal interphalangeal joints for six or more weeks.
4. Symmetric joint swelling.
5. Hand roentgenogram changes typical of rheumatoid arthritis that must include erosions or unequivocal bony decalcification.
6. Rheumatoid nodules
7. Serum rheumatoid factor by a method positive in less than 5% of normals.

2) These criteria have been presented by the ARA Rheumatoid Arthritis Criteria Subcommittee in abstract form for discussion.

3) Arnett FC, Edworthy S. Block DA, et al: The 1987 revised ARA criteria for rheumatoid arthritis. Arthritis Rheum 30:S17, 1987.

1) The material in Tables 4-1 and 4-3 are reprinted with permission from the "Primer on the Rheumatic Diseases" Ninth edition 1988 pp. 316–318. Pub.: The Arthritis Foundation, Atlanta, Georgia.

TABLE 4-2
NEW YORK CRITERIA FOR THE DIAGNOSIS OF RHEUMATOID ARTHRITIS

Rheumatoid Arthritis is present if criteria 1 and 2 plus either 3 or 4 are met

(1) History of an episode of three painful limb joints. Each group of joints, i.e., proximal interphalangeal joints, is counted as one joint, scoring each side separately.

(2) Swelling, limitation of motion, subluxation and/or ankylosis of three limb joints. Necessary inclusions: (a) at least one hand, wrist or foot; (b) symmetry of one joint pair. Exclusions: (a) distal interphalangeal joints; (b) fifth proximal interphalangeal joints; (c) first metarsophalangeal joints; (d) hips.

(3) Radiographic changes (erosions).

(4) Serum positive for rheumatoid factors.

TABLE 4-3
CRITERIA FOR DETERMINATION OF PROGRESSION OF RHEUMATOID ARTHRITIS AND OF FUNCTIONAL CAPACITY OF PATIENTS WITH THE DISEASE

Classification of Progression of Rheumatoid Arthritis

Stage I, Early

*1. No destructive changes on roentgenographic examination

2. Roentgenologic evidence of osteoporosis may be present.

Stage II, Moderate

*1. Roentgenologic evidence of osteoporosis, with or without slight subchondral bone destruction; slight cartilage destruction may be present.

*2. No joint deformities, although limitation of joint mobility may be present.

3. Adjacent muscle atrophy

4. Extraarticular soft tissue lesions, such as nodules and tenosynovitis may be present.

Stage III, Severe

*1. Roentgenologic evidence of cartilage and bone destruction, in addition to osteoporosis

*2. Joint deformity, such as subluxation, ulnar deviation, or hyperextension, without fibrous or bony ankylosis.

3. Extensive muscle atrophy

4. Extraarticular soft tissue lesions, such as nodules and tenosynovitis may be present.

Stage IV, Terminal

*1. Fibrous or bony ankylosis

2. Criteria of stage III

*The criteria prefaced by an asterisk are those that must be present to permit classification of a patient in any particular stage or grade.

Classification of Functional Capacity in Rheumatoid Arthritis

Class I: Complete functional capacity with ability to carry on all usual duties without handicaps

Class II: Functional capacity adequate to conduct normal activities despite handicap of discomfort or limited mobility of 1 or more joints

Class III: Functional capacity adequate to perform only few or none of the duties of usual occupation or of self care

Class IV: Largely or wholly incapacitated with patient bedridden or confined to wheelchair, permitting little or no self care

TABLE 4-4
THERAPIES APPROPRIATE TO THE VARIOUS STAGES OF RHEUMATOID ARTHRITIS

Therapy	*Disease Stage* 1	2	3	4
Patient Education	—	—	—	—
Non-Steroidal Anti-Inflammatory Drugs	—	—	—	—
Intra-Articular Steroids	—	—	—	—
Rest, Physical and Occupational Therapy	—	—	—	—
Psychosocial Support and Counseling	—	—	—	—
plus				
Anti-Malarial Drugs and/or Oral or I.V. Steroids		—	—	—
and/or				
Surgery		—	—	—
Intra-Muscular Gold or D-penicillamine			—	—
or				
Azathioprine			—	—
or				
Experimental: Methotrexate, plasmapheresis				—

CHAPTER 5

OSTEOARTHRITIS

Itzhak A. Rosner, M.D.
Roland A. Moscowitz, M.D.

DEFINITION

Osteoarthritis (OA) is unique among the rheumatic diseases in that, both clinically and pathologically, it is a condition which is exclusively restricted to involvement of the joints of the body. In contrast, rheumatoid arthritis (RA) and virtually all the other rheumatic diseases have a major systemic or non-articular component. Clinically, OA is characterized by the gradual development of pain and limitation of joint motion in association with brief joint stiffness and the absence of prominent joint inflammation. Its specific pathology parallels the clinical presentation; major lesions are located in the articular cartilage and its adjacent bone rather than in the synovium or synovial fluid. To emphasize the relative lack of joint inflammation in this disease, it is also known as osteoarthrosis. The term degenerative joint disease is also used because degeneration of articular cartilage is the prominent pathological change of the disorder. At present, thus, the terms osteoarthritis, osteoarthrosis and degenerative joint disease are used interchangeable. Clinically, although usually a benign disease, osteoarthritis may produce major joint degenerative changes and cause serious disability.

Osteoarthritis represents a number of disease varieties or subsets which present with similar clinical and pathologic alterations, rather than one specific disorder. The individual disease subsets may each represent the evolution of separate processes, with their specific etiologies, along a common pathogenic pathway. These develop into a joint disorder which, in its broadest outline, is recognized as OA, but where the different etiologies responsible leave their distinctive feature upon each subset of the disease. The disease is classified as primary (idiopathic) when it occurs in the absence of any known underlying predisposing factor. Secondary OA is defined as that form of the disease which has an overt, underlying local or systemic cause contributing to its etiology. Some of the causative factors may be mechanical, metabolic or inflammatory. (See Table 5-1). The distinctions on which this simple classification is based may, at times, be artificial, however. Studies on OA of the hip for example, show that many cases of "primary" OA are actually secondary to anatomic abnormalities that result in articulating surfaces that no longer conform to each other and thus lead to premature cartilage degeneration, such as congenital hip dysplasia and slipped capital femoral epiphysis of childhood. Various forms of the disease such as primary generalized OA, erosive inflammatory OA, diffuse idiopathic skeletal hyperostosis and chondromalacia patellae are sufficiently different with respect to clinical, pathologic and roentgenographic findings to be considered distinct symptom complexes. Alternatively, these symptom complexes may not represent disease subsets but may merely reflect one end of the clinical spectrum of disease severity of osteoarthritis in its various forms.

PATHOGENESIS

As cartilage is the site of major pathology in OA, pathogenic factors have been sought within the cartilage itself. Early in the development of OA, even before gross or histologic lesions are apparent, the articular cartilage matrix, the ground substance between the cells which constitutes up to 90–99% of the tissue, demonstrates increased water content and other alterations in its biochemical makeup. These changes are particularly notable in proteoglycans, large molecules which together with collagen make up the major organic component of the cartilage matrix. Also the chondrocytes, the cells of cartilage, display altered metabolism at the earliest stages. This is manifest as increased proliferation of the chondrocytes, increased proteoglycans and collagen synthesis and also increased activity of cartilage degrading enzymes produced by these cells.

Despite apparent reparative efforts by articular chondrocytes, the osteoarthritic process is soon followed by the loss of articular cartilage. Minimal surface disruptions with only fibrillation of the surface are followed by the development of deep clefts into the cartilage, as well as broad and deep ulcerations; and eventually, the entire articular surface is denuded down to subchondral bone. The hallmark of the pathology of osteoarthritis is its focal nature. This latter finding is reflected in the diagnostic X-Ray findings which often show loss of the cartilage space in only portions of involved joints.

In association with cartilage degeneration other changes take place in the bone immediately below the cartilage, at the articular cartilage margins and in the synovial membrane. The bone below the cartilage will frequently demonstrate microfractures and reactive bone formation as a result of altered biomechanics; and hyaluronic acid-filled bone cysts then form, chondro-osteophytes, also referred to as spurs, develop, largely at the margins of the articular cartilage. The mechanism for the formation of these spurs is not clear but seems to involve the presence of joint instability, increased vascularity and inflammation of tissues at the joint margins as well as active bone formation which is stimulated by the abnormal biomechanics of the disturbed joint. Thus, while the process of cartilage degeneration proceeds in OA, there is an active process of new cartilage and new bone formation that occurs largely at the margins of these joints. Occasionally, these projections of cartilage-capped bone are extremely large and cause irritation of surrounding tissues and further joint limitation of motion.

What sets off this pathologic process which results in the lesions of OA is not known. Osteoarthritis is popularly said to be due to "wear and tear" that results from chronic routine use or intermittent abuse of the joints. This view is supported by some epidemiologic data that relates overuse of certain joints to the later development of osteoarthritis. On the other hand, it does not explain the peculiar distribution of some forms of osteoarthritis which spares many frequently used joints, including some weight-bearing joints such as the ankles. Another hypothesis stresses the important contribution of bone to the development of osteoarthritis. Repeated impact sustained by a joint during its use is transmitted to the bone under the cartilage. Microfractures lead to increased stiffness of the bone so that it is no longer able to function properly in absorbing the shock of repetitive impact and impulse loading must now be absorbed by the cartilage itself. The cartilage is unable to handle the additional forces and thus gradually breaks down.

An alternative hypothesis stresses the role of the chondrocytes in the pathogenesis of OA. Since ultimately the articular cartilage is the product of chondrocyte metabolism, any defects in cartilage biochemistry may result from dysfunction of the chondrocytes themselves. Osteoarthritis, then, might be viewed as a disorder of chondrocytes and their ability to maintain the integrity of the tissue via their normal metabolic pathways.

In some subsets of the disease there is also an inherited susceptibility. Hormonal factors may also play a role. Further, primary generalized OA and erosive inflammatory OA occur primarily in postmenopausal women. Their development at a time when the circulating levels of estrogen decline has suggested a causative or permissive role for sex hormones in their pathogenesis. The development of OA in acromegaly, similarly, has suggested that subclinical growth hormone abnormality may also lead to "idiopathic" OA.

The role of inflammation in the development of OA has come under increasing study. Synovia from established cases of OA often show evidence of low grade inflammation. This inflammation has been attributed to cartilage wear particles and degradation products and to crystals such as calcium pyrophosphate dihydrate and calcium hydroxyapatite, which may originate within cartilage. Inflamed synovium may act directly upon cartilage by production of enzymes and other chemical mediators which may degrade the cartilage matrix or, indirectly, by production of factors which stimulate the degradative action of chondrocytes on their own matrix.

Much attention has been directed to the relation between aging and OA. Anatomical and epidemiologic studies have suggested that OA is recognized with increasing frequency in older individuals. On the other hand, there is evidence that the biochemical changes of aging cartilage differ significantly from those alterations seen in OA. Whether aging changes in cartilage constitute a necessary prerequisite for the development of osteoarthritic changes or whether aging merely represents a further opportunity for the accumulation of pathology which ultimately results in the development of OA is unclear.

EPIDEMIOLOGY

Osteoarthritis is the most prevalent rheumatic disease. It is virtually universal in its occurrence in all vertebrate animal species throughout history including dinosaurs. Among humans it occurs in all races. Given sufficient longevity virtually all individuals can be demonstrated to have evidence of osteoarthritis before their death. An X-Ray survey conducted by the United States public health service in 1962 suggested that approximately 20% of adult Americans were afflicted. Of these, only one of eight were symptomatic. The most striking feature of the prevalence of OA is its increasing presence with age. As defined by X-Ray, there is a rate of 4% among persons in their early 20's, increasing to 85% of individuals in their eighth decade of life. Similarly, in autopsy studies pathologic changes of OA have been detected as early as the second decade of life and by age 40, nine out of ten people have such pathologic changes in the weight-bearing joints. Despite X-Ray and pathologic evidence of presence of the disease, under age 45 few people exhibit any symptoms. Among the older age groups, however, where OA is almost universal, 20% of patients have sufficient significant symptoms and disability from their disease so as to require medical attention. The disability resulting from OA and the cost of treatment of this disorder, particularly total joint replacement, imposes an enormous economic cost to society. Surveys have shown that of all the rheumatic diseases, osteoarthritis, particularly degenerative disease of the spine, has the greatest socioeconomic impact.

When surveyed generally, so as to include all clinical presentations and all ages, men and women are equally effected by OA. The pattern of involvement differs between the sexes at various ages however. Under the age of 45, the prevalence among men is greater, typically with the involvement of few joints, predominately hip OA. Over the age of 55 years, the prevalence of the disease is greater in women. The disease in women tends to be more generalized with frequent involvement of the distal interphalangeal, proximal interphalangeal and first carpometacarpal joints of the hands. Objectively, postmenopausally the disease in women appears to be more severe. Women also appear to have more symptoms with their arthritis than men.

Osteoarthritis is found with equal prevalence in all racial groups investigated. Apparent racial differences in the distribution of joint involvement in OA, can in many instances, be attributed to variations in occupation and life-style. Differences in certain predisposing factors which may have a genetic basis, such as congenital subluxation of the hip, may also influence the rate of the development of the disease. For example, studies of Chinese have documented a lower incidence of hip osteoarthritis as compared to Caucasians. One suggestion for this apparent racial influence on the development of osteoarthritis may be found in the culturally determined habit of squatting among the Chinese. This may permit the hip joint to be protected by being frequently put through the extreme range of motion required for adopting this position. In another study in the United States, however, the prevalence of OA of the hips was noticeably greater in white populations and relatively decreased in black and American Indian populations. On the other hand, relatively little difference in the occurrence of OA of the knees has been found among ethnic groups. As noted earlier, hereditary factors are important determinants in the development of Heberden's nodes and these occur rarely in the black populations of South Africa, Nigeria, Liberia, and the United States.

The role of specific genetic factors in the development of OA in general has been difficult to evaluate because of the extremely high prevalence of the disorder. Investigators have attempted to dissect out the contribution of hereditary factors to the development of OA by focusing on subsets of the disease. Earlier work suggested that susceptibility to the development of Heberden's nodes, which are seen more frequently in women, is transmitted by a single autosomal gene, dominant in females and recessive in males. More recently, workers in England, have examined the role of genetic factors in generalized OA and have concluded that it appears to have a polygenic mode of inheritance.

Studies have examined the role of obesity, body somatotype and bone density in the development of OA. While some of these studies have suggested that obesity is not a factor in the induction or aggravation of OA, other studies have demonstrated that obesity disposes to increased frequency of OA involving weight-bearing joints and, interestingly, nonweight-bearing joints such as the sternoclavicular and distal interphalangeal joints. Experimental studies have also suggested that obesity in humans is related to OA not only by its biomechanical stress effects, but also as a result of basic metabolic changes in cartilage such as may be related to the intake of saturated versus unsaturated fat in the diet.

Clinical observations have also suggested that the prevalence of OA is greater in stout individuals described as endomorphic mesmorphs than in thin ones with features of ectomorphism. Reduction in bone mass, with the associated reduced stiffness of the bone as seen in osteoporosis, has been thought to increase the shock absorbing capacity of bone. Reduction in OA in association with osteoporosis has, therefore, been ascribed to the protective effect of osteoporotic bone on articular cartilage against excessive mechanical impact stress. Ligamentous laxity, on the other hand, has been thought to have an increased positive association with joint degeneration.

Along with the endogenous factors described above, exogenous and environmental factors have been investigated as to their relationship to OA. While climate has not been consistently related to the development of degenerative joint disease, occupational and sports activities have been implicated. Osteoarthritis occurring in the shoulders and elbows, both atypical joints of involvement, have been noted in bus drivers and foundry workers, respectively. In another study of women working in a weaving factory, a pattern of hand and finger lesion involvement that could be directly related to the work activity performed by each individual, was noted, with the joints most repetitively used being most involved. While a number of studies have suggested that OA is seen more frequently in soccer players, these were based on the presence of osteophytes alone. When OA criteria are based on loss of cartilage space, as seen on X-Ray, there is less evidence that exercise is harmful. Similarly, no relationships could be demonstrated for pneumatic hammer-drilling to arthritis of the elbow, competitive long distance running to arthritis of the knee, and hips or knee arthritis to sky diving.

CLINICAL ASPECTS

Joint pain is the major symptomatic manifestation of OA in contrast to the chronic inflammatory arthropathies where persistent stiffness is the most prominent symptom. The pain involves the joints diffusely and is often referred to the surrounding musculoskeletal structures. It is frequently described as toothache-like in quality. A further distinction from the joint pain of inflammatory arthritis is that the patient with OA experiences primarily "use" pain. While moderate use of an involved joint may somewhat relieve the stiffness of a primarily inflammatory arthritis, motion at an involved osteoarthritic joint promotes joint pain. As the disease progresses, pain may be felt in the osteoarthritic joint at rest. Night pain is frequently a symptomatic marker for end-stage OA, usually correlating pathologically with marked degeneration of the articular cartilage. Note that the pain in osteoarthritis must arise from the joint capsule, subchondral bone or other periarticular structures since cartilage has no nerve supply, and is thus, insensitive to pain. Further, especially during "acute flares," OA is associated with synovitis with its cardinal signs of joint line tenderness and synovial fluid accumulation. As noted earlier, this inflammation frequently represents a secondary phenomenon induced by cartilage breakdown products or in response to previously deposited calcium pyrophosphate or hydroxyapatite crystals. Joint stiffness on awakening and after inactivity is also a common complaint of OA but rarely persists for more than 15 minutes. In general, the disease is distinguished from the inflammatory arthropathies by the absence of constitutional symptoms and the prominence of local symptoms, instead. With disease progression, limitation of joint motion becomes a problem of increasing proportion for the OA patient. This joint limitation initially results from the pain associated with joint motion and the accompanying periarticular muscle spasm. Eventually, it reflects the irreversible structural damage produced by the degenerative process.

On examination, enlargement of the affected joint is readily noted. This may occur secondary to spur formation, reactive synovial proliferation and increased synovial fluid quantity. At this point, the enlargement is described as firm or rubbery in character and is to be distinguished from the bogginess of markedly inflamed tissues. At the late stages of the disease this joint enlargement progresses to gross deformity and subluxation due to cartilage loss, collapse of subchondral bone, formation of bone cysts and gross bony overgrowth. As the patient gets worse, the pain on passive motion and a restricted range of joint motion are prominent findings. Chronic restriction of joint motion is frequently manifest in joint contractures.

In primary OA there is a specific and characteristic pattern of joint involvement. In the hands, there are involvement of the distal interphalangeal, proximal interphalangeal as well as the carpometacarpal joints. Significantly, and quite useful in the differential diagnosis of primary OA from other disorders, the metacarpophalangeal joints, wrists, elbows and shoulders are relatively spared. In the spine, the cervical and lumbar regions are involved predominately. Within the spine, osteoarthritic changes occur both at the intervertebral disc articulations as well as the apophyseal joints. In the lower extremities, the hips and knees as well as the first metatarsophalangeal joints are sites of typical involvement while the ankles are rarely involved, except in diabetics or massively obese individuals. In addition, the acromioclavicular joint and temporomandibular joint are occasionally involved.

Heberden's nodes are one of the most common and readily recognizable manifestations of primary OA. Clinically, these are defined by firm enlargement of the distal interphalangeal joints of the digits, often with associated flexion, medial and lateral deviation of the distal phalanx. In some cases, they are associated with small gelatinous cysts along the dorsal aspects of the joints.

Pathologically and roentgenographically, they represent cartilaginous and bony enlargement as well as osteophyte formation in joints involved with an aggressive, sometimes markedly erosive, degenerative process with associated intense localized inflammation. Occasionally these lesions appear suddenly with prominent manifestations of inflammation such as redness, swelling and tenderness and intense pain. These nodes are usually multiple, most often begin after age 45 and affect women much more frequently than men. Similar nodes may be seen in the proximal interphalangeal joints where they are called Bouchard's nodes. Yet, in X-Ray surveys of hands, the most frequently affected joint in OA is the first carpometacarpal joint. As the first carpometacarpal joint anchors the thumb, osteoarthritic involvement of this joint frequently results in significant functional impairment with grasping function of the hand limited and painful. Clinically, first carpometacarpal joint involvement in OA is characterized by a "squared" appearance with prominence of the base of the thumb secondary to bony and inflammatory enlargement of the joint.

The knee joints are frequently affected in primary OA with resulting impairment in walking. As the pathology of OA is typically focal in nature, and the knee anatomically and functionally may be divided into three compartments: the medial femorotibial, lateral femorotibial and patellofemoral compartments; it is useful to localize the clinical findings. Typically, there is disproportionate involvement of the medial compartment of the knee leading to medial deviation of the joint (genu varus) with associated instability. Prominent involvement of the patellofemoral joint will frequently result in impaired stair walking or bending and squatting; all functions that involve repeated flexion-extension of the knee with concomitant muscular exertion. Because of the pain associated with joint motion, relative disuse of the joint follows and is accompanied by muscle atrophy about the knee. With progressive osteoarthritic involvement, a flexion contracture of the knee frequently develops. This may lead to functional shortening of one lower extremity and result in the total disruption of the normal biomechanics of gait. Clinically, this leads to associated low back and hip pain due to abnormal compensatory stresses imposed by the primary OA of the knee.

Hip joint OA is frequently insidious in onset with patients first presenting a limp. Pain is typically felt in the groin, frequently with radiation along the inner aspect of the thigh into the knee. Pain may also radiate to the buttock or low back region. Examination is usually required to localize the problem to the hip joint itself. The cardinal finding is one of restricted range of motion, with internal rotation limited at the earliest stages of the disease, but soon followed with limitation of external rotation and flexion of the hip. With more advanced disease, the hip is generally maintained in a flexion-adduction contracture. On examination, the entire lower extremity is found to rest in external rotation. It is the hip contracture which is generally responsible for the functional shortening of the extremity and the gait abnormality. Patients experience pain of full weight-bearing. The flexion contracture of the hip frequently imposes a compensatory curvature of the spine which is then associated with additional severe backache. Patients also frequently complain of pain on turning while in bed and laying on the affected side. This is usually clinically apparent as tenderness over the lateral thigh representing a trochanteric bursitis which frequently accompanies the hip joint disease.

Degenerative changes of the spine may occur in each of the three distinct articulations of the vertebral bodies including the intervertebral discs, the posterior joints of Lushka and the posterior apophyseal articulations. These degenerative changes of the spine are seen most frequently in the areas of maximal spine motion at the apices of the normal lordotic and kyphotic curves of the spine, about C5 in the cervical region, T8 in the thoracic spine and at the L3-4 in the lumbar region. As the intervertebral discs differ from all of the other joints where OA is described, in that they are composed of fibrocartilage rather than hyaline cartilage and true synovial joints are not present, the specific term of spondylosis is reserved for degenerative changes at these articulations. On the other hand, degenerative changes which occur at the apophyseal joints are classified as true OA. In spondylosis, however, the findings are quite similar to that of OA in peripheral synovial joints. As the intervertebral discs degenerate and frequently herniate outside the borders of their normal confinement, there is narrowing of the intervertebral disc spaces and reactive sclerosis of the vertebral body end plates. Osteophytes develop secondarily at the margins of the vertebral end plates and usually project laterally before they curve somewhat in a vertical direction. These spurs are typically most prevalent anteriorly where by their sheer size they may impinge on other structures. In the cervical spine, large osteophytes may give rise to symptoms of dysphagia and respiratory tract symptoms.

The symptoms of spinal OA include localized pain and stiffness as well as radicular pain. The origin of the localized pain is unclear. Typically the pain is related to activity and markedly improved by rest. As the intervertebral discs are aneural, the pain has been thought to originate in paraspinal ligaments, joint capsules and periosteum. Secondary spasm of the paraspinal musculature is induced near the site of joint pathology. In many cases, this secondary muscular spasm may be the predominant cause for pain and disability of an affected individual, and its relief may improve the patient's function markedly though the OA persists.

The radicular pain accompanying spinal OA is due to nerve root compression. This may result from impingement on the root by posterior osteophytes that intrude into the foraminal space, lateral prolapse of a degenerated disc compromising the neural root or by foraminal narrowing from apophyseal joint subluxation. Pressure on the nerve roots may cause severe radicular pain in a typical dermatomal distribution, parasthesias frequently reported as burning, tingling or numbness, and deep tendon reflex or muscle motor changes in the distribution of the compromised root. Though such pathology may occur anywhere throughout the spine, restriction of the symptoms to the body region innervated by the particular involved nerve root can permit relatively precise clinical localization of the site of spine involvement. For example, in the lumbosacral area specific neurologic symptoms and findings in the lower extremity help to define the specific root involved; L3 or L4 roots may be associated with a diminished or absent patellar reflex while an absent ankle jerk indicates S1 root involvement; sensory alteration along the anteromedial aspect of the leg is consistent with L4 root irritation, while L5 lesions product changes at the anterolateral aspect of the leg and medial aspect of the foot and S1 compression results in changes at the posterolateral aspects of the calf and lateral foot; weakness of the foot and great toes dorsiflexion suggests L5 dysfunction.

While nerve root irritation may occur with OA at any level of the spine there are other clinical manifestations peculiar to degenerative disease of the cervical or lumbar spine, the areas of most frequent involvement. In the cervical spine, for example, myelopathy or vascular compromise to the brain may be associated with degenerative disease. In both of these instances osteophyte compression of the extraarticular structures is responsible for the clinical syndrome. Posterior spurs or protruded discs may result in direct compression of the spinal cord, or may indirectly produce a central cord syndrome via impingement and restriction of blood flow through the anterior spinal artery. Similarly, basilar artery insufficiency may result from compromise of the vertebral arteries as these vessels course through the cervical vertebral foramina to the brain. In addition, a less common syndrome of osteoarthritis of the atlanto-axial joint has also been described. This condition may be present with symptoms of occipital pain, stiffness of the shoulder and parasthesias of the fingers.

Two additional syndromes described in association with lumbar spine OA have been noted. A cauda equina syndrome may be present when there is multiple involvement of lumbar roots below the level of L1 where the spinal cord ends. Because of the multiple roots involved and the bilateral nature of the lesion, the symptoms and findings are poorly localized and frequently attributed to spinal cord or vascular insufficiency. With multiple sacral root involvement, urinary and rectal sphincter dysfunction may be present. Another syndrome of the lumbar spine recognized with increasing frequency in older individuals is that of spinal stenosis. Its clinical presentation is quite similar to that of lumbar spondylosis with low back and lower extremity pain typically worsened by exercise along with sensory and motor power changes in the lower extremities. Clinically the syndrome is distinguished by its occurrence in somewhat older individuals; its involvement of multiple, occasionally bilateral nerve roots and its characteristic presentation as a "neural claudication" syndrome. Except for those individuals whose spinal stenosis is the result of congenital narrowing of the spinal canal, the syndrome is usually due to combined anatomic abnormalities with prominent ligamentous hypertrophy, multiple degenerative spurs, herniated discs and spondylolisthesis.

LABORATORY FINDINGS

Osteoarthritis is further distinguished from other arthropathies by the absence of associated diagnostic laboratory abnormalities. The major reason for performing laboratory studies is to exclude the presence of other rheumatic diseases. While the diagnosis of OA is primarily based on clinical findings, that is a consistent history and physical examination as well as supportive X-Ray data, laboratory studies may be useful. For example, evidence for primary hyperparathyroidism with its associated calcium pyrophosphate dihydrate crystal deposition disease or Paget's disease of the bone, two causes of secondary OA, may be obtained via screening blood studies. Measurement of the level of acute phase reactants may also be used to exclude the presence of systemic inflammation which would tend to indicate the presence of a primary inflammatory disorder.

The performance of arthrocentesis, the aspiration of excessive joint fluid and subsequent synovial fluid analysis in OA is performed with the same rationale as other laboratory studies. That is, an effort is made to exclude other primary inflammatory arthropathies and to define the presence of associated conditions which may lead to secondary degenerative joint disease. The typical joint fluid in primary OA is non-inflammatory with a minimal increase in cells, good viscosity and low protein. As associated crystal deposition disease is not uncommon especially in advanced cases, calcium pyrophosphate dihydrate or calcium hydroxyapatite crystals are sometimes seen. Synovial histology in primary OA is non-diagnostic, being essentially normal in the early disease and only demonstrating non-specific inflammation in advanced disease.

Because of the current lack of an objective laboratory parameter which is pathognomic or highly diagnostic of the disease research efforts have been made to analyze joint constituents for a marker of OA. Such studies have revealed the presence of Type II collagen fibers in synovial fluid while immune complexes have been detected in the cartilage itself, but not in the synovial fluid. Unfortunately, these studies have no clinical applicability at this time.

X-RAY APPEARANCE

The X-Ray appearance of a joint consistent with OA is supportive but not sufficient evidence for the diagnosis of OA as the cause of the patient's joint symptoms. Hence, as a general principle, X-Ray evidence of degenerative disease may be extensive and yet bear little relationship to a given patient's symptoms. On the other hand, severe symptoms may develop, especially in the spine, with relatively minor spur formation or disc herniation in certain critical locations to account for these symptoms. In peripheral joints, the X-Ray appearance of OA may be virtually normal with relatively mild pathology leading to clinical symptoms. As the disease progresses, many gradations of abnormality may be noted. As focal degeneration of articular cartilage constitutes the defining pathology of the disease, it is reflected by joint space narrowing occurring asymmetrically within a joint. Reactive new bone formation occurs early in subarticular areas with increased radiodensity reflecting the bony sclerosis (eburnation). In advance disease, bone cysts, also known as geodes, are seen as well-circumscribed lucent areas in periarticular bone. In end stage disease, gross joint deformity, subluxation and the appearance of loose bodies may be seen.

Osteophytes are usually present in osteoarthritis and because they are seen as well-defined projections of radio-opaque density beyond the normal contours of the bone, hence are obvious on X-Ray. Though osteophytes are usually regarded as manifestations of OA, the use of this feature alone in diagnosis has been questioned. In some studies, the presence of osteophytes in joints correlated with aging and did not necessarily signify the presence of clinical OA. Thus, it has been suggested that the X-Ray diagnosis of OA should be based on findings suggestive of structural abnormalities in cartilage, such as decreased joint space, or changes in subchondral bone such as cysts and eburnation. Further, OA may be differentiated from inflammatory arthropathies by the relative absence of juxtaarticular osteopenia. Also, fusion of a joint, which is late stage in erosive inflammatory arthropathies, is rarely seen even in end-stage osteoarthritis.

Since characteristic X-Ray findings are usually the only objective support for the diagnosis of OA, these studies are frequently performed to corroborate the clinical impression. In many peripheral joints, routine posterior-anterior and lateral views are sufficient to demonstrate the findings. In the cervical and lumbar spine where nerve root irritation is a frequent clinical problem, degenerative changes involving the intervertebral neural foramina are best evaluated with the additional use of oblique views. These same views also profile the apophyseal joints and thus aid in their evaluation. Since much of the disability of spinal OA relates to impingement on neural structures, myelography may be of help in localizing the site of pathology when symptoms are severe and surgery is contemplated. Because of its high resolution and capacity for evaluating soft tissue structures as well, computed, axial tomography (CAT) studies are assuming greater importance in the diagnosis of spinal OA. This technology is particularly helpful in the evaluation of spinal stenosis and lumbar facet disease.

At present, diagnostic evaluation of disc herniation and lumbar spine pathology in general, is significantly enhanced when utilizing the radiocontrast of myelography with the resolution capabilities of computerized tomography. The recent introduction of magnetic resonance imaging (MRI) has proven extremely useful.

X-Ray study of the hands on routine posterior-anterior views is particularly revealing in defining the pattern of joint involvement in osteoarthritis, with classical involvement of the first carpometacarpal joint and proximal as well as distal interphalangeal joints. The finding of degenerative changes at the metacarpophalangeal joints or the wrist is immediately suggestive of a secondary OA. Most likely secondary to a systemic or metabolic disease. Interestingly, although Heberden's nodes may feel quite hard on examination, only minimal spur formation may be present on X-Ray evaluation, suggesting that the enlargement noted clinically consists of soft tissue and cartilage.

In evaluating OA of the hip, the anterior-posterior X-Ray view of the pelvis profiles the acetabular-femoral articulation and also offer information on the sacroiliac joints, symphysis pubis and pelvic bones. In OA of the hip, focal degeneration of the articular cartilage frequently leads to superior-lateral migration of the femoral head in relation to the acetabulum. This is differentiated from primary inflammatory disease of the hip where the femoral head migrates medially due to the diffuse circumferential loss of articular cartilage. In advanced degenerative disease, the entire floor of the acetabulum may be displaced medially by the head of the femur so that it bulges into the pelvis. This finding is referred to as protrusio acetabuli.

Because of the multi-compartmental nature of the knee, special X-Ray views are often helpful in evaluating this joint. Anterior-posterior views of the knees, with the patient weight-bearing, allow a more representative demonstration of functional joint space narrowing and bring out the associated tibial deviation in relation to the femur, either medially (varus) or laterally (valgus). Tunnel views, anterior-posterior views taken with the knee in flexion, allow better identification of loose bodies, intra-articular spurs, changes on the femoral condylar surfaces and loss of the joint space not otherwise seen on the routine anterior-posterior view. The skyline or Hughston views taken above the tibial-femoral joint allow a more detailed and direct study of the patello-femoral compartment. As OA is a focal disease, X-Ray of contralateral peripheral joints are helpful in evaluating observed degenerative changes.

VARIANT FORMS OF PRIMARY OSTEOARTHRITIS

Primary Generalized Osteoarthritis

In the early 1950's Kellgren and Moore described a subset of primary OA with diffuse and symmetric polyarticular disease suggestive of a systemic disorder. This form is seen predominantly in perimenopausal women. Typically, the joints involved include the distal and proximal interphalangeal joints, first carpometacarpal joints, other peripheral joints including the knees, hips and metatarsophalangeal joints and the spine. Other characteristics of this form of the disease include its onset with an acute inflammatory phase preceding the chronic articular symptoms. Advanced cases show X-Ray changes greatly in excess of the clinical findings, with profuse osteophyte formation. Diffuse deposits of calcium pyrophosphate dihydrate are frequently demonstrated in these more severely involved joints. Whether this form of OA represents a distinct entity, or simply represents one end of the clinical spectrum of the disease is still being debated.

Erosive Inflammatory Osteoarthritis

This variant form of primary OA is atypical because of the intense joint inflammation found, leading to the relatively rapid erosion of joints and occasionally resulting in ankylosis of previously eroded joints. This variant is similar to the primary generalized form of the disease in its tendency to occur in post-menopausal women. The distal interphalangeal and proximal interphalangeal joints and rarely the metacarpophalangeal joints of the hands represent sites of the most frequent involvement. Typically, painful inflammatory episodes may occur for years until the affected joints become deformed, but relatively asymptomatic. In the acute phase of the disease tender and painful gelatinous cysts are seen at involved joints. The clinical presentation with inflammation and swelling, laboratory studies, synovial pathology and X-Ray findings suggest that this disorder may represent an interface between non-inflammatory OA and RA.

Chondromalacia Patellae

Inclusion of this degenerative disorder of the cartilage of the patella among the subsets of OA is also controversial. This condition is unusual in its frequent occurrence among younger individuals, some in their teens, and in being potentially reversible. Though histologically the changes of chondromalacia are identical to those seen in early osteoarthritis, this pathology may represent the final common pathway through which the articular cartilage of the patella responds to repeated mechanical trauma, conditions which predispose include lateral subluxation of the patella, primary meniscal disease, knee laxity or abnormal patellar positions. In some young people, this condition may be a precursor to the development of true patello-femoral OA however.

Diffuse Idiopathic Skeletal Hyperostosis (DISH)

This condition is frequently included among the variants of osteoarthritis though the recently defined specific criteria for this condition by Resnick and co-workers specifically excludes intervertebral disc space narrowing, the presence of disc vacuum phenomenon (seen in degenerating discs) or vertebral body marginal sclerosis as part of the disease. Thus, this condition is included here as a form of OA because of the presence of osteophytes as prominent pathological findings. In other forms of OA, however, osteophytes occur in the context of degenerative disease of the articular surface, while in this variant the diagnosis according to the above criteria, cannot be made reliably in the presence of degenerative disease of the intervertebral discs. Other criteria for the diagnosis of DISH include "flowing" ossification along the antero-lateral aspect of at least four contiguous vertebral bodies and the absence of findings of spondylitis such as sacroiliac joint erosions, sclerosis or fusion and apophyseal joint ankylosis. Also, unlike other forms of OA where the pathology is restricted to the joints, extra spinal manifestations have been described in this variant including irregular new bone formation or "whiskering," large bone spurs in periarticular locations such as the olecranon process and calcaneus, along with prominent ligamentous calcification. In fact, ossification along the spine involves the anterior longitudinal ligament and peripheral disc margins. There is a curious predilection for involvement of the side of the spine opposite to the location of the thoracic aorta. The exuberant and diffuse calcification and spur formation noted in this disorder has lead to the suggestion that it represents a generalized "ossifying diathesis."

The cause of this variant of OA is unknown. Abnormal glucose tolerance tests and frank diabetes mellitus appear to be over-represented among patients with DISH. There have been suggestions that patients with this disorder have the genetic marker HLA-B27 present to a greater extent than expected, but this poorly reproduced finding may represent the degree of diagnostic confusion of this entity with spondylitis. There have also been suggestions that the condition is related to increased levels of vitamin A or fluoride.

PROGNOSIS IN PRIMARY OSTEOARTHRITIS

The outlook of patients with primary OA is extremely variable. Conventional wisdom and earlier epidemiologic studies correlated increased incidence and severity of the disease with age and suggested that the disease progresses chronically and inexorably to joint destruction. There is, however, a significant body of data that suggests that osteoarthritis is not inevitably progressive. In general the long term outlook is favorable and disability uncommon. Some studies suggest, in fact, that disease severity is not significantly worse in the elderly after the age of 65. Further evidence is to be found in the observation that

X-Ray changes of OA are common in the general population, and yet bear little relationship to the musculoskeletal symptoms reported. Prognosis of the disease relates to some extent to the specific joints involved. Involvement of the interphalangeal joints of the hand, for example, though associated with intermittent pain and moderate deformity, usually leads to relatively little limitation of essential hand function. In the knees or hips, on the other hand, occasionally there is rapid progression of the disease with substantial impairment of ambulation. The knees, in particular, may become deformed with medial or lateral deviation of the tibia in relation to the femur. In the spine, severe symptoms and neurologic sequelae may occur, depending on the specific site of involvement.

SECONDARY OSTEOARTHRITIS

The term "secondary osteoarthritis" may be applied whenever degenerative joint disease occurs secondarily or concomitantly with a clearly identifiable primary disorder. Causes of secondary OA may be either local or systemic in nature. A diagnosis of secondary OA is particularly to be considered when the disease appears at a relatively early age in its onset or involves joints not typically affected in primary OA.

The most common local factor frequently associated with the subsequent development of degenerative joint disease is trauma. The trauma may occur as a single specific event such as fracture, aseptic necrosis or torn meniscus. On the other hand, chronic trauma as related to certain occupations, with overuse or abuse of a given joint, may be associated with the development of osteoarthritis. Another type of chronic local trauma may be that imposed by developmental abnormalities such as hip dysplasia.

Systemic metabolic and endocrine disorders, probably through their effect on cartilage metabolism, are associated with OA. Most of these disorders also predispose to the deposition of calcium pyrophosphate dihydrate crystals in the cartilage and this further compromises the articular cartilage leading to the development of a degenerative arthropathy. Similarly, in metabolic disease where there is excessive accumulation of minerals and by-products of intermediary metabolism, a similar effect is produced. In alkaptonuria (ochronosis), homogentisic acid deposits in connective tissue, primarily fibrocartilage. Thus, the disease is associated primarily with degenerative joint disease of the intervertebral discs of the spine; though peripheral arthritis is seen occasionally in late disease. In hemochromatosis, excess iron deposits in all parenchymal tissues. Recent studies have shown that degenerative joint disease may be the most common clinical manifestation of hereditary hemochromatosis, occurring in 20–50% of patients, frequently relatively early on in their disease. In hemochromatosis, degenerative changes of the second and third metacarpophalangeal and metatarsophalangeal joints is particularly characteristic, though other joints may be involved. Calcium pyrophosphate dihydrate deposition is noted frequently. Similarly, in Wilson's disease, a condition characterized by excessive retention of copper, OA is noted at an earlier age than commonly seen in primary disease.

The endocrinopathies are also generally associated with an increased incidence of degenerative disease. Hypothyroidism and diabetes mellitus are associated with an increased incidence of calcium pyrophosphate dihydrate deposition in joints, with the secondary development of OA. Separately, diabetes in association with neuropathies frequent in this disorder may dispose the development of joint degeneration. Presumably the loss of proprioceptive mechanisms, joint instability and other mechanical dysfunction is uncorrected by the normal protective mechanisms of the joint leading to recurrent trauma, degeneration and eventual fragmentation and disorganization of the joint. Possibly, because of the above described mechanism, the ankle, which is usually spared in idiopathic OA may be involved with joint degeneration in diabetes. Acromegaly, a pituitary disorder of growth hormone hypersecretion, results in the excessive growth of articular cartilage and the development of peripheral and spinal OA. Excessive cartilage growth with increased thickness of the articular cartilage is responsible for the characteristic X-Ray finding of wide joint spaces in the setting of degenerative joint disease in this disorder. Increased levels of parathyroid hormone, whether primary or secondary, are further associated with cartilage damage, usually in the setting of calcium pyrophosphate dihydrate crystal deposition.

As noted above, calcium pyrophosphate dihydrate deposition in articular cartilage is a frequent accompaniment of secondary OA due to a large number of metabolic and hormonal disease states. In addition, it is frequently noted in association with primary generalized OA and in conditions of joint laxity. These crystals are also found in neuropathic degenerative arthropathies such as with diabetes mellitus, syphilitic neuropathy (tabes dorsalis) and spinal cord tumors or malformations. Even in the context of presumable idiopathic primary OA, more severe and destructive arthropathy is frequently associated with calcium pyrophosphate dihydrate crystal deposition. It is this impressive collection of the association of calcium pyrophosphate dihydrate deposition and degenerative disease which has fueled the controversy as to whether subclinical deposition of these crystals may, in fact, be responsible for "primary osteoarthritis."

In addition to the above, a large number of relatively uncommon causes have been identified as leading to secondary OA including repeated intra-articular injections of adrenal corticosteroids and severe cold injury, occurring prior to epiphyseal closure. The signs and symptoms, laboratory findings and X-Ray abnormalities related to secondary OA are generally quite similar to those seen in the primary form of the disease, except where they reflect the presence of the primary disease itself. Clinically, where crystal deposition is a major factor, inflammation plays a more prominent role. The management of patients with secondary OA is similar to that outlined below for patients with the primary form of the disease. Unfortunately, once joint degeneration is set in motion, even if there is correction or amelioration of the underlying disease process, the osteoarthritis process usually continues to progress independently.

TREATMENT

An important element of the management program of any patient with OA is education of the nature of his/her disease. Frequently, simple reassurance as to the benign nature of the condition is sufficient to enable the patient to live with his/her disease without the need for special treatment. Furthermore, an understanding by the patient of the pathology, prognosis and goals of treatment in OA enhances the patient's compliance with the therapeutic program, especially where it may involve changes in life-style or occupational activity.

There is no specific medical treatment for osteoarthritis and therapeutic efforts are largely empiric and supportive in nature. Major therapeutic efforts are directed at correcting some of the mechanical dysfunction which may initially cause and then exacerbate the further degeneration of joints in osteoarthritis. As symptoms are largely related to the use of involved joints, programmed rest or immobilization via splinting of joints offer significant symptomatic relief. Mechanical advantage is gained in various joints by use of specific modalities adapted for the particular joint involved. In the case of degenerative joint disease of the cervical spine, this is accomplished by use of a cervical collar for immobilization, or cervical traction to relieve the pressure on neural roots. In the low back, temporary use of lumbosacral spine support may restrict motion and maintain posture so as to reduce nerve root irritation. The effective management of acute flares of lumbar degenerative disease frequently requires strict adherence to bedrest and the adjunctive use of local heat, analgesia and muscle relaxants. In lower extremity OA the use of a cane to share some of the load-bearing function of the involved hip or knee joints will result in relative rest of the affected joints.

In addition, patients are urged to modify their life-styles so as to reduce excessive joint stress by changing the nature and pace of their activities. For example, utilization of long-handled tools when doing house cleaning or gardening chores may protect joints such as the lumbar spine and knees.

Alteration in vocational tasks and the choice of avocational activities may also be needed.

While use of mechanical aides may have usefulness in short term relief of joint symptoms, long term mechanical advantage is gained in osteoarthritic joints by the performance of appropriate exercises. These exercises, in the case of hip and knee joints, are aimed at relieving the adduction and flexion contractures which complicate the development of OA. In addition, in the knees, exercises often performed isometrically strengthen the muscles which move the joint and thus result in improvement of function. In lumbar spondylosis, exercises to increase pelvic tilt results in enlargement of vertebral foraminal spaces with relief of nerve root irritation.

At the current state of the art, the role of pharmaceuticals in the treatment of osteoarthritis is largely limited to use of analgesics and anti-inflammatory agents to promote pain relief and lessen secondary inflammatory responses. For minimal symptoms of OA where pain relief is necessary, the use of simple analgesics may be sufficient. As pain is often due to the secondary associated inflammation, frequently, more effective pain relief is achieved via the use of nonsteroidal anti-inflammatory agents rather than simple analgesics. Generally, doses somewhat lower than those used in primary inflammatory arthropathies such as RA are quite efficacious in ameliorating the symptoms of OA. When focal "flares" with a large inflammatory component occur, intra-articular steroid injection, used judiciously and infrequently, may be effective in rapidly reducing the symptoms. This use of intra-articular steroids is somewhat controversial however. There is no controversy on the other hand, on the lack of utility and contra-indication of the use of systemic steroids in the treatment of osteoarthritis. When the disease progresses and severe rest pain and night pain are experienced, great care must be taken to avoid the use of narcotic analgesics.

Once adequate trials of rest, physical therapy and the use of analgesics as well as anti-inflammatory medications has been attempted, and yet the patient is severely disabled by pain there remains a surgical option. In the treatment of spinal OA where symptoms are largely neuropathic in origin, the aims of surgery are vertebral stabilization via fusion, especially in the neck, and surgical relief of irritation of the spinal nerve root via laminectomy, foraminotomy or disc removal. In OA of the hands, surgery is rarely indicated, except in the case of the first carpometacarpal joint where excision arthroplasty affords excellent pain relief with relatively little loss of function. In some medical centers aggressive surgical treatment of hip and knee osteoarthritis has been pursued in cases of early to moderate disease where focal disease is prominent. In these cases, osteotomies are performed, resulting in realignment of the articulating surfaces with redistribution of forces away from the site of greater pathology to more normal tissues.

In the treatment of OA of the hip and knee, patients once relegated to loss of ambulation and possible use of a wheelchair can today be offered total joint replacement. In osteoarthritis, replacement of the diseased joint with an artificial prosthesis is, in a sense, "curative." This is the case in OA because in this entity the disease is entirely restricted to the joints. The major indication for joint replacement is pain relief. In osteoarthritis, especially with hip involvement, total joint replacement affords the patient not only pain relief, but the possibility of significant functional improvement.

SUGGESTED READINGS

Ehrlich G.E.: Inflammatory osteoarthritis. I. The clinical syndrome. *J. Chronic Dis.* 25:317–328, 1972.

Gardner, D.L.: The nature and causes of osteoarthrosis. *Br. Med. J.* 286:418–424, 1983.

Howell, D.S.; Altman, R.D.; Pita, J.C., *et al:* The pathogenesis of osteoarthritis. In *Current Concepts,* Scope Publication, 1983.

Kellgren, J.H.; Moore, R.: Generalized osteoarthritis and Heberden's nodes. *Br. Med. J.* 1:181–187, 1952.

Moskowitz, R.W.: Clinical and laboratory findings in osteoarthritis, Ch. 102. In McCarthy, D.J., ed.: *Arthritis and Allied Conditions,* 11th ed. Lea and Febiger, Philadelphia, 1989.

Resnick, D.; Shaprio, R.F.; Wiesner, K.B., *et al:* Diffuse idiopathic skeletal hyperostosis (DISH) (Ankylosing hyperostosis of Forestier and Rotes-Querol). *Semin. Arth. Rheum.* 7:153–187, 1978.

Roberts, S.; Burch, T.A.: Prevalence of osteoarthritis in adults by age, sex, race and geographic area. United States 1960–62. (National Center for Health Statistics: Vital and Health Statistics. Data from the National Health Survey.) U.S. Public Health Service Publication No. 1000, Series II, No. 15, 1966. Washington, D.C. U.S. Government Printing Office.

TABLE 5-1
CLASSIFICATION OF OSTEOARTHRITIS

Primary
Idiopathic
Generalized Osteoarthritis
Inflammatory Erosive Osteoarthritis
Chondromalacia Patellae
Diffuse Idiopathic Skeletal Hyperostosis
Secondary
Local Determinants
Acute Trauma (Fracture, Torn Meniscus)
Chronic Trauma (Occupational or Sports Activity)
Developmental (Joint Dysplasia, Osteochondrosis)
Septic Arthritis
Avascular Necrosis
Hemarthrosis (Hemophilia)
Inflammatory Arthritis (Rheumatoid Arthritis)
Steroid Injection
Frostbite
Bone Disease (Paget's Disease)
Neuropathic Arthropathy (Diabetes Mellitus, Syphilis)
Systemic Determinants
Endocrine (Acromegaly, Hyperparathyroidism)
Metabolic (Ochronosis, Pseudogout)
Joint Hypermobility
Hereditary

CHAPTER 6

SYSTEMIC LUPUS ERYTHEMATOSUS

Joyce Z. Singer, M.D.
Ellen M. Ginzler, M.D.

INTRODUCTION

Systemic lupus erythematosus (SLE) is a chronic syndrome with an unusual diversity of clinical and immunological abnormalities. The syndrome is characterized by inflammatory changes in virtually any organ of the body. The hallmark of this disease is its uniqueness. Every patient has an individual constellation of symptoms, physical findings, and laboratory abnormalities. This range of possible manifestations may result in misdiagnosis of SLE as epilepsy, schizophrenia, rheumatoid arthritis, allergies, inflammatory bowel disease and many other illnesses.

Systemic lupus erythematosus is seen primarily in women of childbearing age. It occurs more frequently in blacks than whites in this country, with a sex ratio of one male to each nine females affected. The prevalence of systemic lupus in San Francisco was calculated to be 1 in 700 women in the age group of 15 to 64. Among black women of the same ages, the prevalence was 1 in 245. It has been estimated that 500,000 to 1,000,000 Americans have systemic lupus with 50,000 new cases diagnosed each year. Thus, SLE, once thought to be a rare disease, is probably more common than multiple sclerosis, muscular dystrophy and leukemia.

ETIOLOGY

SLE is the classic example of a disease of immune origin, thought to result from an overactive, self-destructive attack of immune cells on body tissues. In fact, current concepts of the pathogenesis of SLE suggest that it is not a disease of immunologic hyperactivity, but rather one of immunodeficiency. It has been postulated that a decrease in numbers and/or function of suppressor T-lymphocytes is responsible for abnormal immunologic regulation, resulting in a failure of recognition of self and a loss of immunologic tolerance. As a consequence, autoantibodies are produced.

The autoantibodies produced in SLE appear to mediate the tissue injury which leads to the clinical expression of disease. In some instances, the antibody may be directly cytotoxic to tissues or cells, such as lymphocytotoxic antibodies. More often, tissue injury is the final result of the deposition of immune complexes, which result from the interaction of self antigens and autoantibodies, in turn producing an inflammatory response. Tissue infiltration by inflammatory cells attracted to the area of damage results in further injury.

In some features of SLE, knowledge of the histopathologic lesion allows for an understanding of the nature of the clinical disease manifestations, and provides a basis for formulating therapy. The renal pathology, for example, appears to be the result of immune complexes containing immunoglobulin and complement, deposited within the basement membrane of glomerular capillary walls. Damage to the glomerulus allows leakage of red and white blood cells and protein into the urine, and may eventually result in a deterioration of renal function.

The clinical features of lupus central nervous system involvement are much more difficult to correlate with the histologic appearance. In some patients, deposition of immune complexes has been demonstrated in the brain at autopsy. Nevertheless, the most common features of lupus cerebritis, namely seizures and organic brain syndrome, are generally accompanied by the absence of abnormalities in the electroencephalogram, cerebrospinal fluid examination, brain scan, or computer tomography of the brain.

PREDISPOSITION

Genetics

Despite much research, the etiology of SLE remains unclear. It is likely that both an environmental exposure and a genetic predisposition are necessary for disease expression. This concept has been strengthened by studies with several genetically distinct species of mice which all developed spontaneous lupus-like syndromes (e.g., the NZB/W, BXSB, and MRL/1 strains).

The evidence for a genetic predisposition to SLE in humans is strengthened by family studies. Numerous kinships have been described with multiple causes of SLE present. Up to 12% of patients with SLE have a close relative with the disease. Twin studies have shown a significant concordance of presentation of SLE among monozygotic pairs.

Human leukocyte antigen (HLA) typing of patients with SLE and their family members has provided further insight into the genetic tendency to develop this disorder. The major histocompatibility complex, known as HLA in humans, is a complex of genes located on chromosome number 6 that contains the genetic code for cell-surface molecules involved in the recognition of foreign antigens. A subdivision of this gene complex, known as HLA-D or HLA-DR produces proteins expressed primarily on macrophages and lymphocytes. The proteins are intimately involved in the control of the immune response. The expression of the specific types HLA-DR 2 and HLA-DR3 on the lymphocyte membrane is significantly increased in SLE patients as compared to normal control subjects.

Studies of SLE families have also revealed defects in the complement system. Numerous kindreds have been described with inherited deficiency of various complements components. To date, the deficiencies reported to be associated with SLE include: C1q, C1r, C1s, C2, C4, C5, C6, C7, C8 and C1 esterase inhibitor.

Environment

Genetics alone cannot explain the occurrence of SLE. Even in families with definite genetically determined characteristics, no clearly defined pattern of inheritance of SLE has been established. Many individuals with known genetic risk factors do not develop SLE. This is most clearly demonstrated in Block's studies of monozygotic (identical) twins, only 69% of whom were concordant for the development of SLE. Environmental factors must play a role in the 31% of discordant pairs.

In addition, more than fifty case reports of complete C2 deficiency are in the literature, but only about one third of these patients have SLE. Family studies of non-twin siblings with SLE have shown long intervals between age of onset of the disease (average 9 years) as compared to short intervals between actual onset (3 years). Also, autoantibodies such as antinuclear and lymphocytotoxic antibodies can be found in unaffected nonconsanguinous household contacts of SLE patients. These points suggest that environmental factors are of importance in triggering SLE in a susceptible individual.

Viruses and many other environmental factors have been associated with the expression of SLE. Medications, hormones, vaccinations, cosmetics, foods, trace metals, pets, urban environment, ultraviolet radiation, chemicals and trauma have all been implicated. The case reports of possible environmental triggers are many, but evidence of the relative importance of any of these factors has not been established.

Hormonal

Explanations have been sought for the marked preponderance of SLE in women. Abnormalities of estrogen metabolism have been found in males and females with SLE, and more recently androgen abnormalities have been described in females with SLE. In addition, families have been described with first degree relatives of SLE patients having abnormalities of estrogen metabolism.

CLINICAL SYNDROME

Systemic lupus erythematosus can affect virtually every part of the body, and as previously emphasized, the manifestations are unique to the individual. Constitutional signs and symptoms, such as fatigue, malaise, anorexia, weight loss and fever are common varying with the level of disease activity.

Musculoskeletal

Joint disease is present at some time during the course of SLE in about 90% of patients and is the presenting complaint in about one half. Arthralgias alone may be present or true arthritis with joint inflammation and swelling may occur. The joints most commonly involved include the small joints of the hands and feet, knees, wrists and ankles. Most SLE patients have a non-deforming arthritis such that the bones and joints appear normal on X-Ray. However, it is also possible to see bone erosion on X-Ray, indistinguishable from those of rheumatoid arthritis. Inflammation of tendons and ligaments is also a common finding in SLE and can lead to joint laxity.

Myositis (inflammation of muscles) occurs in about one-third of SLE cases. It may be mild or even subclinical, manifested only by increases in serum creatine phosphokinase or other muscle enzymes. However, in some cases, myositis may be the predominant clinical feature with incapacitating weakness of the neck and proximal extremities with muscle atrophy.

Skin

Skin disease occurs in about 85% of SLE patients. The types of skin manifestations are numerous and most are not pathognomic of SLE. The most classical SLE manifestation is the malar or butterfly rash. This is an erythematous, sometimes scaly rash over the cheek and bridge of the nose. A diffuse erythematous rash is also common, often present in sun-exposed areas of the body (photosensitivity), but can be found over the entire body.

Discoid lupus lesions are found in 15–20% of SLE patients. They are most often seen on the face, scalp and external ears, but occur on the palms, soles and trunk as well. These skin lesions begin as erythematous patches with progress outward, often leaving a well-demarcated scar with skin thinning, dilated skin capillaries and plugging of hair follicles.

Vasculitis (inflammation of blood vessels) involving the skin can lead to erythematous, tender nodules on fingers and toes as well as skin ulcers on the ankles. Ulcers are also common on mucosal surfaces in the mouth and nose. These ulcerations may be asymptomatic or very painful.

Alopecia is seen in 40–60% of SLE patients. It can be caused by scarring of the scalp from discoid lupus lesions. Hair loss from normal scalp can be seen in a patchy or generalized pattern and is frequently associated with disease activity.

Renal Disease

Kidney involvement is clinically evident in 50–70% of patients and is potentially the most serious manifestation. Renal involvement is detected by red and white blood cells and protein in the urine. In more severe cases, decreasing kidney function may occur as demonstrated by worsening creatine clearance. High blood pressure may be a sign of active kidney disease or it may be the result of damage to the kidneys from previous disease activity. Although there may be some discrepancies, the severity of kidney involvement seen on biopsy usually parallels the severity of clinical and laboratory abnormalities. The renal involvement may remain mild or may progress to irreversible kidney failure necessitating chronic hemodialysis or renal transplantation.

Nervous System

Neuropsychiatric manifestations occur in as many as 60% of patients with SLE. One of the most common central nervous system features is grand mal seizures. Electroencephalograms in these patients are often abnormal, showing paroxysms of non-focal increased activity. Grand mal seizures alone do not confer a poor prognosis.

Organic brain syndrome is another common central nervous system feature. Although it frequently occurs in the presence of other evidence of disease activity, intellectual function may remain impaired or continue to deteriorate even as other active disease features become quiescent. It may be difficult to distinguish organic brain syndrome in an SLE patient from a primary psychiatric disturbance, medication side effects, i.e., steroid-induced psychosis, or emotional response to the stress of having a chronic illness. Chronic organic brain syndrome carries a poor prognosis, with about 50% mortality in five years.

Aseptic meningitis presents in an SLE patient with fever, headache and stiff neck. It is critical to consider that a patient with these symptoms may have infectious meningitis or even a central nervous system hemorrhage.

Cerebral visual disturbances may occur in up to 20% of SLE patients. These include unformed hallucinations, such as bright lights, formal hallucinations, blind spots, complete or localized areas of blindness.

Cerebral vascular accidents occur in SLE, with resultant loss in neurologic function. These vascular accidents may be caused by active inflammation of blood vessels in the brain during acute exacerbation of SLE, as a result of severe hypertension, often accompanying kidney involvement, or from accelerated atherosclerosis secondary to old vasculitis, or as a complication of steroid therapy. Similar involvement of the spinal cord may occur, such that the cord can become inflamed (transverse myelitis), leading to paraplegia and loss of control of the bladder and bowels. Peripheral nervous system involvement may result in sensory deficits, usually in the extremities. Patients with this problem most often complain of paresthesis in the hands or feet.

Heart

Cardiac disease is common in SLE. About 20% of patients have evidence of pericarditis with chest pain and/or effusion. Approximately 25% of patients develop myocarditis. Clinically these patients exhibit increased heart rates, and may develop arrhythmias or even congestive heart failure.

Myocardial infarctions occur in SLE patients in greater than expected incidence for the age group involved. Pathologic examination of hearts of SLE patients dying of myocardial infarctions reveal premature coronary atherosclerosis. As with cerebrovascular disease, the cause of this accelerated atherosclerosis may be inflammation of coronary vessels or side effects of long-term steroid therapy.

Pulmonary

The most common pulmonary manifestation of SLE is pleuritis occurring in approximately 60% of patients. Inflammation of the pleura is usually associated with fluid accumulation in the pleural cavity and presents with chest pain aggravated by deep breathing and coughing.

The lung tissue itself may be involved with an acute pneumonia-like illness which may be mild and transient, or may progress to hemorrhage in the lungs leading to death. Chronic lung involvement with pulmonary fibrosis and progressive dyspnea on exertion also occurs.

Gastrointestinal

Non-specific gastrointestinal symptoms occur in up to 50% of patients with SLE. Vasculitis can occur in the blood vessels supplying the small and large intestines. This is often heralded by bloody diarrhea. Colonic perforation due to vasculitis can lead to death.

Hematologic

Hematologic abnormalities in SLE can manifest as low counts of any of the blood cells. The most common blood abnormality seen is a non-specific anemia attributable to chronic disease. However, decreased numbers of red blood cells, white blood cells and platelets can occur due to immune destruction. Blood clotting abnormalities are also seen in SLE patients and must be ruled out before an SLE patient undergoes surgery.

Vasculature

Vasculitis (inflamed blood vessels) occurs in many organs, with the clinical manifestations depending upon the organ(s) involved. Vasculitis involving the vessels leading to the extremities can cause gangrene due to interference with blood supply. Amputation may be necessary in a few patients. The vasculitis involving skin, lungs, gastrointestinal tract, heart and central nervous system has been discussed in previous sections.

Raynaud's phenomenon is present in 20–40% of SLE patients. It is characterized by spasm of the blood vessels of the extremities, most often in response to cold or stress. Clinically Raynaud's phenomenon presents as a three phase color change from white (vasoconstriction) to blue (cyanosis) to red (hyperemia) often associated with pain. Raynaud's phenomenon may be mild and completely reversible, however, with long-standing disease, it can progress to chronic narrowing of the involved vessels, with secondary tissue loss, pitting ulceration and distal necrosis.

Laboratory

Numerous laboratory abnormalities occur in SLE, some disease specific and others non-specific. Already described include abnormalities in blood cell counts, urine analysis, blood clotting parameters and renal, heart and muscle chemistries. Elevation of the erythrocyte sedimentation rate is a non-specific indicator or inflammation and its level is often helpful in following disease activity.

DIAGNOSES

The American Rheumatism Association has established criteria for the diagnosis of SLE. The revised 1982 criteria are listed in Table 6-1. To fulfill the diagnosis of SLE by this standard at least four of the eleven must have been present at some time during the patient's history. The criteria were selected by computer analysis for their specificity and sensitivity. Some newer potentially useful factors were not included in the criteria because of lack of information. The diagnosis of SLE in the individual patient may be made without fulfilling these criteria based on other significant evidence such as a consistent renal biopsy or multi-system disease with autoimmune features. There criteria are not established to be absolute but rather to develop a uniform language among physicians for patient diagnosis and research.

MANAGEMENT

The management of systemic lupus must be individualized for each patient. As has previously been emphasized, no two lupus patients are alike and thus, therapy should reflect each patient's particular problems.

The ultimate goal of therapy is to keep the lupus patient as well as possible with as few complications from therapy as can reasonably be achieved. In addition to the medications which will be discussed, emphasis must be placed on the multidiscipline approach to patient care. A patient with SLE frequently will need care from many medical specialties such as neurology, orthopedics, nephrology, cardiology, pulmonary, psychiatry, hematology, obstetrics and gynecology, gastroenterology and dermatology, in addition to care from a rheumatologist or primary care physician. The allied health professional is important to the team approach since many lupus patients require physical therapy, occupational therapy and nutritional advice. Emotional and social service support are also frequently necessary for patients and their families in dealing with a chronic illness with an unpredictable course.

All health professionals caring for SLE patient should be involved in patient education. Patients familiar with patterns of their own disease course will more readily recognize early disease flares and understand possible complications of therapy. Education should include advice regarding nutrition. While many diets stressing vitamins or specific foods have their proponents, the best recommendation is generally for a well-balanced diet, taking into account the special needs of patients with problems such as hypertension or renal failure. SLE patients with Raynaud's phenomenon should protect themselves from cold exposure by not handling cold objects and by wearing warm clothing. If a history of photosensitivity is obtained, the patient should be instructed to avoid sunlight by wearing protective clothing with long sleeves and big hats, or to use good quality sunblocks on exposed skin.

Medical treatment of SLE is based upon the possible achievement of two goals, to relieve clinical symptoms and reverse tissue inflammation and damage. Some SLE patients with mild disease or with disease in remission require no therapy. Treatment of the patient with mild SLE should be directed at the specific disease manifestations present. Salicylates are the first drug of choice for arthralgias, transient arthritis and fever. When salicylates are ineffective or not tolerated due to side effects, such as epigastric pain, the non-steroidal anti-inflammatory drugs may be beneficial. Occasionally, chronic synovitis unresponsive to these agents develops. The anti-malarial drug hydroxychloroquine has been used in these patients, as well as for those with chronic fevers. Chronic skin rash should be treated first with topical steroid preparations, sometimes requiring occlusive dressings. Cutaneous vasculitis of the fingertips, palms and soles may improve with topical steroids but, at times, the tissue necrosis may be reversed only with oral steroid therapy.

A number of manifestations of active lupus cause considerable morbidity but usually do not result in permanent debilitating sequelae. These cases of moderately severe SLE include serositis, myositis and hematologic features, such as hemolytic anemia and thrombocytopenia. These manifestations generally respond to corticosteroid therapy. Steroids should be used in the lowest dose possible to control the disease manifestations.

Some of the potentially very severe manifestations of SLE include central nervous system and renal disease. Central nervous system features, such as aseptic meningitis, respond well to steroid therapy. Grand mal seizure, however, are best treated with anti-convulsants. Organic brain syndrome frequently progresses to dementia despite steroids, which may be tried in acute cases, but should be rapidly tapered if improvement is not readily apparent. Functional psychosis may improve with psychotropic drugs alone, but steroids may be required in addition.

Aggressive therapy with high-dose corticosteroids is generally well accepted in attempting to reverse severe renal disease. The value of other immunosuppressive agents is controversial. There are two potential points in the management plan at which their use might be contemplated. They are added to steroid therapy during acute exacerbations of lupus which are either unresponsive to very high doses of steroids, or responsive only to doses producing unacceptable toxicity. Cyclophosphamide, either orally or intravenously, may result in acute improvement, but studies suggest that long-term survival, especially of patients with nephritis is unchanged. Immunosuppressive agents may also be useful as maintenance therapy during periods of disease remission to prevent subsequent flares. The most commonly used drug for this purpose is azathioprine. Despite aggressive therapy with steroids and immunosuppressive drugs, some patients with nephritis will rapidly progress to uremia. Others will slowly develop increasing renal insufficiency in the absence of other evidence of SLE activity. Hemodialysis or renal transplantation should be considered rather than continuing drug therapy.

Focal central nervous system involvement resulting from vasculitis may either be life-threatening or lead to catastrophic irreversible damage. Intracerebral or subarachnoid bleeding may cause focal neurologic deficits, or sudden death. High-dose intravenous steroids or cyclophosphamide may, at times, reverse these processes, but no controlled studies of their efficacy have been published.

Plasmapheresis is an experimental and very expensive technique under investigation for the treatment of SLE. This procedure involves circulating blood through a machine which removes plasma, but returns blood cells to the patient. In theory, plasmapheresis removes the circulating immune complexes responsible for tissue damage. Although reports conclude that it may be possible to acutely improve a patient's immediate status, long-term benefits of plasmapheresis remain unclear.

COMPLICATIONS OF THERAPY

The possible side effects of therapy must be considered when choosing medication for a patient. Corticosteroid therapy is associated with significant toxicity. Infection is common in steroid-treated patients, with the incidence of bacterial infections rising about eightfold in patients receiving more than 40 mg of prednisone per day. In patients who already have compromised renal or cardiac function the fluid and sodium retention induced by steroid may result in intractable edema or hypertension. Steroid-induced diabetes mellitus, myopathy and psychosis may complicate the treatment of active lupus. Long-term steroid use frequently leads to osteoporosis and its secondary complications such as vertebral collapse and chronic bone pain. The specific toxicity of immunosuppressive agents may be difficult to distinguish from that of steroids since they are often used together. Azathioprine may produce leukopenia, and in rare cases, its use result in bone marrow failure, which may be fatal because of infection or hemorrhage due to thrombocytopenia.

Similarly, cyclophosphamide has been associated with leukopenia, bone marrow failure and an increased incidence of common and opportunistic infections. It is also associated with the development of alopecia, hemorrhage cystitis and amenorrhea secondary to ovarian failure. An increased incidence of tumors has been suggested with the use of all immunosuppressive agents. However, the most reliable documentation has been in association with cyclophosphamide, where lymphomas and bladder carcinoma, as well as other solid tumors have been seen.

ASEPTIC NECROSIS

Aseptic necrosis occurs in about 10% of SLE patients and is due to interference of blood supply to the affected bones. The hip is the most common joint affected, but the condition can also involve the knee, shoulder and elbow. The X-Ray of the bone involved may initially be completely normal or reveal only subtle bone changes. With advanced disease, there may be severe arthritis of the joint next to the affected ones and collapse of the involved bone segment. The earliest symptoms are hip pain on weight bearing. This may progress to pain at rest, with inability to internally rotate or flex the hip. The development of aseptic necrosis has been thought to result from chronic steroid therapy. However, correlation with either the duration or total dose of steroids has been poor. The best correlation appears to be with the total duration of SLE itself, independent of its specific disease manifestations or the level of disease activity.

Acute management of this problem includes rest and analgesics. Bone marrow decompression procedures have been shown to reduce pain, but the long-term outcome of this procedure is unknown at present. Incapacitating pain or inability to function are indications for total joint replacement.

PREGNANCY

Pregnancy in a patient with SLE is an important consideration, especially since systemic lupus is primarily a disease of women of child-bearing age. Fetal loss is common in SLE patients. In one study, 126 out of 613 pregnancies in SLE patients ended in spontaneous abortion. Stillbirth and premature birth also occur with greater frequency than would be seen in healthy women. SLE patients also commonly have babies born small for gestational age.

Neonatal lupus is rarely seen in babies born to mothers with systemic lupus, and is presumable due to transplacental transfer of maternal antinuclear antibodies. Some of the possible features of this syndrome include a diffuse rash, thrombocytopenia and serologic abnormalities. In most cases the disease stops within three to six months. Recently an association has been established between congenital heart block in infants and serologic abnormalities (anti-Ro antibodies) in the mothers.

There is considerable controversy concerning the effects of pregnancy on the course of SLE. It has been our experience that SLE patients with active renal disease and/or hypertension do poorly when pregnant, with an increased rate of fetal loss and toxemia of pregnancy. However, for other SLE patients, the effects of pregnancy on disease activity are unpredictable. Some patients remain well while pregnant, while others may have severe disease flares. A recent study revealed no increase in the number of flares in 35 pregnant lupus patients when compared to age-matched nonpregnant SLE controls.

All women of child-bearing age with SLE should be educated about the possible risks of pregnancy. SLE patients with active renal disease and/or hypertension are likely to have significant pregnancy-associated problems and should not become pregnant. In addition, patients who have serious manifestations of SLE or require potentially teratogenic drugs should avoid pregnancy. Even when a pregnancy is not contraindicated, education about potential difficulties such as fetal loss and neonatal SLE should be discussed. During pregnancy, an SLE patient should be managed both by a rheumatologist and an obstetrician experienced in the care of high risk pregnancy.

COURSE

The course of systemic lupus is variable. Some patients have mild disease with rash, arthralgias and serologic abnormalities and may never require hospitalization. Other patients may have a malignant course and die of multiple organ failure shortly after diagnosis. It is more typical, however, to have exacerbations of SLE at variable intervals, often at the same season of the year. These flares may be precipitated by stress, menses, infection, sun exposure, etc. Frequently, flares are mimetic such that a patient with a flare consisting of leukopenia, fever and arthritis is likely to report the same manifestations during subsequent exacerbations. However, SLE can be unpredictable with subsequent flares of varying severity and new manifestations.

PROGNOSIS

Mortality in SLE has decreased, but remain appreciable. A 1954 study reported 50% mortality after four years. Estes and Christian followed 150 patients over eight years and reported 36% overall mortality in 1970. A multicenter study in 1982 reported an overall 20% thirteen year mortality among the original SLE patients. In this study mortality was 10% at one year, 23% at five years and 29% at ten years from diagnosis. Most deaths in these series were from active kidney disease or infection.

Age at onset of disease does affect prognosis. The elderly tend to have a relatively mild disease course. In contrast, children under the age of sixteen are reported to have higher morbidity and mortality than adults. This may reflect the increased incidence of renal disease in younger SLE patients.

Increased survival in the more recent series may to some extent reflect better understanding of the disease course and its response to treatment. However, the improved statistics may also be explained by recognition of milder cases of SLE with an inherently better survival. It is also likely that advances in antibiotics and anti-hypertensive therapy as well as the increased availability of services, such as hemodialysis, play a role in the improved outlook for SLE patients.

SUGGESTED READINGS

"Systemic lupus erythematosus," *Primer on the Rheumatic Diseases,* 8th edition. 1983:49–59; Rodnan, G.P., Schumacker, H.R., eds. Atlanta: Arthritis Foundation.

Rothfield, N. Systemic Lupus Erythematosus: Clinical Aspects and Treatment, Ch. 67 in Arthritis and Allied Conditions. McCarty D.J., Ed. Lea & Febiger, Phila., 11th edition, 1989.

Ginzler, E.M., Blumenthal, D.R. "Renal involvement in SLE: Clinical and Pathological Spectrum." *The Kidney and Rheumatic Diseases*. Bacon, P.A., Handler, N.M., eds.; 1982:3–20. London: Butterworth Scientific.

Block, S.R., Winfield, J.B., Lockshin, M.D., D'Angelo, W.A., Christian, C.L. Studies of twins with systemic lupus erythematosus. *Am J Med* 1975; 59:533–52.

Fesse, W.J. Systemic lupus erythematosus in the community. *Arch Intern Med* 1974; 134:1027–35.

Ginzler, E.M. Treatment of systemic lupus erythematosus. *Primary Care* 1978;5:149–57.

Small, P., Mass, M.F., Kohler, P.F., Harbeck, R.J. Central nervous system involvement in SLE. *Arth Rheum* 1977;20:869–78.

Hall, R.C.W., Stickney, S.K., Gardner, E.R. Psychiatric symptoms in patients with systemic lupus erythematosus. *Psychosomatics* 1981;22:15–24.

TABLE 6-1
1982 REVISED CRITERIA FOR THE CLASSIFICATION OF SYSTEMIC LUPUS ERYTHEMATOSUS

1. Malar Rash
2. Discoid Rash
3. Photosensitivity
4. Oral Ulcers
5. Arthritis
6. Serositis
   a. Pleuritis or
   b. Pericarditis
7. Renal Disorder
   a. Proteinuria greater than 0.5 grams/24 hours or
   b. Cellular casts
8. Neurologic Disorder
   a. Seizures or
   b. Psychosis
9. Hematologic Disorder
   a. Hemolytic Anemia or
   b. Leukopenia less than 4000/mm^3 or
   c. Lymphopenia less than 1500/mm^3 or
   d. Thrombocytopenia less than 100,000/mm^3
10. Immunologic Disorder
   a. Positive LE cell preparation or
   b. Positive anti-DNA antibodies or
   c. Positive anti-Sm antibodies or
   d. False positive test for syphilis
11. Antinuclear antibody

CHAPTER 7

GOUT

Tsai-Fan Yu, M.D.

INTRODUCTION

Gout is a disease of kings and king of diseases. It is a disease that commands great attention by clinicians as well as the laity. Victims of gout are proud of their eminence and their over-indulgence.

The earliest clinical description of gout is attributed to Hippocrates (460–370 B.C.), although it is likely that the Egyptians knew about it much earlier. A large mass in the great toe of an elderly male, presumably a tophus, was discovered among archeological artifacts in upper Egypt. Several prescriptions deciphered in the Ebers Papyrus (1500 B.C.) contain crocus and saffron herb, from which colchicine is derived.

The association of uric acid and gout became known in 1776, when Karl Wilheim Scheele, a Swedish apothecary, reported that urinary stones were not, as generally believed, calcareous in nature alone, but consisted predominantly of a previously unrecognized organic acid, uric acid. About that time, William Hyde Wollaston, a nephew of William Heberden, isolated uric acid from a gouty tophus from his own ear. In 1793, Murray Forbes extended Wollaston's observation when he speculated that gout might be associated with an increased concentration of uric acid in the body. Forbes also confirmed Scheele's conclusion that the chief constituent of urinary calculi was an acid, which was present normally in urine and could be precipitated by the addition of muriatic acid.

Sir Alfred Baring Garrod (1819–1909), the father of modern day concepts of gout, set forth his views in a series of ten propositions on the true nature, or essence, of gout. He was the one who introduced the famous thread test, in which uric acid crystals from evaporated serum adhered to a fine thread.

THE ORIGIN AND DISPOSITION OF URIC ACID

Uric acid is formed from several metabolic pathways. Exogenously, it may be derived from ingested preformed nucleoproteins, nucleic acids and nucleotides.

Endogenously, it is degraded from the nucleic acids and nucleotides synthesized in the body. Another pathway of uric acid formation is the direct synthesis from simple carbon and nitrogen compounds, such as glycine, glutamine, aspartate, bicarbonate, ammonia, etc., without intermediary formation of nucleic acids. Whereas in most mammals, uric acid is converted to allantoin by the enzyme uricase; in man, it is the final product of purine metabolism due to the absence of uricase.

Under normal circumstances, about two thirds of eliminated uric acid is excreted by the kidney. The remaining one-third is disposed of by the intestinal tract. In hyperuricemic man, the extrarenal disposal is proportionately greater. Of interest is that the bacteria flora in the intestinal tract possess uricase and therefore can degrade uric acid.

Very little uric acid is bound to plasma proteins under physiological conditions. Thus, it is safe to assume that serum uric acid is completely filtered through the glomeruli of the kidneys. Between 98–99% of all uric acid thus filtered is reabsorbed. Hence, the uric acid in urine is derived from renal tubular secretion.

Most of the weak organic acids affect uric acid excretion by competing with it for transport by the renal tubules. Lactate, hydroxybutyrate and acetoacetate are examples of some endogenous metabolites which inhibit renal tubular secretion of uric acid. Drugs like salicylate or phenylbutazone may give rise to either urinary retention, or increased excretion of uric acid, depending upon the drug concentration in the renal tubules. Diuretics such as chlorothiazide, chlorthalidone, ethacrynic acid and furosemide may be uricosuric when administered in acute studies. In chronic use, these drugs tend to cause retention of uric acid if the accompanying depletion of extra-cellular fluid volume is not corrected.

VARIANTS OF GOUT

Almost all those having gout are hyperuricemic, but hyperuricemia does not always indicate that one must have gout. A person who inherits the metabolic defect which produces an excess of uric acid may never develop gout. But, of course, a hyperuricemic state increases the risk of developing gout.

Primary Gout

Gout is considered to be mainly a disease of males. The male to female distribution in general is approximately 95:5. Since females usually develop gout after menopause, it is of interest to note that in those with onset of gout beyond 65 years of age, the female incidence is as high as 20–40%. Familial transmission of gout is considered to be polygenic and multifactorial.

Acute gouty arthritis

The onset of acute gouty arthritis is usually sudden and the pain is excruciating. Thomas Sydenham (1624–1689), a famous English physician, had his own onset of gout at age 30. He had severe acute gouty arthritis and kidney stones. His treatise on gout written in 1683 was subsequently translated from Latin to English in 1717. Part of the description of an attack of acute gouty arthritis, based on his personal experience is quoted as follows:

> "He goes to bed and sleeps well, but about two o'clock in the morning, is waked by the pain, seizing either his great toe, the heel, the calf of the leg, or the ankle; this pain is like that of dislocated bones . . . the pain is first gentle, but increases by degrees . . . till towards night it comes to its height . . . sometimes resembling a violent stretching or tearing of these ligaments, sometimes gnawing of a dog . . . the part affected has such a quick and exquisite pain, that it is not able to bear the weight of the cloths upon it . . . there are a thousand fruitless endeavors used to ease the pain, by changing the place continually, whereupon the body and the affected members lie, yet there is no ease to be had."

Acute gouty arthritis is frequently monoarticular, but polyarticular involvement does not necessarily rule out the possibility of gout. About 70% of patients have their first attack at the first metatarso-phalangeal joint, although other peripheral joints are not spared. When axial joints are involved, some other diagnosis should be considered.

The criteria of making a diagnosis of acute gouty arthritis depends on the history, clinical characteristics of an acute joint and hyperuricemia (serum uric acid: >7 mg/dl). Identification of uric acid crystals in synovial fluid confirms the diagnosis.

Tophaceous gout

While acute gouty arthritis is episodic and painful, tophaceous gout is a slowly progressive condition. It is due to a positive uric acid balance from excessive production and/or impaired renal excretion of uric acid. The development of urate deposits in joints or tissues, termed tophi, is related to the degree of hyperuricemia and the duration of gout. Tophi are rarely present in patients whose serum uric acid is less than 8 mg/dl. When the serum uric acid exceeds 11 mg/dl, many tophi may be present. Similarly, the incidence of tophi is low if gout has been present for less than five years. As the duration of gout increases, more patients become tophaceous.

Tophus at the helix of the ear is a favorite site for early urate deposition. Tophi are frequently found at joints most susceptible to recurrent acute attacks, such as the first metatarso-phalangeal, the ankles, the fingers, the wrist and the elbow joints. Atypical locations are the shoulders, sterno-clavicular, acromio-clavicular as well as the knee, hip, sacroiliac or the vertebral joints. Attacks at these atypical locations are very rare. Some urate crystals may infiltrate within the tendon sheaths. This may occur beneath the transverse carpal ligament, compressing the median nerve with the development of carpal tunnel syndrome. Joint stiffness and aching, which may be confused with acute gouty arthritis, may occur in early stages of tophaceous formation. In the advanced stages, joints may be destroyed, resulting in ankylosis, with flexion deformities suggestive of chronic deforming rheumatoid arthritis. Some joints may look like hypertrophic degenerative arthritis. In other cases, tophaceous deposits and degenerative arthritis may co-exist. At the first metatarso-phalangeal joint, a bunion may look like a tophus. On the other hand, a tophus may develop within the deformed area. Tophus and degenerative arthritis may be found in the same knee joint. Hence, degenerative arthritis does not preclude tophaceous deposits and vice versa. Demonstration of uric acid crystals in aspirated synovial fluid makes the diagnosis definitive.

A huge tophus may break through the skin forming discharging sinuses. At times, secondary infection may set in. Such grotesque pictures of tophi were frequently seen before the era of the modern anti-gout therapy (Figure 7-1).

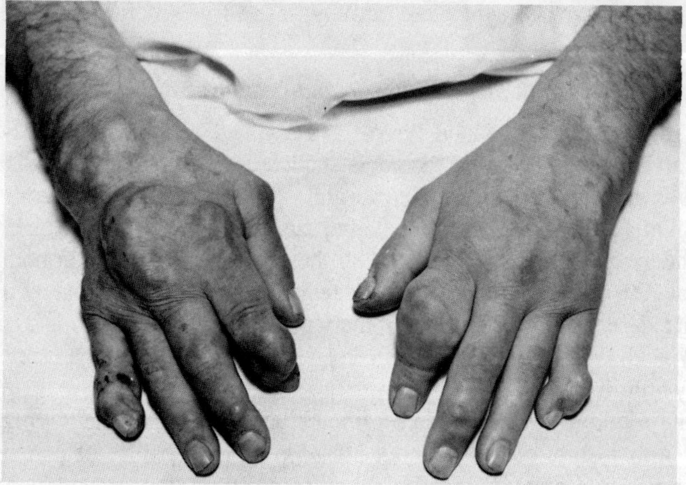

Figure 7-1: Deforming Tophi of the Hands

Secondary Gout

Gout secondary to enzyme abnormalities

The most extreme degree of excessive purine synthesis found in human subjects is associated with a genetic deficiency of the enzyme hypoxanthine-guanine-phosphoribosyl transferase (HGPRT). The gene for HGPRT is x-linked, hence, the deficiency state occurs in males only. Lesch-Nyhan syndrome patients, with complete absence of HGPRT, usually show compulsive self-mutilating behavior, such as biting away of the lips and tongue and amputating the finger tips. They are spastic, choreoathetotic and mentally retarded. In partial, HGPRT deficiency abnormal neurological manifestations are absent. Overproduction of uric acid along with recurrent kidney stones and gout at young age occurs. Serum uric acid is usually over 15 mg/dl and daily urinary uric acid excretion is in excess of 1–2 gm.

Type I glycogen storage disease due to glucose-6-phosphatase deficiency is a rare hereditary disease of childhood. In such patients, the hyperlacticacidemia and ketonemia cause renal retention of uric acid, which leads to hyperuricemia and eventually gout. Such patients also show overproduction of uric acid as determined by increased incorporation of glycine-1-14C into uric acid. Thus, the pathogenesis of gout here is due to both overproduction and under-excretion of uric acid.

Another enzyme deficiency which leads to gout and hyperuricemia is heredity fructose intolerance. This disease is characterized by deficient phosphofructoaldolase. In a few families, gout is due to enhanced phosphoribosyl pyrophosphate synthetase activity, instead of a deficiency in enzyme activity.

Gout associated with blood dyscrasia and neoplastic diseases

The most common blood dyscrasias associated with gout are polycythemia vera and myeloproliferative disorders and less frequently leukemias. Different types of anemias, coagulation defects and various neoplastic disorders, such as Hodgkin's disease, multiple myeloma, etc. may also, at times, give rise to secondary gout. Gout associated with these conditions occurs in both sexes. About 10% of these gouty patients are female and the onset of gout, as a rule, is about a decade after the onset of primary gout. Acute gouty arthritis sometimes is atypical; kidney stones and tophi frequently precede the first attack of acute gouty arthritis.

In primary gout, the mean serum uric acid is approximately 9 mg/dl and daily urinary uric output is about 500–600 mg. Only 30% of patients with primary gout excrete more than 800 mg/day. But in gout secondary to blood dyscrasia, however, serum uric acid is frequently more than 10 mg/dl, and uric acid excretion frequently exceeds 1 gm/day unless renal function is impaired. The hyperuricemia and hyperuricosuria are further exaggerated when chemotherapy is underway.

Gout secondary to lead intoxication

Chronic lead poisoning is frequently associated with progressive kidney damage. Hyperuricemia is accompanied by decreased uric acid excretion in urine. Sometimes clinical gout develops. Lead mobilization test using EDTA (Ethylene diamine tetra-acetic acid) is considered to be a very sensitive test for the diagnosis of lead poisoning. The three day urinary excretion of lead after EDTA may be doubled in patients with gout and a history of lead exposure, as compared to gouty patients without lead exposure. This condition is sometimes referred to as "saturnine gout."

KIDNEY STONES (NEPHROLITHIASIS)

Most stones in the urinary tract are calcium oxalate, or calcium oxalate mixed with calcium phosphate. About 10% of stones are composed of uric acid. Causal relationship between gout and urinary stones was known as early as Galen's time in the second century, A.D. Nephrolithiasis occurs in 20–25% of patients with primary gout and in as many as 50% of patients with secondary gout from blood dyscrasia. Of these, pure uric acid stones occurs in 80%, calcium stones in 14% and mixed calcium and uric acid stones in 5%.

Uric acid, a weak acid has a pKa of 5.75, which means that 50% is ionized in a solution of pH 5.75. At plasma pH of 7.4, uric acid is virtually completely ionized, thus it exists as its sodium salt. Free uric acid is sparingly soluble even less so than its sodium salt. The solubility of uric acid in urine at pH 5.0, is only about 60 mg/L. It is increased to 200 mg/L at pH 6.0; and further increased to 580 mg/L at pH 7.0.

Urine collected from patients with gout under fasting conditions or after meals is unduly acid. A pH of 5.0 or less occurs in almost 50% of these patients, even more acid in those with uric acid stones. While urinary ammonia excretion is less than that in non-gouty controls, the uric acid excretion is much more. Stones occur in less than 20% of gout patients whose uric acid excretion in urine is less than 600 mg/day. Stone incidence increases to 50% when urine uric acid excretion exceeds 1 gm/day. When uric acid forms aggregates of crystals in acid urine, the rate of growth is exaggerated if the urine volume is reduced, as in systemic dehydration. Thus, hyperuricosuria, low urine pH and reduced urine volume are undoubtedly predisposing factors for stone formation.

Some patients develop renal colic only once and others repeatedly. The symptoms of renal colic, of course, may also vary according to the size of the stone and the location in the urinary tract. A silent stone may sit in the kidney without causing any symptoms, only to be found incidentally. On the other hand, a stone may be caught at a strategic location obstructing the urinary tract and causing inflammation in the surrounding tissue. With urinary tract infection, some stones may be transformed into a struvite stone with a uric acid nidus.

Recurrent stones of varying sizes, even without infection, may sometimes cause proteinuria, azotemia and renal damage. As renal damage progresses, hyperuricemia becomes worse and hyperuricosuria disappears. Such patients usually form more tophi.

HYPERURICEMIC NEPHROPATHIES

Acute hyperuricemia, as in blood dyscrasia patients, especially after cytotoxic therapy, may lead to extreme hyperuricosuria and acute hyperuricemic nephropathy. Acute or short term hyperuricemia produces lesions in Henle's loop of the kidney. In uncomplicated gout, chronic hyperuricemia may be present for years without diminution of renal function. With aging, increased incidence of hypertension, cardiovascular disease and diabetes may enhance adverse effects on the kidneys. Chronic persistent hyperuricemia is not necessarily associated with any renal lesion, but in association with vascular conditions the following may occur: glomerulosclerosis; Henle's loop degeneration and regeneration; renal interstitial inflammation and fibrosis, and arterial vascular degeneration. Urate deposition as tophi or tubular obstruction with urate crystals in kidney is not too commonly observed. In patients with inborn enzyme defects, the lesions of abnormal urate deposition are more noticeable, and so are the various vascular complications. Saturnine gout usually presents with proteinuria and a distinctive renal convoluted proximal tubular degeneration with acidophilic intra-nuclear inclusions. The renal vascular changes may be progressive with ultimate development of nephrosclerosis, indistinguishable from other forms of nephropathy.

URIC ACID IN SERUM, URINE AND SYNOVIAL FLUID

The mean serum uric acid concentration in non-gouty males varies between 5.0 and 7.0 mg/dl and that for females is usually 1.0 mg/dl less. Serum uric acid may be elevated by drugs, such as some diuretics (Chlorothiazide) or anti-tuberculosis drugs (Isoniazid, Pyrazinamide, etc.).

The identification of uric acid crystals in synovial fluid aspirated from an acutely inflamed joint makes a definitive diagnosis of acute gouty arthritis. The needle-like crystals of monosodium urate may be seen under regular light microscope if the condenser is turned down. The crystals may be free in the fluid or within polymorphonuclear leukocytes. By using a polarizing light microscope with a red plate compensator in place, uric acid crystals show up as yellow needles when parallel to the plane of the compensator and blue when viewed at right angles (negatively birefringent).

TREATMENT

The important measures for the treatment of gout are directed to acute gouty arthritis, chronic urate deposition in the joints and kidneys and the associated medical conditions.

Drug Therapy

Acute gouty arthritis

The duration of an untreated attack is not predictable. If proper treatment is initiated early in the course, dramatic relief may soon take place. There are several effective drugs which may be employed.

Colchicine: May be used either orally or intravenously. If given orally, one may start with 1.0 mg, followed by 0.5 mg every two hours. Stop medication when nausea, vomiting or diarrhea set in. Frequently an attack may be terminated before the onset of gastrointestinal symptoms appear. Colchicine is to be avoided in patients with abnormal intestinal conditions.

Intravenous Colchicine: May be given if oral therapy is contraindicated. The injection must be carefully and slowly given to avoid leakage from the vein. Colchicine, not to exceed 2.0 mg diluted in 10–20 ml of saline, may be used. Do not repeat more than once however. Frequently, one does not need a second injection if the first is given early during the attack.

Phenylbutazone: 200 mg three or four times a day after meals for two to three days, together with 1.0 mg of oral Colchicine a day, is an alternative treatment. It is gratifying to see that many patients can get over a severe acute attack after taking less than eight doses. Nevertheless, Phenylbutazone should not be used in patients with blood dyscrasia, cardiac failure or peptic ulcer.

Indomethacin: 25.0 mg three times with Colchicine 0.5 to 1.0 mg a day for four to five days is effective without many undesirable side effects. Dosage exceeding 100 mg a day may cause gastric irritation and dizziness.

ACTH (Adrenocorticotrophic Hormone): In severe gouty arthritis, it is advisable to use ACTH intramuscularly. For prompt action, use the lyophilized preparation 80–100 units in a few ml of saline as the first dose. It may be tapered gradually and given two to three days as ACTH gel. Aqueous ACTH intravenously given, is reserved for severe cases only.

Prevention of recurrent acute gouty attacks

As mentioned, acute gouty arthritis is episodic. However, intervals between attacks usually get shorter and symptoms become more severe as time goes on. By using colchicine, 0.5 to 1.0 mg daily, recurrent attacks of gout can be effectively prevented in the majority of the patients. The side effects of colchicine at this dosage are minimal. At higher doses, colchicine is toxic and arrests cell mitosis. Co-existence of associated medical conditions, dietary indiscretion or sudden changes in body weight may offset the beneficial effect of colchicine prophylaxis.

Chronic gout

For satisfactory results, it is imperative to have a negative uric acid balance. To accomplish this one must decrease the rate of uric acid production and/or increase the rate of its excretion. Prior to 1950, rigid dietary restriction was more or less the only measure to affect the uric acid balance. In the early 1950's, gouty tophi were unexpectedly made to disappear by protracted use of uricosuric agents. When allopurinol appeared in the 1960's, a new tool was added to prevent the formation of tophi and to reduce the size of tophi already formed.

Drugs Which Increase Uric Acid Excretion. Probenecid and sulfinpyrazone are two potent uricosuric agents currently available. By inhibiting the tubular re-absorption and secretion of uric acid, both uricosuric agents increase the urinary uric acid thus reducing the serum uric acid. The usual dosage of probenecid is 1.0 gm a day and 200 to 400 mg/day in divided doses for sulfinpyrazone. It is always advisable to start the drug with sub-optimal dosage to watch for possible hypersensitivity. As a starting dose for probenecid, use 0.5 gm/day; for sulfinpyrazone, use 100 mg/day. The dosage may be increased after one to two weeks. As long as the optimal dosage is maintained, the excess uric acid is being mobilized.

Since both drugs promote uric acid excretion, neither is suitable for use in patients with kidney stones. Both are ineffective in patients with renal insufficiency. But for tophaceous patients with satisfactory renal function, either drug should be very helpful. Side effects are relatively low if the dosage is not excessive. Sulfinpyrazone may sometimes depress the bone marrow. It is important to have dosage carefully adjusted and blood counts frequently checked. The most common side effect of both drugs is gastrointestinal discomfort, which may be overcome by taking the drug after meals.

Allopurinol: A Drug Which Modifies Uric Acid Production. Allopurinol inhibits the formation of uric acid from its precursors, hypoxanthine and xanthine, by blocking the enzyme xanthine oxidase. Thus, its action is on the liver unlike that of the uricosuric agents which act on renal tubular transport. Since its action does not depend on kidney function, allopurinol is effective in patients with renal insufficiency.

Surgical Intervention

In recent years, extensive disfiguring tophi are rarely seen due to the use of potent drugs. However, vestiges of chronic deforming gout may still be occasionally observed. Among these patients may have severe gout with renal insufficiency; some fail to adhere to protracted medical regimen, and some may not get the expected drug benefit due to interactions with drug therapy for other associated medical conditions. Joint deformity may become much worse after the disappearance of the tophi originally occupying those joints. Thus, surgical intervention may be useful for removal of a sequestrated tophus which impedes the joint motion despite protracted medical therapy. In cases of carpal tunnel syndrome or tarsal tunnel syndrome, decompression of the nerves will give symptomatic relief if the diagnosis is properly made. And finally, arthroplasty for the destroyed joint(s) is an important way to achieve better stability for weight-bearing and better joint mobility.

Medical Management for Patients with Kidney Stones

General principles involve adequate hydration, maintenance of appropriate urine acidity, control of hyperuricosuria and of secondary infection, if present. Under ordinary circumstances, a fluid intake of two liters a day should be sufficient to produce an adequate amount of urine. However, whenever there is excess loss of fluid through the skin due to vigorous exercise or humid hot environmental conditions, one's fluid intake should be proportionately increased. Under pathological conditions, as in gastrointestinal upsets or during febrile illness, more fluid intake is necessary to maintain the fluid balance.

Optimal urine pH for control of uric acid stones should be maintained between 6.0 and 7.0 since uric acid solubility is greatly increased at pH above 6.0. Adjustment of urine pH may be accomplished by giving sodium bicarbonate 2.0 to 4.0 gm/day. In patients with hypertension, potassium bicarbonate may be used instead. By taking an alkaline ash diet containing relatively more vegetables and less meats, urine pH can be increased to a certain extent.

In most cases, large urine volume and relatively high urine pH prevent recurrence of uric acid kidney stones effectively, except in those with extreme hyperuricosuria and hyperuricemia, related to enzyme abnormalities or blood dyscrasias. In such patients reduction of excessive uric acid in serum and urine can be effectively achieved by means of allopurinol as for tophaceous gout. It is important to remember that uricosuric drugs should not be used in patients with kidney stones.

Sometimes, uric acid may become the nidus for calcium oxalate stones. Chlorothiazide is found to be effective for such stones by diminishing the urinary excretion of calcium. Reduction of oxalate in diet is very important since there is no drug to increase oxalate excretion in urine.

The Role of Diet and Alcohol

There has been a tendency in recent years to neglect dietary therapy for patients with gout since potent drugs are available to correct hyperuricemia and to prevent gouty arthritis. This concept is unfortunately not quite correct. Many patients with gout are not only overweight, but may also have various associated medical conditions requiring careful dietary treatment. From my personal experience with more than 2,000 patients with gout for over three decades, almost half of these patients were hypertensive; approximately 20% had histories of coronary artery disease; 15% had nephropathy, and 8 to 10% had diabetes mellitus or impaired glucose tolerance. In 40% of the patients, there is some abnormality in serum lipids and type IV hyperlipidemia is most prevalent. Overweight, more than 10% of ideal weight, occurred in 42%.

For an overweight gouty man the total calories, as well as fat intake, should be reduced. Low protein intake can be helpful for one with nephropathy. In gout with hypertension or coronary artery diseases, sodium should be reduced as well. In patients with gout and diabetes mellitus, relatively less carbohydrate as well as fat may be preferred depending upon the severity of the diabetes. Thus, dietary treatment of gout is important, particularly in those with associated medical conditions.

Some patients with all good intentions try to reduce their weight by taking a crash diet or fasting. The biochemical changes from such programs are comparable to having a diet containing excessive amounts of fat. The increased catabolism of fat, be it exogenous or endogenous, induces systemic ketosis and ketonuria. In turn, urinary uric acid excretion is dramatically decreased and serum uric acid may be increased to as high as 20–25 mg/dl. The relationship between the accumulation of ketones in the blood to decreased excretion of uric acid by the kidney is usually quite constant. With systemic ketosis, urine pH becomes extremely low, favoring the formation of kidney stones. Frequently, acute gouty arthritis may develop. In short, a gouty man should have a sensible diet which is low in purines; moderate in proteins (not exceeding 80 gm/day); low in fat, high in vegetables, and moderately restricted in calories to 2,000 or less. He should avoid liver, sweetbreads, brains, kidneys, anchovies, sardines, meat extracts or gravies and, likewise avoid dried beans, peas, lentils, asparagus or olives. Sauces, mustards, pickles and other salted foods should be omitted for those who also have uncontrolled hypertension or cardiac insufficiency.

Some gouty sufferers are not only gluttonous, but are also fond of alcoholic drinks. It is well-known that an acute attack of gouty arthritis can be attributed to a taste for drink.

The following is quoted from Gilbert and Sullivan's *Gondoliers:*

> "A taste for drink, combined with gout,
> Had doubled him up forever,
> Of that there is no manner of doubt —
> No probable possible shadow of doubt—
> No possible doubt whatever."

The oxidation of alcohol leads to increased hepatic lactate production and increases lactate concentration in the blood. The elevated blood lactate reduces the uric acid excretion in urine and, in turn, promotes hyperuricemia.

In general, gout can be brought under control with less difficulty if one is moderate in eating and drinking. Further, other medical complications may be avoided.

CONCLUSION

With better understanding of uric acid metabolism and advances in drug development to control hyperuricemia, gout has become an easily manageable disease. Intelligent use of an anti-inflammatory drug dramatically terminates an incapacitating acute attack of gouty arthritis in a few hours. With more meticulous art in using colchicine, the ancient poisonous drug has turned out to be a gem in preventing recurrent gout. Rational use of drugs, which modify the rate of uric acid formation or uric acid excretion, has been able to avoid the formation of tophi and to promulgate its disappearance if already formed. Crippling deformities are not frequently seen any more. Although the incidence of renal calculi is not drastically less, infected stones are hardly seen and surgical intervention is rare.

Nevertheless the nature of gout, particularly that of the episodic acute arthritis, is not clear. Is there any hormonal factor which may influence the sequential reactions in activating an acute attack? Is there any clue that gout is an auto-immune disease?

Incidence of gout with various associated diseases is not on the decline. The management of gout must include the recognition as well as therapy of the associated medical diseases. When anti-gouty drugs are employed in conjunction with drugs for associated conditions, it is imperative to know how the different drugs interact.

Thus, the progress made in understanding pathogenesis and management of gout in the last two to three decades is just a beginning. More vistas will have to be explored. Yesterday's seeds bear some promising seedlings today. More seedlings will be necessary for tomorrow's harvest.

SUGGESTED READINGS

Yu, T.F.; Gutman, A.B. Mobilization of Gouty Tophi by Protracted use of Uricosuric Agents. **Am J Med** 11:765–769,1951.

Rodnan, G.P. A Gallery of Gout, Being a Miscellany of Prints and Caricatures from the

16th Century to the Present Day. **Arth Rheum** 4:27–46,1961.

Yu, T.F. Nephrolithiasis. In Symposium on Gout, **Postgraduate Medicine** 63:164–170,1978.

Talbott, J.H.; Yu, T.F. *Gout and Uric Acid Metabolism.* Stratton Intercontinental Medical Book, Inc., New York 1976.

Yu, T.F.; Berger, L. (editors). *The Kidney in Gout and Hyperuricemia.* Futura Pub. Co., Mt. Kisco, NY 1981.

Kelley, W.N., et al, eds. Textbook of Rheumatology. WB Saunders, Phila., 3rd edition, 1989. Ch. 78.

CHAPTER 8

DIFFUSE CONNECTIVE TISSUE DISEASES

Frederick Swerdlow, M.D.

There are a group of ailments collectively termed "diffuse connective tissue diseases." In this category, the general headings of *scleroderma, vasculitis* and *myositis* each actually refer to a subset of ailments sharing certain clinical features in common but which may actually be different diseases.

SCLERODERMA

Scleroderma or progressive systemic sclerosis is an illness characterized by increased deposits of fibrous tissue often referred to as scar tissue in various organ systems of the body, especially the skin, gastrointestinal tract, heart, lungs and kidneys. This illness occurs most often in women and has a peak incidence between the ages of 30 and 50.

The *cause* of scleroderma is not known. Overproduction of fibrous tissue also known as collagen by fibroblasts has been shown in patients with this illness. In addition, it has been observed that there is diminished capillary blood flow. Whether this decrease in circulation is the cause of the illness or is secondary to the illness is not known. In some patients with scleroderma, abnormalities in the immune system may be demonstrated. For example there is a high incidence of antinuclear antibodies. Other abnormalities have also been demonstrated such as inflammatory infiltrates of cells in affected organs and, abnormalities of fibroblasts, causing them to produce excess collagen. An illness similar to scleroderma may occur in individuals exposed to certain medications as well as to some chemicals present in the environment. Patients who have received organ transplants may develop a syndrome called a graft vs. host reaction, which may resemble scleroderma. As mentioned previously, despite these tantalizing clues, the cause of scleroderma remains unknown.

The illness itself may be a localized problem confined simply to the skin where it may be known as morphea or linear scleroderma. More often, scleroderma is a truly generalized illness with involvement of many of the body's organ systems. Early on, the skin involvement may present with generalized swelling, particularly of the hands similar to fluid retention known as edema. Later, this swelling may give way to generalized tightening of the skin not only of the hands but all over the body including the face and trunk. In almost all patients with scleroderma, there is a sensitivity of the blood vessels in the extremities to cold, known as Raynaud's phenomenon. When exposed to cold, the skin, particularly of the tips of the fingers and toes in patients with Raynaud's phenomenon blanches to a pale color, followed later by a bluish discoloration and still later to a redness. Raynaud's phenomenon may occur as the earliest manifestation of scleroderma and may be present alone for many years before other signs of the disease appear. Most patients with scleroderma experience discomfort in the joints. In some patients, actual arthritis may occur, though the most prominent joint manifestation is flexion contracture and loss of mobility owing to fibrous deposition in the tissue around the joints. Deposits of calcium may also occur within the soft tissue of patients with scleroderma and are referred to as calcinosis. Many patients with scleroderma develop involvement of the gastrointestinal tract, the most common manifestation of which is difficulty in swallowing due to disturbed motility of the esophagus with loss of peristalsis. Loss of muscle tone at the junction of the esophagus and the stomach may permit reflux of stomach acids into the esophagus with inflammation and later stricture formation. This also contributes to difficulty in swallowing and to food sticking behind the breastbone in patients with scleroderma. In such patients one often observes replacement of the normal musculature of the esophagus by fibrous tissue. Lower in the gastrointestinal tract loss of motility of the bowel is often observed and there may be generalized dilatation of the duodenum. Localized outpouching of the colon called diverticula may also be noted on barium enema examination. In association with such diverticula and generalized hypomotility, there may be overgrowth of bacteria within the intestine, which can lead to a syndrome known as malabsorption where nutrients in the meal are not adequately absorbed by the patient leading to weight loss and wasting. The majority of patients with scleroderma ultimately develop lung involvement. Even early on when the chest X-Ray may be normal, one can demonstrate through sophisticated pulmonary function testing abnormalities of lung function. Eventually, infiltrates appear on the chest X-Ray due to increased deposits of fibrous tissue within the lung. In association with such changes, there may be increased pressure within the pulmonary blood circulation, i.e. pulmonary hypertension. Pulmonary hypertension may exert a significant strain upon the heart. Lastly, pulmonary involvement with scleroderma seems to be associated with an increased incidence of both bronchiolar and alveolar cell cancers. Dysfunction of the heart in scleroderma may also be a consequence of fibrosis of the muscle of the heart leading to so-called cardiomyopathy. Inflammation of the outer lining of the heart, known as pericarditis, with the development of fluid surrounding the heart, known as pericardial effusion, may also occur. Kidney involvement in scleroderma is not uncommon. When it becomes clinically apparent, it is usually associated with severe hypertension, which is difficult to control and may at times lead to rapidly progressive kidney failure. Myositis characterized by muscle weakness and inflammation occurs in some patients with scleroderma and will be discussed in more detail later.

An overall more benign type of scleroderma has been clinically recognized for many years and is characterized by deposition of calcium in the soft tissues, Raynaud's phenomenon, dysfunction of the esophagus, tightening of the skin in the fingers known as sclerodactyly and dilatation of blood vessels in the skin known as telangiectasias. These entities make up the so-called CREST syndrome, which is generally held to be a more slowly progressive type of scleroderma, though sometimes also associated with pulmonary hypertension.

Laboratory abnormalities in scleroderma may include anemia, as is often observed in patients with chronic illness but may also be a consequence of hemolysis or destruction of blood cells within affected organs. Abnormalities in the urine such as the presence of blood cells (hematuria) as well as the presence of protein often indicate kidney involvement with the disease. In most patients with scleroderma, there are positive tests for antinuclear antibodies and most characteristic of this illness is presence of antibody to the nucleolus. Anti-centromeric antibodies have also been described in a high percentage of patients with the CREST syndrome.

Unfortunately, there is no definitive treatment which has been shown to be effective in all patients with scleroderma. In some patients, the Raynaud's phenomena may be helped by vasodilating drugs. It may be even more important for the patient to simply avoid cold exposure and other environmental agents which are known to cause vasospasm such as tobacco. The gastrointestinal manifestations of scleroderma may be benefited by supportive therapy. Acid reflux from the stomach into the esophagus may be helped by antacids as well as drugs to diminish production of acid by the stomach along with elevation of the head of the bed overnight while the patient is lying down. Malabsorption of nutrients due to overgrowth of bacteria in the gastrointestinal tract may be treated with antibiotics. Kidney involvement, usually associated with severe hypertension, may be helped by treatment with newer anti-hypertensive drugs such as Captopril or Enalapril. In such patients, prior to the use of potent anti-hypertensive drugs, kidney involvement with scleroderma was almost 100% fatal, while the outlook now, for most patients treated early, is more favorable. It has recently been recommended that patients with scleroderma be treated with D-penicillamine, a drug which may inhibit the cross-linking of newly formed collagen, hence possibly preventing the generalized fibrosis noted in the illness. It has been suggested that prolonged treatment with penicillamine may prevent the ultimate internal organ involvement observed in most patients. The use of corticosteroid drugs in scleroderma is generally reserved for patients with severe and persistent joint inflammation or myositis. Because of the possibility of salt retention associated with the use of corticosteroids, blood pressure must be carefully monitored in any patient with scleroderma so treated.

POLYMYOSITIS

Polymyositis is a term describing an inflammatory disease primarily involving the body's voluntary musculature and characterized mostly by muscle weakness. The term myositis is actually descriptive rather than diagnostic and is taken to represent a group of illnesses with diverse clinical manifestations. The following classification is widely used to characterize these illnesses:

Group I Primary idiopathic polymyositis
Group II Primary idiopathic dermatomyositis
Group III Myositis associated with malignancy
Group IV Childhood myositis often associated with vasculitis
Group V Myositis associated with other collagen vascular disease

The cause of the polymyositis syndrome is unknown. In some patients, evidence of infection with toxoplasmosis has been demonstrated. Despite this finding and other efforts to uncover possible viral infections in such patients, no sure primary infectious cause has been discovered. While most patients with polymyositis fail to demonstrate circulating antibodies to muscle, some patients demonstrate a delayed type hypersensitivity to muscle antigens, suggesting an immune mechanism is involved. Recently, evidence of complement activation within blood vessels of patients with myositis has been demonstrated.

A muscle biopsy obtained from a clinically affected area or weak area of the body may demonstrate various changes. The most frequently biopsied muscles are the deltoid or triceps in the upper extremities and the quadriceps and gastronemius of the lower extremities. Typical pathologic changes may include degeneration of muscle fibers, at times be replaced by fibrous tissue, muscle cell destruction, localized or diffuse inflammatory cell infiltrates, variation of sizes of muscle fibers and, at times, vasculitis.

Myositis occurs approximately twice as often in women as men and it is not a rare illness. It has been reported in every age group though it occurs most commonly between the ages of 40 and 60.

The hallmark feature of the disease is muscle weakness. It may gradually develop or present in a fulminant fashion leading to almost complete paralysis. More often, individuals involved with this illness notice gradually increasing difficulty in getting up from sitting and kneeling positions or difficulty raising the arms overhead to perform chores of daily living. When the neck musculature is involved, the patient may have difficulty in holding up his head or raising it from the pillow. Difficulty swallowing (dysphagia) with food sticking high up in the throat owing to weakness of the voluntary muscles of swallowing is a common complaint. At times there may be severe pain in the muscles though usually this is not the case. In patients with longstanding myositis, shortening or contracture of the muscles may occur. In some patients, the muscle inflammation may be accompanied by a skin rash giving the name of dermatomyositis to this condition. In approximately 40% of patients with myositis, a rash will be present. The typical rash is a reddish, dusky eruption present over the front of the neck and anterior chest, at times present also on the dorsal surface of the MCP joints and PIP joints of the hands, along with redness around the nailbeds. At times a rash may be present on the knees and elbows as well. Swelling around the eyes and a rash on the eyelids is unusual but when present, is highly suggestive of a diagnosis of dermatomyositis. Occasionally, true arthritis and Raynaud's phenomenon may be present in patients with myositis. A small percentage of patients with polymyositis will develop lung problems. This is characterized clinically by cough and shortness of breath, and on chest x-ray by an infiltrate in the interstitial area of the lungs.

As previously mentioned, there is an association observed in some patients between myositis and malignant disease, particularly in older patients. Cancer of the lung, prostate, breast, uterus, ovary and gastrointestinal tract are the most commonly reported malignancies. Lymphoma and leukemia have been described as well. Because of this, many physicians feel that it is reasonable to do testing to rule out the presence of malignant disease in patients presenting with myositis, particularly those over the age of 40 and those whose response to treatment is poor.

Laboratory abnormalities which should be looked for in patients suspected of myositis are elevation of the "muscle"* enzymes usually found in the blood. These include CPK, SGOT, SGPT, aldolase and LDH. In almost all patients with myositis, one or more of these enzymes will be elevated. At times, the level of the enzyme may rise or fall antedating a parallel change in the disease state. Another diagnostic test of value is the electromyogram which measures electrical activity of muscle cells. Abnormalities suggestive of myositis include so-called spontaneous fibrillations, complex polyphasic potentials of short duration and repetitive high frequency action potentials. As mentioned above, a muscle biopsy should be performed in every patient suspected of having myositis

---

*"Muscle" enzymes are principally found in heart or skeletal muscle but may leak into the circulation following muscle damage. Principal enzymes tested are creative phosphokinase (CPK), serum glutamate oxaloacetate transaminase (SGOT), serum glutamate pyruvate transaminase (SGPT) and lactic dehydrogenase (LDH). Eds.

looking for signs of muscle cell damage or inflammation.

The mainstay of treatment of the various myositis syndromes is corticosteroids. Usually prednisone in a dosage of 60 mg/day is the starting therapy with the dose lowered if clinical improvement occurs or increased if the patient fails to respond within a period of six weeks. If the illness is not responsive to corticosteroids or if unacceptable side effects develop, other therapeutic agents may be employed including the so-called cytostatic drugs. Methotrexate is the agent which has been most widely used in the past, though azathioprine has been employed more recently. Plasmapheresis has been claimed to be effective in some patients with myositis where all other types of treatment had previously failed.

During the course of therapy serum levels of muscle enzymes may be followed serially in an effort to foretell the ultimate clinical course. Clearly in patients demonstrated to have malignant disease, or to have an associated connective tissue disease, therapy must be directed towards those entities.

VASCULITIS

Vasculitis or inflammation involving blood vessels on both the arterial and venous sides of the circulation is a term characterizing a group of many clinically definable syndromes. With rare exception, the cause of vasculitis in an individual patient is unknown though in certain vasculitis syndromes, the etiology has been defined. The treatment of the various vasculitis syndromes varies and for that reason, syndromes are separated mostly on clinical and pathological grounds. In some cases vasculitis may occur alone while oftentimes vasculitis may develop within the setting of another recognized disease such as scleroderma or myositis. The most commonly encountered vasculitic syndromes will be briefly described below in an effort to demonstrate the wide variety of problems that may be encountered.

Polyarteritis Nodosa

The first vasculitic syndrome to be recognized is now termed polyarteritis nodosa. It is characterized pathologically by inflammation and at times destruction of the entire wall of the inflamed blood vessel, sometimes progressing to scarring and fibrosis of the involved vessel wall. Obstruction of the vessel by a thrombus (clot) with interruption of circulation to the tissues and so-called infarction (tissue death) may occur. Affected blood vessels may dilate with the formation of so-called aneurysms. The inflammatory cells observed within the blood vessel walls of patients with polyarteritis are polymorphonuclear leukocytes. The clinical features of the illness depend upon the site of the blood vessel involvement and the degree of obstruction of blood flow. Kidney involvement is noted in the great majority of cases and may be caused by vasculitis of the renal artery or branching vessels or by glomerulonephritis. In most patients with kidney involvement hypertension is observed. Vasculitis of the heart is noted in approximately 70% of cases and may be characterized by pericarditis or by true myocardial infarction leading to dysfunction of the heart muscle. Gastrointestinal tract vasculitis may present with bleeding into the intestine as a consequence of visceral infarction with or without perforation. Intestinal obstruction may occur and rarely, aneurysms of the abdominal blood vessels may rupture causing massive bleeding. Bleeding into the liver may occur as well. Inflammation of the gall bladder with perforation and inflammation of the pancreas have been observed. A common manifestation of vasculitis is neuropathy, that is dysfunction of nerves which may present as peculiar sensations or loss of muscle function in the extremities. This may be due to actual infarction of the nerve due to interruption of its blood supply. Central nervous system involvement due to abnormalities of circulation to the brain or spinal cord may also occur. Muscle pain is characteristic of vasculitis presumably due to lack of adequate circulation to the muscles of the extremities. Joint pain or frank arthritis may develop. Various skin rashes characterized either as nodules, ulcers or bleeding under the skin may also be observed.

A diagnosis of polyarteritis nodosa depends on a biopsy of an involved organ with proof of inflammation of the blood vessel. Less specifically, angiography may reveal typical changes in the blood vessels such as dilatation or aneurysm formation with variability in the size of the blood vessel lumen. Laboratory abnormalities are often observed including an elevation of the erythrocyte sedimentation rate, elevation of the white blood cell count, increased amounts of circulating gamma globulin as well as the presence of protein and blood cells in the urine when the kidney is involved. The electromyogram is often abnormal owing either to abnormalities of circulation to the nerves or muscles.

The treatment of polyarteritis nodosa, in the past, has mainly been with high doses of corticosteroid drugs, which have been demonstrated to prolong survival in this illness. Immunosuppressive therapy with cyclophosphamide and azathioprine has been used more recently in patients who did not respond to corticosteroids alone or who develop unacceptable side effects from such therapy.

Allergic Granulomatous Angiitis

A syndrome closely resembling polyarteritis but with prominent involvement of the lung including asthma and pulmonary infiltrates was described in 1951. Sinusitis and other allergic features such as hay fever are also frequently observed in this syndrome. Skin manifestations include subcutaneous nodules and purpura often occur. The diagnosis is based upon the demonstration, by biopsy, of granulomatous inflammation of the blood vessels involving arteries, capillaries and veins. Laboratory abnormalities especially an elevated blood cell count with marked eosinophilia is characteristic of this illness. Elevated levels of immunoglobulin E have also been reported. As in polyarteritis nodosa, the mainstay of treatment is corticosteroid drugs, though immunosuppressive therapy with cyclophosphamide and azathioprine has also been used.

Hypersensitivity Vasculitis

This syndrome is presumed to be an immune response to some environmental agent which incites the illness. On biopsy lesions typically occur in post-capillary venules and all of the inflammatory lesions are typically in the same stage of development. Involvement of the kidney, gastrointestinal tract and nervous system is common. Purpuric skin lesions are often observed. In cases where the inciting agent may be a drug, such agents clearly should be avoided. In most cases, however, no inciting agent is noted and treatment with corticosteroids is the mainstay of therapy and is usually effective.

Wegener's Granulomatosis

This disorder is characterized by granulomatous destructive arteritis of the respiratory tract from the nose to the lung and is often accompanied by similar arteritis involving the kidney. Clinically, respiratory involvement may be characterized by a persistent sinusitis and chronic middle ear inflammation (otitis media). Destruction of the tissues of the nose may develop. Lower respiratory tract disease is characterized by cough and pneumonia. Occasionally one may observe involvement of the eyes presenting as drooping of the eyelids, conjunctivitis or inflammation of the deeper layers of the eye. Rarely involvement of the retina may occur. Abnormalities of motion of the eyes called ocular palsies may develop. Kidney disease when present is usually severe progressing to renal failure.

Diagnosis of Wegener's granulomatosis is based on the demonstration of so-called necrotizing granulomatous vasculitis on biopsy either of the upper respiratory mucosa or of the lung tissue itself. In the kidney, glomerulonephritis may be observed with granuloma formation with necrotizing lesions of the renal vessels. X-rays of the sinuses often reveal destructive lesions involving bone. The chest x-ray may show large infiltrates at times with cavitation. Anemia, elevation of the white blood count and an elevated erythrocyte sedimentation rate typically develop. Blood cells in the urine signify kidney involvement and, as mentioned above, renal failure may be observed.

While corticosteroids alone have been used in the past in the treatment of Wegener's granulomatosis, they are of limited benefit and the mainstay of therapy is treatment with cyclophosphamide. In some patients such therapy may actually be curative. A small number of patients who could not tolerate cyclophosphamide or in whom this drug was not effective, have been treated with azathioprine with some success.

Henoch-Schonlein's Purpura

This vasculitic syndrome typically occurs in children and is characterized by purpura (blood spots under the skin), abdominal pain and kidney disease. The lesions often occur several weeks following an upper respiratory illness. When gastrointestinal involvement is present, it is oftentimes associated with severe gastrointestinal bleeding. At times obstruction or perforation of the intestines may occur. Kidney involvement is characterized by the presence of blood cells in the urine as well as protein with the rare development of kidney failure. Scattered purpuric skin lesions which may coalesce are usually present.

The diagnosis of Henoch-Schonlein purpura is based on typical clinical features as well as biopsy of the skin lesions which reveal collections of fragmented polymorphonuclear leukocytes around blood vessels. Kidney biopsy may demonstrate glomerulonephritis, occasionally with scarring. Non-specific laboratory features include anemia, elevated white blood cell count and elevated erythrocyte sedimentation rate. Urinary findings include blood cells and protein in the urine. At times circulating immune complexes containing immunoglobulins have been described in patients with this vasculitic syndrome. Similar immune complexes have been demonstrated in the kidneys of patients.

Treatment of Henoch-Schonlein purpura is often unnecessary as the illness usually remits spontaneously. Corticosteroids have been used particularly in those patients with severe renal involvement. Immunosuppressive therapy with cyclophosphamide and azathioprine has been used in a small number of individuals.

Giant Cell Arteritis

Giant cell arteritis is a disease of unknown cause in which the branches of the arteries originating from the arch of the aorta are prominently involved with a granulomatous or so-called giant cell arteritis. Pathologic sections of the inflamed vessels show infiltration with lymphocytes, macrophages, histiocytes and so-called multinucleated giant cells. Thickening of the inner lining of the blood vessel wall may result in narrowing and occlusion of the vessel lumen.

Clinical features include constitutional complaints such as fever, malaise and weight loss. Many patients have clinical features related to the arteries. Most common are headaches localized to the area of the temporal or occipital arteries. Tenderness and, at times, enlargement of the involved portion of the arteries may be observed. Occasionally, pain occurs in the jaw and tongue while eating and speaking. The syndrome known as *polymyalgia rheumatica* occurs in a large percentage of patients with giant cell arteritis and is characterized by aching discomfort in the muscles, particularly of the upper arms and thighs. Occasionally patients experience sudden loss of vision, often leading to blindness owing to obstruction of the retinal artery or artery to the optic nerve. The illness typically occurs in patients over the age of 50 and should be suspected in anyone with a polymyalgia rheumatica syndrome complaining of severe headache.

The most common and characteristic laboratory abnormality is a highly elevated erythrocyte sedimentation rate usually over 100 mm/hr that occurs in almost all patients. Other findings are anemia, elevated serum globulin concentrations and occasionally elevated enzymes including SGOT and SGPT, along with an elevated alkaline phosphatase.

Corticosteroids are extremely effective as therapy for giant cell arteritis and it has been demonstrated that they can prevent the visual loss attendant on this illness. A starting dose of 60 mg of prednisone/day is usually employed in the treatment of this illness with the dose reduced as the clinical features warrant. Most patients with giant cell arteritis will require treatment with corticosteroids for several years.

Takayasu's Arteritis

Takayasu's arteritis is a rare illness of unknown cause characterized by obliterative arteritis involving the branches of the aortic arch leading to diminished blood flow. Non-specific symptoms such as constitutional complaints with fever and fatigue along with muscle pain are quite common. More specific findings include visual disturbances, and fainting or dizziness due to poor cerebral blood flow. Renal artery involvement is often indicated by hypertension. Cramping of the limb musculature is common in patients with longstanding disease. Pathologically, the illness is characterized by lymphocytic infiltration of the walls of the great vessels. In some patients, scarring fibrotic changes have been observed. This illness occurs eight times more frequently in women than men with a peak age of onset in the 20's. Since the illness involves branches of the aortic arch, the diagnosis may be established by angiogram and blood vessel biopsy is usually not done.

Laboratory abnormalities such as an elevated erythrocyte sedimentation rate and elevated white cell count are characteristic. Although corticosteroids have been used as management for the constitutional manifestations of the illness, there is no convincing evidence of long-term benefit in terms of preventing vascular insufficiency. When hypertension is present, owing to renal artery involvement, it is usually managed conservatively.

SUGGESTED READINGS

Cupps, T.R. and Fauci, A.S. *The Vasculitidies,* Vol. XXI in the series, Major Problems in Internal Medicine, Ed: L.M. Smith Jr. Pub. W.B. Saunders Co., Philadelphia.

Currie, S. *Polymyositis and Related Disorders* in *Disorders of Voluntary Muscle.* Ed: V.N. Watson. Pub. Churchill Livingston, Edinburgh, 4th ed, 1981.

Leroy, E.C. Scleroderma (Systemic Sclerosis), Ch 76 in *Textbook of Rheumatology,* Eds: W.N. Kelley, E.D. Harris, S. Ruddy and C.B. Sledge. Pub. W.B. Saunders Co., 2nd ed, 1985.

Kelley, W.N., et al, eds. Textbook of Rheumatology, WB Saunders, Phila., 3rd edition, 1989, Sec. 9–12.

McCarty, D.J., ed. Arthritis and Allied Conditions, Lea & Febiger, Phila., 11th edition, 1989, Sec. 6.

CHAPTER 9

RHEUMATOID VARIANTS

Harry Spiera, M.D.

Rheumatoid variants refer to a group of inflammatory arthritities which can be distinguished from rheumatoid arthritis. The distinctions are made primarily on clinical, serological and radiographic grounds. The true relationships among these diseases awaits a better understanding of etiology and pathogenesis.

SERO-NEGATIVE SPONDYLOARTHROPATHIES

Sero-negative spondyloarthropathies refers to a group of illnesses which are characterized by chronic inflammatory arthritis which on the basis of certain clinical and serological characteristics, can be distinguished from rheumatoid arthritis. These diseases include principally ankylosing spondylitis, and Reiter's syndrome.

Though one disease is distinguishable from the other, they all have certain features in common. These include male predominance, axial skeleton involvement and absence of rheumatoid factor (RF), hence the term sero-negative. They will be considered individually.

Ankylosing Spondylitis

Ankylosing spondylitis (AS) was once called rheumatoid spondylitis, implying that it was the same disease as rheumatoid arthritis. One reason for this was that the histopathology of AS was similar to that of RA, a disease of unknown etiology and pathogenesis, and some patients with this disease manifested peripheral joint involvement similar to that seen in RA.

On the basis of certain clinical and laboratory distinctions (Table 9-1) spondylitis was clearly distinguished from rheumatoid arthritis and is now called ankylosing spondylitis. Other names used in the literature include Marie-Strumpel's spondylitis and Van Bechterew's disease.

As noted above, AS is a disease of unknown etiology and pathogenesis. It affects men predominantly and often begins in the 3rd to 5th decade of life. It is characterized by severe lower back pain which eventually evolves to affect the entire axial skeleton including the lumbar, dorsal and cervical areas. The patient often complains of morning stiffness and in contrast to patients with degenerative disc disease and mechanical back problems, may feel systemically ill. Moreover, gelling phenomenon and easy fatigability are usually present. Up to 25% may have peripheral joint involvement. As with most other chronic rheumatic diseases of the joints, there are often exacerbations and remissions and the course is quite unpredictable. In the majority of instances, the disease "burns itself out" wherein the patient may be left with spinal stiffness and abnormal x-rays but there is no longer active inflammatory disease.

AS is often complicated by extraarticular manifestations. Eye involvement includes iritis and uveitis. Non-infectious prostatitis is sometimes present. A small proportion of patients with chronic AS get heart involvement manifested by aortic regurgitation. This can lead to severe heart failure. Amyloidosis (a disease in which there are abnormal protein deposits in various tissues of the body) is occasionally seen. There seems to be an association between AS and inflammatory bowel disease, both ulcerative colitis and Crohn's disease.

There are characteristic X-Ray findings. Sclerosis and narrowing of the sacroiliac joints bilaterally are almost always found. In the absence of sacroiliac involvement, the diagnosis of AS is difficult to establish. There may be calcification of the spinal ligaments and an ascending pattern of changes in the facet joints of the lumbar, dorsal and cervical spine. In the far advanced patient, there may be the so-called "bamboo spine" wherein the entire spine is calcified and fused into one unit.

Laboratory findings tend to be non-specific. They include an elevation of sedimentation rate and oftentimes a mild anemia. Autoantibodies such as RF and ANA are not found in any greater frequency than they are in the general population. Between 80 and 90% of patients with AS have the HLA-B27 antigen as opposed to about 8% of the general population. This finding does not have great diagnostic specificity but has theoretical importance in regard to the etiology and pathogenesis of AS.

The diagnosis of AS must be considered in any young man manifesting back pain, particularly when there are systemic features such as morning stiffness and easy fatigability. An important clue to the diagnosis is that sometimes pain is alleviated with activity as opposed to mechanical pain which gets worse with increasing activity.

The important findings on physical examination are loss of motion in the lumbar area, loss of chest expansion and limitation of motion of the cervical spine to rotation and extension. In the far advanced patient with a totally rigid "poker" spine with dorsal kyphosis and the forward-going head, the diagnosis is quite simple. However, in the early patient with only back pain and fatigue, a high index of suspicion is necessary. The diagnosis is best established by the finding of bilateral sclerosis of the sacroiliac joints.

There is no specific treatment for AS. The mainstays are non-steroidal antiinflammatory agents which are usually far more effective in AS than they are in RA. Particularly effective are indomethacin and phenylbutazone. However, because of the relatively serious toxicity attributed to phenylbutazone, it is rarely used. Corticosteroids are often ineffective and are not particularly helpful in the majority of patients. Furthermore their long-term use is associated with significant side effects. However, in the rare patient they may be of value. The "disease modifying agents" such as gold, penicillamine and azathioprine, which are often used in RA have no place in the management of AS.

The second mainstay of treatment in the patient with AS is physiotherapy. Most crucial is a good exercise program to insure maintenance of posture and preservation of motion. Also important are breathing exercises in which the patient is encouraged to use in the intercostal muscles for respiration. This is an attempt to preserve pulmonary function as the maintenance of the motion at the costovertebral joints will aid in respiration. One of the complications of late AS is loss of costovertebral motion and the patient becomes entirely dependent on diaphragmatic breathing. The therapist should train the patient in a home program and make sure that he maintains his exercise program on a daily basis.

Though some patients with AS go on to severe spinal deformity with progressive kyphosis and limitation of motion of their entire spine, the majority of patients do quite well in that the inflammatory disease remits. If the patient has maintained his posture, he will usually continue to function reasonably well. It is the impression of many investigators that the work record of patients with AS is quite excellent.

Reiter's Syndrome

Reiter's syndrome is an illness characterized by four major manifestations. These include arthritis, conjunctivitis, urethritis and muco-cutaneous abnormalities. The etiology and pathogenesis are unknown but in most instances it follows either a non-specific urethritis or Shigella dysentery. Any of the clinical manifestations may predominate in the individual patient. In the majority of instances, however, the most prominent and disabling problem relates to the joints. The patient will often complain of pain in his heels and feet with swelling of the small joints of the feet. There may be involvement of the upper extremities and generally asymmetric involvement of the major joints such as knees, wrists, ankles and elbows. It may be associated with extreme toxicity and high fever. In progressive cases there is often spinal involvement similar to that seen in AS. The patient may complain of severe prostatitis or urethritis or there may be some sterile pyuria and tenderness of the prostate gland. In the female, cystitis may occur and occasionally only trigonitis, which can be diagnosed on cystoscopy. Eye involvement is usually manifested by a conjunctivitis though, at times, the deeper layers of the eye can be involved. Muco-cutaneous lesions include a variety of findings including a scaly rash about the penis referred to as a circinate balanitis. There may be a thickening and keratinization at the bottom of the feet referred to as keratoderma blenorrhagicum which may resemble pustular psoriasis. Dystrophic nail changes may be found. At times the patient may have painless mouth ulcers of which he may not even be aware.

In the patient with the full-blown syndrome of Reiter's disease, recognition is usually easy, particularly if it occurs after some type of venereal infection. However, in some patients, the various manifestations appear at different times or may be very subtle. Thus the changes may have to be specifically sought after such as the mucous membrane lesions. Conjunctivitis may be extremely mild and the urethritis manifested only by a sterile pyuria.

Laboratory findings are non-specific. There may be a leukocytosis. Sedimentation rate is usually elevated and no abnormal autoantibodies are found. As with AS, the HLA-B27 antigen may be found in 70–90% of patients with Reiter's syndrome. Again this has no diagnostic specificity as 8% of Caucasian males also have this antigen. The x-ray findings usually do not occur until later in the course and they may include sacroiliac changes which may be asymmetrical and changes in the spine. In the peripheral joints there may be joint space narrowing, erosions and, at times, bony ankylosis.

The treatment of Reiter's syndrome is primarily symptomatic with use mainly of non-steroidal antiinflammatory agents. Also physiotherapy, range of motion exercise and rest are important to maintain range of motion of the joints. The conjunctivitis and skin lesions are treated topically. The urethritis normally does not require treatment, though bacteriological culture is necessary to make sure that it is not of infectious origin. Most physicians will treat the early patient with a course of a broad-spectrum antibiotic.

The clinical course of patients with Reiter's syndrome is variable. At one time it was believed that the majority of patients had a self-limited disease and the arthritis would just get better. However, as more patients are being studied, it is apparent that many patients with Reiter's syndrome go on to a deforming disease that remains either chronically or intermittently active.

In patients who have chronic progressive disease, there have been some literature reports on the use of immunosuppressive agents but this approach must still be regarded as being somewhat experimental and should be left to the specialist.

REACTIVE ARTHRITIS

Reactive arthritis refers to a type of arthritis that occurs after a specific infection but where the organism is not detectable in the involved joint. In that sense rheumatic fever which follows a streptococcal infection and yet is not due to a demonstrable streptococcal infection in the joint, and Reiter's syndrome which may follow infection with Shigella and yet is not Shigella arthritis, can be examples of this phenomenon. However, the diseases most commonly referred to as reactive arthritis follow infection with Salmonella and Yersinia. The resultant arthritis is a polyarthritis, usually affecting large joints and tends to be self-limited. Many patients who are positive for the HLA-B27 genome demonstrate features consistent with AS. There are no diagnostic serological or radiographic features. Treatment is usually with the use of non-steroidal antiinflammatory agents. Reactive arthritis following Yersinia is found far more frequently in the Scandinavian countries than in the United States.

Though not numerically common, this group of illnesses may serve as a model for the more common chronic inflammatory diseases in that in a genetically predisposed host, a specific infection can lead to a chronic non-infectious inflammatory disease. This may prove to be the mechanism by which an infectious agent may be the cause of RA.

PSORIATIC ARTHRITIS

Psoriatic arthritis refers to a type of inflammatory joint disease which occurs in patients who also suffer from psoriasis. Psoriasis is characterized by the development of thick scaly skin which can involve many different parts of the body. It has been recognized for many years that patients with psoriasis are predisposed to the development of different forms of inflammatory joint disease in higher incidence than in a population without psoriasis.

Several different types of arthritis are seen in patients with psoriasis. Typical AS and RA in such patients may represent the coincidence of two diseases. However, there is a distinctive type of arthritis which seems unique to patients with psoriasis which is usually called psoriatic arthritis.

Classic psoriatic arthritis is characterized by an asymmetrical synovitis with a predilection for the distal interphalangeal joints of the hands and feet. There is often involvement of other joints in an asymmetrical fashion. Rheumatoid factor and other serologic abnormalities are absent and the only laboratory abnormality is usually an elevated sedimentation rate. Subcutaneous nodules do not occur. Such patients do not manifest the multi-system complications often seen in RA such as vasculitis, lung disease or Sjogren's syndrome.

Many patients have nail changes associated with psoriasis such as stippling and hyperkeratosis. In most patients, psoriasis is present before the onset of arthritis though in some the onset is approximately coincident. In some patients, the arthritis may precede the psoriasis. This may lead to diagnostic confusion. Usually the psoriasis is clinically obvious but at other times may be subtle and the patient himself is unaware that he has psoriasis, believing that he has no skin disease or, possibly, "dandruff." The psoriasis must be actively sought for as part of the physical examination, particularly in the scalp, behind the ears, the periumbilical area, over the elbows, in the pubic area and the perianal region. Nail involvement must also be carefully sought.

Diagnosis is made on the basis of the clinical findings of asymmetric arthritis with particular involvement of the distal interphalangeal joints of the hands and feet in a patient with psoriasis who has no rheumatoid factor. The sedimentation rate may be elevated. As in other inflammatory diseases of the joints, x-ray changes do not occur until the inflammation has been present for a period of time. Though X-Ray changes are not specific, there are some characteristic features which help the clinician and radiologist distinguish psoriatic arthritis from other types of inflammatory joint disease. Synovial fluid examination reveals high white cell count but not the low complement or RF activity characteristic of rheumatoid arthritis.

The treatment of psoriatic arthritis in many ways resembles the treatment of rheumatoid arthritis. Aspirin and non-steroidal antiinflammatory agents form the pharmacological mainstay of treatment. Though not well documented by prospective double-blind studies the clinical impression is that the new non-steroidal antiinflammatory agents are much more effective in psoriatic arthritis than are aspirin and its derivatives. In my experience, meclofenamate is often particularly effective in this group of patients for pain relief.

If the disease becomes progressive with erosive, destructive changes, then "disease-modifying drugs" are often used. Gold is used most frequently. Penicillamine seems to have no place in the management of psoriatic arthritis and the use of the antimalarial agents is controversial. There has been some fear that the use of antimalarial agents may exacerbate psoriasis though one prospective study failed to verify this concern. Dermatologists have been using methotrexate for the treatment of severe psoriasis for many years. Oftentimes this treatment is extremely effectively for the arthritis as well. This is also true of azathioprine. The use of methotrexate and azathioprine in the treatment of psoriatic arthritis should be reserved to clinicians who have experienced with their use. In patients with severe disease, corticosteroids may play a role. Physical therapy with particular emphasis on range of motion exercises is as important in the treatment of the patient with psoriatic arthritis as it is with any patient who has chronic inflammatory joint diseases.

The prognosis of psoriatic arthritis tends to be quite good in most patients. Many remit spontaneously and retain an excellent functional status. Some patients, however, go on to severe crippling and deforming disease. In its worst form, psoriatic arthritis can result in what is called "arthritis mutilans" in which there is severe destructive joint change in the hands and feet resulting in severe deformity.

Both psoriasis and its associated arthritis are characterized by spontaneous exacerbations and remissions. However, the exacerbations and remissions of these two conditions do not necessarily coincide. Corticosteroids and methotrexate, are both useful for the treatment of both arthritis and psoriasis but, in most cases, treatment of the two conditions are independent of each other.

Since the etiology and pathogenesis of psoriasis and arthritis are unknown, the basis for their association remains unclear. It is not known whether the two are caused by the same agent or agents or by susceptibility factors common to both. There is no firm data indicating that genetic factors predispose patients to these conditions.

JUVENILE RHEUMATOID ARTHRITIS

The most common and most important rheumatic disease of children is juvenile rheumatoid arthritis (JRA). Its prevalence is unknown but there are estimates that there may be as many as 200,000 children with JRA in the United States; thus it is one of the major chronic diseases of children. Its etiology is totally unknown. Autoimmunity is probably an important pathogenetic factor, although the evidence for immunologic abnormalities is somewhat less convincing than in the adult variety. Serological abnormalities, when present, are not specific. Thus JRA is primarily a clinically defined entity, referring to a child under the age of 15 years with a persistently swollen joint lasting for at least six weeks, in whom other causes for synovitis can be excluded.

The disease can present in a number of different ways and a variety of classifications have been proposed. The classification most widely accepted recognizes three forms:

I. Systemic Onset JRA
II. Pauciarticular Onset JRA
III. Polyarticular Onset JRA

Other proposed classifications have suggested that factors such as histocompatibility antigens, serological abnormalities and x-ray changes be included in the classification. Much further work is required before an entirely satisfactory classification is accepted. This will depend on a better understanding of the etiological and pathogenetic factors.

The systemic onset group is often the most difficult to identify. These children typically present with systemic features such as fever, skin rash, lymphadenopathy, serositis, splenomegaly, and anemia. Joint signs and symptoms may not occur until later in the course of the disease. The diagnosis really cannot be made in the absence of arthritis; therefore the patients are often subjected to extensive diagnostic studies. For example, I have seen one child who had recurrent life-threatening pericardial effusion requiring repeated pericardiocentesis. The child also had fever and anemia for two years until the first inflamed joint appeared. Of the three forms, the pauciarticular is the most common. In this type the knees and ankles are the most commonly involved joints although virtually any joint can be affected. A skin rash occurs less frequently than in other forms. Systemic features are less common and prognosis seems to be better than in other forms. Most children with pauciarticular disease remit and achieve good functional status. Of particular interest is that young girls with pauciarticular disease and positive antinuclear antibodies seem to have a relatively high incidence of iridocyclitis. Though all children with JRA require monitoring for iridocyclitis, this group requires the most careful surveillance.

The polyarticular form most resembles the adult variety of rheumatoid arthritis. These children are most likely to have positive tests for rheumatoid factor in their sera and are more likely to go on to erosive and crippling disease.

The most common laboratory abnormality is an elevated erythrocyte sedimentation rate. Positive tests for RF are seen in only about 20% of cases. With special techniques for "hidden" RF a positive incidence as high as 80% has been reported. However, these techniques are difficult and do not lend themselves to routine clinical use. Positive tests for ANA are found in up to 60 to 70% of patients but this finding is too nonspecific to be of diagnostic value. Anemia is commonly found and is usually the anemia of chronic disease, with no other distinctive features. In the systemic onset group, leukocytosis often is seen. Antistreptolysin-0 titers often are elevated but probably is irrelevant to the disease and may reflect the high incidence of streptococcal disease in childhood. Agammaglobulinemia and hypogammaglobulinemia sometimes are seen in children with JRA and possibly define a separate subgroup.

As indicated previously, the diagnosis of JRA depends principally on the presence of persistent synovitis in the absence of other causes of joint disease.

Treatment is often complex and may involve a number of different disciplines. There are no known "cures" though many patients remit. Goals of treatment are relief of pain and preservation and restoration of joint function. In most patients, aspirin is the drug of choice for analgesic purposes and for its antiinflammatory effect. In addition to the usual problems of tinnitus, nausea and vomiting, and gastrointestinal upset, elevations of transaminase enzymes (SGOT and SGPT) are common in children with JRA treated with aspirin. Serious liver disease is very infrequent.

Of the large variety of nonsteroidal antiinflammatory agents other than aspirin that have been introduced, most have not been approved for use in children. The exceptions are tolmetin sodium and naproxen. Other agents such as sulindac, ibuprofen, fenoprofen, meclofenamate, and indomethacin are not currently approved for use in children in the United States.

Therapeutic exercises to maintain range of motion are prescribed early to prevent the flexion deformities that can occur very rapidly in children. Circular plaster and prolonged immunobilization is avoided whenever possible as these children are prone to develop ankyloses quite rapidly.

Patients are encouraged to stay within their peer group and live as normal and active a life as possible.

Corticosteroids are avoided whenever possible. Their use is reserved for life-threatening or severe systemic disease. In addition to the well-known adverse effects of corticosteroids, their use in children may result in serious growth disturbances.

Aspirin, tolmetin sodium, and even corticosteroids, though effective for analgesia and for reducing inflammation, do not alter the natural history nor prevent progression of the disease. Therefore, when JRA is chronic and progressive with resultant joint destruction, an attempt is made to induce a remission of the disease. The two major agents used for this purpose are gold and penicillamine. These are potentially toxic agents from which serious side effects can occur. These include nephritis, marrow suppression, stomatitis, dermatitis, and liver dysfunction. There are not much data available as to the use of the antimalarials in JRA. Cytostatic agents such as cyclophosphamide and azathioprine usually are avoided.

Orthopedic surgery is often of great help. The most common procedures done are hip replacement, soft tissue releases, and synovectomy. The last was much more popular a number of years ago when it was felt by some that it would prevent destructive joint disease. However, as more data have accumulated, it seems that synovectomy has only a temporary ameliorative effect on the course of the disease.

Children with JRA are monitored periodically by their ophthalmologists in an attempt to detect early iridocyclitis. The iridocyclitis of spondyloarthropathy seems to be more benign than the iridocyclitis of JRA.

The prognosis of JRA usually is good. Mortality seems to be related to the development of secondary amyloidosis with consequent renal failure. This problem seems to be far greater in Europe than in the United States. The reasons for this difference are not clear.

As of this date no etiological agent or agents have been identified, though many studies have been done in an attempt to find an infectious agent. JRA seems to be associated with hypogammaglobulinemia, IgA deficiency and other immunodeficiency syndromes.

In essence our understanding of JRA is on a descriptive clinical level. Treatment is supportive and empiric and, when necessary, corrective surgery is done. Fortunately most children tend to remit and have a good prognosis.

POLYMYALGIA RHEUMATICA

Polymyalgia rheumatic (PR) though strictly speaking not a 'rheumatoid variant' is included here. It is a clinical entity occurring mainly in the elderly. It is characterized by severe pain and stiffness of the shoulder and hip girdle associated with marked fatigue, morning stiffness and a gelling phenomenon. The onset is usually acute and the patients fairly rapidly evolve into a severe pain condition. In the classic form there is no evidence of joint swelling or redness though on occasion, joint swelling has been described in association with this syndrome. Some people believe that this and a type of rheumatoid arthritis in the elderly where there is diffuse swelling of the hands and negative RF may be the same disease. There is an association between PR and cranial arteritis though in the vast majority of patients with PR who do not have clinical evidence of cranial arteritis, do not seem to be at risk for the complications of cranial arteritis. On physical examination the patients are uncomfortable, often have tenderness of the muscles and have limitation of motion of the shoulders and hips. They have no joint swelling or rash. On laboratory examination they have a markedly elevated sedimentation rate but have no abnormal antibodies in their sera. There are no characteristic x-ray findings though the majority of patients with PR because of their age, have evidence of osteoarthritis of their cervical spine and in the lumbar spine. The patients respond dramatically to small doses of corticosteroid and often, within hours of starting the first dose of prednisone, are asymptomatic. If a patient has coincident headache, swollen, tender temporal arteries, visual disturbance or jaw claudication then they must be considered as at least potentially having cranial arteritis and the appropriate studies done and treated with higher doses of corticosteroids. All patients with PR must be made aware of the possible association with cranial arteritis and report to the doctor any severe headache or visual disturbance that may occur. Usually the patient's clinical response to small doses of steroids is dramatic and no specific physical therapy is necessary. However, if the illness has gone on for a period of time, there may be limitation of motion of the shoulders and hips and they may require range of motion exercises to restore normal mobility.

This illness is usually self-limited and most patients require treatment for about two years. In contrast to the arthritic diseases no residual joint impairment results.

There are many other diseases which are complicated by arthritic manifestations. Included among these is an acute arthritis associated with inflammatory bowel disease e.g. Crohn's disease and ulcerative colitis. Childhood leukemia may present with joint problems. Sickle cell anemia, and Whipples disease are other examples. Details are beyond the scope of this chapter but can be found in standard rheumatological texts.

SUGGESTED READINGS

Ankylosing Spondylitis edited by J.H. Moll, Churchill Livingstone, Edinburgh, 1980.

Spiera H. Polymyalgia Rheumatica in Rheumatic Diseases: Diagnosis and Management. Editor: W.D. Katz, M.D. J.B. Lippincott Company, Philadelphia, 1977.

Reiter's Syndrome (Reactive Arthritis) by Sharp, J.T. in Arthritis and Allied Conditions. Daniel McCarty, Editor, 10th Edition, Lea & Febiger, Philadelphia, 1983.

Juvenile Rheumatoid Arthritis. Calabro J.J., Chapter 51 in Hollander, Arthritis and Allied Conditions. Daniel McCarty, Editor, 10th Edition, Lea & Febiger, Philadelphia, 1983.

Psoriatic Arthritis: Michet, C.J. and Kahn, D.L. in Textbook of Rheumatology, Wm. N. Kelley, et al. eds. Philadelphia. W.B. Saunders, 3rd edition, 1989, ch. 61.

TABLE 9-1
SOME DISTINCTIONS BETWEEN ANKYLOSING SPONDYLITIS AND RHEUMATOID ARTHRITIS

	Ankylosing Spondylitis	*Rheumatoid Arthritis*
Sex Distribution	Overwhelmingly male	Mostly female
Peripheral Joints	25%	100%
Axial Skeleton	100%	Infrequent
Nodules	Extremely rare	20%
Eye Complications	Uveitis, iritis	Episcleritis
Urethritis	Common	Rare
Aortic Regurgitation	10%	Rare
Radiographic Changes	Sacroiliac sclerosis, and ligamentous calcifications	Erosions, joint space narrowing
Rheumatoid Factor	Same as general population	60–80%
Genetic	HLA-B27 90%	DR-4
Pharmacologic Treatment	NSAID's	NSAID's, corticosteroids, gold, Penicillamine antimalarials

CHAPTER 10

BONE DISEASE

K.T. Rajan, M.B., Ph.D.

INTRODUCTION

This chapter will review various facets of bone disease including natural history, pathophysiology, medical complications and therapy. The principal diseases relevant to rheumatology are: osteoporosis, osteomalacia and Paget's disease.

Bone disease is more common than generally recognized and probably affects a large percentage of the population all over the world. It spans the entire age spectrum, but is usually seen in middle and older age and occasionally in early adult life. A disease like osteoporosis (loss of mineral material) often goes unnoticed until it is picked up by chance at the onset of some acute condition like fracture or collapse of bone. Similarly Paget's disease of bone is often picked up during radiography for some other reason or after finding a raised serum alkaline phosphatase level in routine biochemical screening. There may be geographical variations; for instance, Paget's disease is often seen in European countries while osteomalacia is more often seen in the Third World countries where dietary factors and other illnesses may precipitate the condition. At one time it was considered that osteomalacia was uncommon in an affluent society, however, due to the growth of an aging population there is an increasing incidence of this condition.

Remodelling of Normal Adult Bone

Bone is a specialized form of connective tissue which is hard because of deposition of mineral substance within a soft organic matrix. It is composed predominantly of various calcium salts of which phosphate and carbonate are in abundance. In the normal adult skeleton there is hard compact cortical bone and spongy or cancellous bone, which is found in vertebra (back bone), flat bone (skull, pelvis) and ends of long bones. Most, if not all, bone disease may result from abnormalities in the remodelling process.

The principal bone cell types are the osteoblasts (bone laying), osteoclasts (bone resorbing) and osteocytes (the function of which is not clear). All play a role in the final outcome of the disease process. The sequence of events in remodelling of normal adult bone can been summarized as: activation, resorption, reversal, formation and mineralization. There is a particular time course for each of these phases which is influenced by hormones, Vitamin D, steroids, ions and mechanical stress. There is an equilibrium between resorption and formation—but the relationship changes with age and sex. Interpretation must take account whether transient or steady state conditions prevail. This is of importance when assessing the effect of treatment.

In general, the plasma level of alkaline phosphatase and urinary excretion of hydroxyproline usually reflect the osteoblastic and osteoclastic activity respectively. Skeletal balance results from a coupling between resorption and repair. In health, resorption is always followed by repair.

In summary then, osteoclastic bone destruction has a significant organization, with each area of osteoclastic activity being normally followed by proliferation of osteoblasts and new bone formation.

Biochemical Changes

Laboratory measurement of selected biochemical parameters may be of help in assessing physiological bone activity and in establishing diagnosis. Thus, activity of the enzyme alkaline phosphatase in serum is frequently elevated in osteomalacia and Paget's disease due to osteoblastic activity. Enhanced osteoclastic activity leading to collagen breakdown as seen in Paget's disease is marked by increased urinary concentration of the amino acids hydroxylysine and hydroxy proline. Measurement of serum ions, calcium and phosphate is of considerable utility. Typically they are decreased in osteomalacia. However, due to bone loss, urinary levels are increased. Measurement of Vitamin D and its metabolites may be helpful, as decreased levels are sometimes seen in osteoporosis and more commonly in osteomalacia.

Bone Examination

X-Ray changes may be pathognomonic of Paget's disease and are also useful in the detection of osteoporosis and osteomalacia. The whole skeleton may be involved or an isolated bone only may be affected. In many instances the patient may be asymptomatic and the abnormality detected during radiography for some other condition.

In the bone scan technique, radio-isotopes are administered intravenously and then after a given time, the whole skeleton is scanned using a gamma scintillating camera. For this purpose, labelled ethane-1-hydroxydiphosphonate fluorine-18-gallium (-67) and technetium (-99) have been found useful. If the bone turnover is high, the affected bone traps larger amounts of the radioisotope.

Bone biopsy may be useful in diagnosis of bone disease and also may indicate response to treatment. Quite often a co-existing disease like osteomalacia associated with Paget's disease, which may not have been suspected on clinical grounds, may be unmasked.

OSTEOPOROSIS

This disease is marked by reduction in the bone mass per unit volume with a normal chemical composition and histology. The biochemical parameters are also normal. This is by far the most common and important bone disease, and may be associated with a variety of other diseases.

Incidence

Osteoporosis is a condition of the elderly and is most common in women and more prevalent in Caucasians. In the U.S. clinical signs of osteoporosis have been reported in one-quarter of all white women at sometime in their lives. By the age of 85, about eight to ten percent of all women develop vertebral fractures. In the United Kingdom, 25 percent of all women over sixty show radiographic evidence of osteoporosis. The increased incidence of hip fractures in the elderly has been attributed to osteoporotic changes.

Aetiology

A small negative balance in calcium over a period of time can be cumulative and lead to osteoporosis. In "menopausal syndrome" oestrogen deficiency can result in excessive bone resorption while bone formation rate is normal. However, in many patients there is more than one factor contributing to the onset of the condition.

(1) Age: There is a decline in bone mass with aging and this is much more common in women than in men.

(2) Hormones, Vitamins and Drugs: The level of oestrogens falls at menopause and bone becomes more sensitive to the action of parathormone (PTH) and 1,25, dihydroxy cholecalciferol. Oestrone is produced by the adrenal glands and its levels falls during menopause. The sensitivity of bone to the resorbing action of PTH is increased as the oestrogen level falls. Deficiency of Vitamin D metabolism may be associated with decreased calcium absorption.

Levels of the hormone, calcitonin are usually 25 percent lower in women than in men, and it has been suggested this may be important in initiating osteoporosis in women. Furthermore, decreased calcitonin and response to calcium infusion has been reported in post-menopausal women with osteoporosis.

Corticosteroids and heparin have been associated with osteoporosis. This disease is often a feature of high dose steroid administration and is seen in Cushing's syndrome. In diabetes, insulin deficiency may impair bone formation. In thyrotoxicosis, where there is excessive thyroxine circulating, there is direct resorption of bone occurring, which could lead to fractures of long bones.

Immobilization often leads to osteoporosis and Sudeck's atrophy. Prolonged immobilization of fractures often results in local osteoporosis. It is considered that there is increased urinary excretion of calcium with bone loss more common in weight bearing bones.

(3) Dietary: There is no direct evidence that decreased calcium intake results in osteoporosis, though it is quite conceivable that low calcium intake or high calcium losses may be a significant risk factor. There is some evidence that increased protein intake may predispose to osteoporosis.

(4) Heredity: In a number of disorders, a family history may be useful in arriving at a possible diagnosis. Osteogenesis imperfecta, homocystinuria, Marfan's syndrome, Menkes syndrome, Ehlers-Danlos syndrome, Werner-Rothmund syndrome, all may be associated with osteoporosis.

(5) Other Factors: In races where women continue to work till old age, osteoporosis is uncommon. In these situations there may be adequate exposure to sunlight, exercise and, as a consequence, increased dietary absorption of calcium. The bone disease, multiple myeloma is also associated with osteoporosis.

Diagnosis

Symptoms are usually due to bone collapse and fracture commonest in the spine, and the dorsal and upper lumbar regions. It is not unusual for patients to fracture their femurs after a trivial fall. Wedging of the vertebra results in angulation of the back. Loss in height can be marked. The rib cage gets crowded. Bone histology is of limited value, though this may help in excluding Paget's disease or osteomalacia. Diagnosis of osteoporosis is primarily by exclusion. There are no biochemical abnormalities except in immobilized patients who may have a raised calcium.

Treatment

Improvement can be aided by adequate nutrition and mobility. Physiotherapy can preserve bone mass. Increased mobility and strengthening the muscles can encourage patients to continue to lead active lives. Supportive treatment by providing spinal corsets and analgesics may be helpful. In the elderly, hydrotherapy may encourage early mobilization especially following fractures of femur or vertebral collapse.

It has been suggested that 1.2 g of calcium taken orally daily (e.g., in a quart of milk) may be advisable. Vitamin D may help where oral intake is low. Daily supplements up to 1,000 I.U. is reasonable. If malabsorption exists then larger doses up to 10,000 I.U. daily may be indicated. Salmon calcitonin administered with a calcium supplement of 1.2 g per day may produce an increase in calcium absorption and bone mass.

Anabolic steroids and androgens are effective in hypergonadal males. They may also help in reducing bone resorption.

It has been noted that prevalence of osteoporosis is much less in areas with high fluoride intake in the water. Sodium fluoride with calcium supplementation is often helpful.

There is considerable evidence that oestrogen therapy administered within the first year following menopause can significantly reduce bone loss and retard osteoporosis. However, in later years the efficacy of oestrogen replacement remains unproven. When oestrogen are used, the increased risk of uterine cancer must be considered.

Osteoporosis may be easier to prevent than treat. The general principles of prevention include a well-balanced diet with adequate calcium intake, particularly in the younger years. Regular weight bearing exercise is helpful. Smoking should be avoided. In women with early menopause, either natural or surgical oestrogen replacement should be considered. Osteoporosis in many cases is preventable and treatable. In those with this disease, there may be long periods of remission and it may be possible to prevent fracture by energetic mobilization of the patients. Health education is vitally important.

OSTEOMALACIA

The essential feature of this disease is delayed mineralization of cartilage and bone. If the condition presents during the periods of growth affecting the epiphyses, then it is termed rickets; whereas the term, osteomalacia is used in the adult where the epiphyses is fused.

Aetiology

Causes of this disease may be classified as follows:

(1) Vitamin D deficiency caused by
   - (a) Inadequate exposure to the sun
   - (b) Inadequate intake, which may be either true dietary deficiency or malabsorption, i.e., as in sprue, Crohn's disease and surgical removal of bowel.

(2) Vitamin D resistant osteomalacia is a rare form of rickets which responds only to very high doses of Vitamin D.
(3) Renal tubular defects are characterized by impaired urinary acidification leading to renal stone formation as well as osteomalacia. In the rare condition of Fanconi's syndrome where there is urinary loss of calcium or phosphate, osteomalacia may occur.
(4) Renal osteodystrophy: In uremic bone disease of long duration, osteomalacia and rickets can occur, depending on the age of onset of the disease.
(5) Drug-Induced osteomalacia: There are many drugs which may induce this disease when used for prolonged periods. These drugs include: diphosphonates, sodium fluoride, phenobarbitone and diphenyl hydantoin. Excessive alcohol intake has also been associated with osteomalacia.
(6) Calcium deficiency may be due to dietary deficiency. Usually the elderly are at risk. A similar condition is seen in immigrants, especially in the United Kingdom, where clothing habits together with the indoor existence of the female reduces the rate of synthesis of Vitamin D.

Diagnosis

Pain

The patient may complain of generalized bone pain especially in long bones or may present with fractures. The pain is usually on weight-bearing and hip pain due to pseudo-fractures, is common. Certain movements may be painful, especially rising from the sitting position or negotiating stairs. Often there is sudden onset of symptoms not associated with obvious injury. Manual compression of the rib cage, legs or pelvis produces pain. In a child, bow legs or known knees may be noticeable. There may be recession of the ribs at the attachment of the diaphragm and enlargement of costal cartilages. Even the skull may be very thin and soft. When calcium levels go down significantly, tetany may result. It is uncommon to see rickets in the western countries. However, in the East and Far Eastern countries, there is still a high incidence of this condition.

Muscular pain and weakness are frequently seen. The reflexes are diminished resulting from myopathy due to Vitamin D deficiency. The gait is frequently waddling due to proximal weakness.

Biochemical Changes

Serum calcium levels tend to be low, but are more variable if secondary hyperparathyroidism is present. Vitamin D levels are typically reduced and in consequence, phosphate levels are also low.

The product of calcium and phosphate concentration, (Ca) x (P), is reduced, and as a consequence, there may be decreased mineralization. It is important to note that in children, plasma phosphate levels tend to be higher. However, the plasma calcium x phosphate product is generally below 30 in children with rickets and below 25 in adults with osteomalacia.

Levels of alkaline phosphatase are usually raised as is the concentration of parathormone. Absorption of calcium and phosphate are usually reduced. Bone turnover is increased and there may be increased collagen in urine as determined by measuring 24-hour hydroxyproline levels.

Radiological Changes

In rickets, the epiphyseal line disappears. In long bones, cartilage widens and the distal end of the bone becomes cupped and ragged. Ossification centers may be absent and there may be fractures. The pathogenic features of osteomalacia consist of symmetrical pseudo-fractures of the pelvis and long bones. In the absence of treatment they may be visible for months. It has been suggested that these occur in places which represent the sites of entry of nutrient arteries supplying the bones. One of the commonest features especially in children, is bending of bones. There may be generalized loss of cortical bone and occasionally subperiosteal resorption of the phalanges, as a consequence of secondary hyperparathyroidism. The X-Ray of the spine is unlike that in osteoporosis. The density of the spine is often normal and this may be due to an increase in the total amount of trabecular bone and as a consequence of secondary hyperparathyroidism.

The density of the spine is often normal and this may be due to an increase in the total amount of trabecular bone and as a consequence, the mineral content of the spine may actually be greater than normal.

Treatment

Primary deficiency can be easily corrected by administration of Vitamin D, e.g., ergocalciferol. Patients lacking exposure to sunlight or those with dietary deficiency due to religious or other reasons may present problems.

In gluten-induced malabsorption enteropathy, a gluten free diet is needed. However, initially parenteral calciferol may be necessary. Obviously in those cases where osteomalacia is alcohol or drug induced, the removal of the offending substance is desirable.

In general, rickets and osteomalacia are easily identifiable and treatable conditions. Biochemical and radiological investigations help in diagnosis and in monitoring response to treatment.

PAGET'S DISEASE

This is a slow progressing bone disorder affecting patients in their middle life and predominantly affecting the skull and long bones of the lower extremity. Sir James Paget presented a series of five cases illustrating the above features to the Medical and Chirurgical Society of London in 1877, which was published in the Transactions. In the last decade considerable information regarding the disease has been gathered.

Incidence

The overall incidence is about four percent and rises progressively to eleven percent in the seventh decade. Men are slightly more commonly affected than women in a ratio of 4:3.

Familial clustering has been reported in several instances. Up to 20% of patients have a family history of the disease. Paget's disease is more common in the United Kingdom, the United States, New Zealand, Australia, France and Germany. It is rare in Japan, the Indian subcontinent, Middle East and Africa. In North America, the disease is equally common among both black and white populations. Although it is uncommon among the North American Indians, there are prehistoric skeletons discovered in Wisconsin and the Illinois River Valley region showing the effect of Paget's Disease. A parietal bone found in an ancient Egyptian tomb is thought to have been affected. It has been suggested that Beethoven suffered from the disease, which was ultimately responsible for the deafness in his later life.

Aetiology

There have been numerous hypotheses, but none of these have been proven or commonly accepted. Some believe that the disease may be due to a slow virus infection. Evidence in favor has been demonstrated by electron microscopy. Sustained viral antibody titres against measles virus have been reported in a few patients. However, no virus has been isolated.

Sarcomatous change is thirty times more frequent in patients with Paget's disease over the age of 40. It has therefore been suggested that the disease is neoplastic in origin. However, patients usually live to a ripe old age and the disease remains localized and is not invasive.

The blood supply to the bone is significantly increased and following response to treatment the vascularity diminishes. It is likely to be a consequence rather than the cause of the disease.

As calcitonin administration diminishes the activity of the disease, a deficiency of this hormone has been postulated as the cause of the disease. However, blood calcitonin concentration are within normal range in patients affected with the disease.

Diagnosis

The majority of patients are asymptomatic and are discovered accidentally when radiography is being carried out for other purposes. Occasionally a raised alkaline phosphatase level found during biochemical screening alerts one to the possibility of the disease. Many patients may present with a complication of the disorder. Lethargy and fatigue may be presenting symptoms in severe disease. Pain is a common presenting symptom. This is seen mainly in weight bearing bones. Pain is often worse in bed at night when the limbs feel warm due to the increased blood flow.

Deformity

Long bones may be large and deformed especially if the tibia or femur are affected. Skull deformity is common, the patient complaining of having to buy different sizes of hats due to progressive increase in the size of the skull vault. Progressive loss of hearing, vision, hemifacial spasm and trigeminal neuralgia may result over a period of time. Vertebral involvement with collapsed vertebra may lead to back pain especially when the lumbar vertebra are involved. Facial deformities may rarely result in ocular problems. More often replacement of dentures may be required. Shortness of breath and chest pain due to left ventricular hypertrophy and ischaemia may be evident.

Biochemical Changes

In Paget's disease, the alkaline phosphatase is usually raised, acid phosphatase may also be elevated. Due to the increased turnover of nucleic acid, uric acid is often raised. Twenty-four hour urinary hydroxyproline measurements give a good index of the activity of osteoclasts. Hydroxylysine levels are also elevated and this may be a more accurate index of collagen degradation. Estimation of serum and urine calcium and phosphate levels are not useful.

Bone Studies

The X-Ray changes are pathognomonic of the disease. The skull is thickened with typical "cotton wool" appearance. Areas of new bone formation can be seen. The pelvis shows enlargement of the affected bone with coarsened trabecular pattern and irregular patchy sclerosis. The long bones may be enlarged and deformed, most commonly, the tibia and femur, although almost any bone may be affected.

Skeletal scan with bone seeking radioisotopes have been used, e.g., labelled ethane 1-hydroxy-diphosphonate, labelled with radio-technetium or gallium. An increased uptake of the labelled material is seen, and is a more accurate method of assessing the activity of the disease. Response to treatment can be monitored in this way.

Bone biopsy is rarely necessary. If needed, it can be carried out under a local anesthetic usually from the iliace bone. Hyperactive osteoclasts and osteoblasts with excessive bone resorption paralleled by excessive bone formation is evident.

Treatment

Paget's disease is a common disease. It is asymptomatic in the majority of patients. When there is bone pain, effective treatment is available and the long-term results are encouraging.

Calcitonin inhibits bone resorption by inhabiting overactive osteoclasts. Porcine or salmon calcitonin are normally used but can be substituted by synthetic human calcitonin if there are hypersensitivity reactions. There is a high incidence of antibody formation, but this rarely causes resistance to treatment. Relief of pain usually begins two to six weeks after starting treatment. Maintenance therapy may be necessary for up to twelve months.

Diphosphonates inhibit bone resorption and mineralization by binding crystals and inhibiting their growth and dissolution. Treatment is maintained for at least six months, with periodic monitoring of calcium and alkaline phosphatase. The possibility of osteomalacia developing during treatment should be considered. At times, combinations of calcitonin and diphosphonate are employed.

Cytotoxic agents such as Mithramycin and actinomycin D are rarely used. Analgesics are an important adjunct of treatment. Indomethacin is often quite helpful.

Surgical therapy is occasionally employed particularly when osteoarthritis of the hip is present. Osteotomy may correct bone deformity.

SUGGESTED READINGS

Caplan, A.L. Bone Development and Repair. Bioessays 6:171–175, 1987.

Handy, R.C. *Paget's Disease of Bone: Assessment and Management,* Praeger Publishers, London, 1981.

Kelly, V.N.; Harris, E.D.; Ruddy S.; and Sledge, C.B. (Eds.) *Textbook of Rheumatology.* W.B. Saunders Company, Philadelphia, 3rd edition, 1989. Metabolic Bone Disease. Ch. 98, Hahn T.J.

Nordin, B.E.C. *Metabolic Bone and Stone Disease.* Churchill Livingstone, Edinburgh, 1973.

Osdoby, P.; Krukowski, M.; Oursler, M.J.; and Salino-Hugg, T. The Origin and Development of Osteoclasts. *Bioessays* 7:30–34, 1987.

Resnick, D. and Niwayama, G. *Diagnosis of Bone and Joint Disorders,* Vol. 4 Sec. XIII, Metabolic Disease, W.B. Saunders, Publishers. Philadelphia, 1987.

Stanbury, S.W.P., Torkington, G.A., Lunar, D.H., Adams, Praenic, de Silva and Taylor, C.N. Asian Rickets and Osteomalacia: Patterns of Parathyroid Response in Vitamin D Deficiency. Proceedings of Nutrition Society 34, 777, 1975.

CHAPTER 11

LOCAL MUSCULOSKELETAL CONDITIONS (Bursitis, Tendinitis, Trauma and Sports Injuries)

Burton L. Berson, M.D.

Injuries to joints and soft tissues, as well as inflammatory conditions are relatively common in our health-oriented, sports-minded society. Problems which we encounter vary according to the nature of the individual (age, sex, physical status), the sport (contact, non-contact, endurance), the mechanism of injury or overuse pattern, equipment and other variables. Injuries are classified as acute or chronic. Acute injuries are treated in the first 48 to 72 hours by the "RICE" regimen of *R*est, *I*ce, *C*ompression and *E*levation. Chronic conditions require modification of activity, medical or physical therapy to alleviate the cause of the problem, then rehabilitation to restore the part to its prior normal functional state. The entire limb and person must be thoroughly rehabilitated.

The stability of joints varies according to the anatomical and functional needs. Ligaments, which are cord-like thickenings of the joint capsule made up of dense collagen fibers running in the same direction and possessing great tensile strength and poor vascularity, are the prime static stabilizers. Ligamentous support for the shoulder is relatively weak because of the great mobility required for motion. Stability is thereby sacrificed and dislocations are more common than in any other major joint. Conversely, the hip joint provides necessary stability for the torso and must have powerful ligamentous protection, making dislocation extremely rare. Ankle ligaments are the most frequently sprained in athletics, and knee ligaments the most seriously injured.

Muscles and tendons which cross the joint afford dynamic stability and protection, while providing motion by contraction and relaxation. Tendons are made up of dense collagenous tissue with poor vascularity, and often an overlying sheath. Muscle on the other hand has good vascularity and healing powers and consists of contractile (muscle fiber) and non-contractile (connective tissue) elements.

Bursa are clefts in the connective tissue between muscles, tendons, ligaments and bones. They are closed sacs lined by synovium similar to a joint, and may in some cases be continuous with a joint through an opening (e.g. the popliteal bursa of the knee joint). They facilitate the gliding of muscles or tendons over bony or ligamentous prominences. Bursae, because they are subjected to repetitive movement and frictional irritation, are frequent sites for inflammation (bursitis), and degenerative changes leading to calcification within the sac, both of which may result in pain and loss of motion.

TENOSYNOVITIS, TENDINITIS AND BURSITIS

Tenosynovitis is inflammation of the synovium surrounding a tendon. It is usually due to strain from overuse, direct blow or infection. The inflammatory reaction in the normally avascular synovium with oversecretion of synovial fluid and fibrin causes "sticky" adhesions between the tendon and its surroundings which may result in an adhesive tenosynovitis in the chronic stage, as is seen in late stages of bicipital tenosynovitis and frozen shoulder. Constrictive tenosynovitis caused by thickening of the walls of the tendon sheath with narrowing of its lumen so that the tendons cannot slide through it, is the other sequela of tenosynovitis. This results in a snapping or triggering seen most commonly in the flexor tendons to the fingers at the level of the distal palm.

Tenosynovitis in the acute state can be diagnosed by pain on function and crepitation caused by adherence of the tendon to the synovium. Treatment is rest, local heat, or ice if very recent, and anti-inflammatory medication with judicious steroid injections if necessary. The chronic problems pose more therapeutic difficulties, and require diligence in a physiotherapeutic regimen, to surgical intervention.

Tendinitis and bursitis occur frequently about the shoulder. Due to the bony anatomy of the shoulder girdle, impingement on soft tissues resulting in rotator cuff tears and inflammation occur. The rotator cuff, especially the supraspinatus tendon which has been shown to have a poor blood supply at this region, is impinged between the acromion and the greater tuberosity of the humerus when the arm is elevated or abducted as in throwing, tennis service, or swimming. The subacromial or subdeltoid bursa which is superficial to the rotator cuff may become inflamed, fluid-filled due to synovial secretion, and degeneration with calcium formation may develop. The biceps tendon at the shoulder is avascular, similar to the supraspinatus tendon and is subject to involvement in this condition. The chronic irritation leads to an inflammatory response or tendinitis and microscopic tears with repeated trauma over time which progresses to full-thickness rotator cuff tears and degenerative bony changes.

Active and passive range of motion must be assessed. With a full-thickness rupture of the rotator cuff, in addition to abductor weakness there is a restricted range of active shoulder motion with maintenance of good passive mobility. This is in contrast to chronic bicipital tenosynovitis resulting in an adhesive capsulitis or frozen shoulder in which both active and passive range of motion is restricted. Modification of the motion in the athletic activity that contributed to the impingement syndrome will be necessary once the inflammatory reaction is resolved and the motion and strength restored. In far-advanced cases, surgery in the form of a limited resection of the anterior acromion and repair of the rotator cuff may be necessary.

Achilles tendinitis is another example of attritional changes developing in a poorly vascularized tendon subjected to repetitive overuse. The development of microtears and inflammation in a degenerative tendon in middle-aged athletes may result in a complete Achilles' tendon rupture. This end-stage may be prevented by corrective measures instituted earlier in the form of protection with a heel lift or cast, and physiotherapy to strengthen and stretch the involved tendon.

Another very common form of tendinitis is so-called "tennis elbow" or lateral humeral epicondylitis. This is another overuse syndrome which occurs at some time or other to one-third of tennis players; is directly related to age and frequency of play and is usually due to an improper backhand. The pathologic anatomy appears to be development of microscopic tears in the common wrist extensor tendons at the elbow due to repetitive overuse and improper stroke execution. A chronic inflammatory response then develops within these micro-tears that resembles granulation tissue and exacerbates tissue separation if not successfully treated.

Most patients with lateral epicondylitis have never touched a tennis racket. Activities of daily living, such as dish-washing, turning door knobs, typing, and carpentry to name just a few can produce the same pathologic changes of tennis elbow. Tenderness to palpation is present over the lateral epicondyle and pain is increased by fist-clenching and extension of the wrist against resistance. Passive stretching of the extensor muscle origin by forced pronation of the forearm with flexion of the wrist is an important diagnostic test.

Treatment of the acute tennis elbow is much more successful than that of the chronic condition. Activities that cause pain should be eliminated and the extremity rested. The use of a wrist splint to prevent excessive wrist motion in writing, typing, and other daily activities may be helpful. Stretching exercises are important to prevent as well as treat the acute and chronic condition. Ice and anti-inflammatory agents are helpful in reducing local symptoms. Hydrocortisone injections should be reserved for refractory cases and used judiciously. Multiple injections can lead to tendon atrophy and rupture.

Healing is complete when there is no pain with full return of motion, strength and endurance. Prevention of recurrence requires avoiding the overload forces which occur with the improper tennis stroke, especially the backhand. Muscle-strengthening exercises for the entire extremity are necessary. A two-handed backhand almost guarantees against developing a tennis elbow.

Some bursae are situated over bony prominences and become irritated as a result of direct pressure. The olecranon bursa of the elbow may become distended due to pressure on the point of the elbow. Though initially a traumatic inflammation, secondary infection may develop because of its superficial location. This requires aspiration, antibiotics, and drainage. Gout may also cause an olecranon bursitis. Prepatellar bursitis often referred to as housemaid's knee, due to localized swelling in the subcutaneous prepatellar bursa, occurs due to the pressure phenomena of constant kneeling. If sepsis has been ruled out by a negative culture, the treatment of the recurrence after the initial aspiration, is with repeat aspiration and steroid instillation with compression bandages. Multiple symptomatic recurrences in athletically-active people may necessitate surgical excision.

Popliteal bursa or Baker's cyst which develops in the back of the knee is generally secondary to intra-articular pathology in the knee which causes a swelling or synovitis. The primary cause might be an inflammatory synovitis due to rheumatoid or psoriatic arthritis, or due to an internal derangement such as a torn meniscus. Treatment then becomes one aimed at curing the primary pathology by medication or synovectomy if inflammatory, or by conventional or arthroscopic surgery if it is mechanical. An arthrogram may be helpful in establishing the diagnosis of popliteal cyst with associated intra-articular pathology such as a torn meniscus.

Common Knee Injuries

The knee sustains the most frequent major injuries of any joint in athletic trauma. An early accurate diagnosis and prompt management are essential in restoring an injured knee to its pre-injury level as rapidly as possible. The knee joint is smoothly integrated, moving in flexion and extension with rotation occurring in the flexed knee only. The powerful quadriceps and hamstring muscles control the motion and dynamic stability. The static stability and coordinated function is controlled by the collateral ligaments on either side, the cruciate ligaments within the joint and the meniscal cartilages separating the femur from the tibia. An injury to any one or more of these important units will upset the smooth integrated function, increasing the stress on the other structures, resulting in uncoordinated or restricted motion, instability or giving-out, swelling and weakness.

The most common athletic injury to the knee is a ligament sprain. Sprains are graded as mild (first degree), moderate (second degree), and severe (third degree) depending on the amount of damage to the ligament fibers. Mild to moderate sprains in which there is no loss of continuity of the ligament will heal with conservative treatment of protection with a cast or brace, then rehabilitation. The mechanism of healing involves an inflammatory response which is subsequently converted to collagenous tissue. A severe or complete ligamentous rupture (third degree) in which there is no continuity of the ligament, results in an unstable joint which usually requires surgical repair as soon as possible. Diagnosis of acute ligamentous rupture immediately after a clipping injury in football or a twisting fall in skiing may be obvious. Instability of the knee may be present in several planes including antero-posterior, medio-lateral and rotatory. Several hours or days after the injury however, swelling, muscle spasm and pain may make accurate assessment of knee stability difficult due to inability to stress the ligaments. In such a case, assuming a high index of suspicion of major ligament rupture by an experienced knee surgeon, examination under anesthesia in the hospital operating room, possible arthroscopy and immediate surgery is justified. With a lower index of suspicion in an athlete, or a severe injury in a sedentary or older individual, a more conservative approach is the rule.

The medial collateral ligament is the most commonly injured ligament due to forceful sideways or rotatory thrust, or contact type of injury. As the rotatory force of the injury continues, the anterior cruciate ligament is ruptured and when the medial meniscus is also torn with further continuation of the stress, the "unhappy triad" results, with an unstable knee. An audible pop with rapid accumulation of blood in the joint are ominous signs of a severe ligamentous injury.

Serious knee injuries are not always the result of contact sports or falls in skiing. Recently we have recognized how frequently ligamentous and meniscal injuries can occur by mechanism of sudden deceleration, especially when combined with internal rotation in the extended knee as when coming down with a rebound in basketball or in gymnastics. The resultant rupture of the anterior cruciate ligament, either isolated or with an associated torn meniscus is more subtle and difficult to diagnose. Testing for ligamentous instability requires experience to determine which knee is unstable and possibly a candidate for surgery.

Usually associated with a ligamentous injury to the knee is a tear of the meniscus or semilunar cartilage. The medial meniscus is injured at least three times more often than the lateral meniscus because it is less mobile. The menisci are very important to the normal function of the knee. In addition to their well-known function as shock-absorbers and synovial fluid distributors, they are stabilizers and weight-bearing structures. The peripheral third of the meniscus has a blood supply from the capsule, therefore, a peripheral detachment or tear of the meniscus in the outer one-third has the potential for healing. A tear in the inner two-thirds of the avascular body of the meniscus, however, as usually occurs in the typical longitudinal "bucket-handle" tear in athletes, does not have the potential for healing because of a lack of blood supply. The mobile fragment of the torn meniscus can slip in and out of the joint and cause "locking" or inability to extend the knee. This is the so-called "trick knee." When it frequently recurs, the articular cartilage becomes eroded and traumatic arthritis develops.

Arthroscopy and arthroscopic surgery have dramatically changed the treatment of mechanical problems of the knee, especially meniscal tears. By means of tiny punctures in the skin instead of large incisions as in conventional surgery, the torn mobile meniscal fragments can be removed with tiny instruments while viewing the procedure on a T. V. monitor via a camera attached to the arthroscope which is placed in the knee joint. A peripheral tear of the meniscus can be sutured to the capsule under arthroscopic control, and there is some very promising experimental work to repair and reconstruct anterior cruciate ligament ruptures, recent and old, via arthroscopic surgery through these tiny incisions.

The importance of the menisci in knee function has been increasingly recognized in recent years. Arthroscopic surgery removes only the damaged portion of the meniscus, preserving the intact, stable rim. This preserves the stabilizing and weight-bearing function of the peripheral rim. Formerly we removed the entire meniscus through a relatively large incision resulting in a lengthy rehabilitation and the frequent development of degenerative arthritis over a period of years. Arthroscopic surgery has reduced the rehabilitation dramatically, allowing immediate ambulation with rapid return to work and sports, and hopefully will reduce the incidence of degenerative arthritic changes in the future.

Although arthroscopic surgery is a proven modality on an out-patient basis for much knee and other joint surgery, most knee surgeons still prefer open procedures for repair and reconstruction of ligament ruptures, if surgery is to be performed. The disability resulting from the anterior cruciate-deficient knee is that of "buckling" or "giving-out." Many of these injuries can be improved by an intensive rehabilitation program concentrating especially on the hamstring muscles and utilizing isokinetic and isotonic methods, as well as by bracing. Others may have to modify their athletic activities which cause the buckling, or undergo reconstructive surgery. Reconstructive surgery is a technically-demanding procedure, usually confined to athletically-active and well-motivated patients who have not improved with conservative treatment. Rehabilitation is prolonged and may last up to one year prior to return to competitive sports. The results in properly selected patients have been good.

Chondromalacia patella is an ill-defined entity referring to anterior knee pain due to patellar cartilage softening (malacia) and patella-femoral incongruity usually secondary to other knee problems such as ligament or meniscal derangements, patella malalignment, subluxation or dislocation. Pain on prolonged sitting and stair-climbing with patella-femoral tenderness and crepitus are characteristic of chondromalacia.

Dislocation of the patella occurs in younger athletes, frequently girls. The history is one of sudden deceleration or change in direction with the knee flexed. The patella dislocates laterally and usually snaps back into place when the knee is extended. By the time the patient reaches the Emergency Room, X-Rays are normal and the only findings are a swollen, anteriorly-tender knee. Occasionally a loose body may appear on X-Ray due to the shearing force as the patella slides over the lateral femoral condyle. If a dislocated patella is not suspected and treated with immobilization, recurrent dislocation may occur with subsequent degenerative changes of the articular cartilage of the patella. Conservative therapy consists of isometric quadriceps progressive resistance exercises and patella-control braces to prevent excessive lateral patellar mobility. Surgery, either arthroscopic or conventional is necessary if there is no response to conservative treatment over a prolonged period of time.

Adolescent knee problems are fairly common in the athletically-active youngster due to repetitive stress on the rapid and unequal growth of bone and soft tissue in this area. "Jumper's knee" is a traumatic inflammatory condition of the extensor mechanism due to forceful constant contractions as in running and jumping in these rapidly growing children. There may be a slight malalignment of the patella, and the undersurface may become malacic. There may be microtears with granulation tissue on the undersurface of the quadriceps or patellar tendons due to inflammation and attempt at repair. Basketball is the frequent cause of the problem. Treatment varies from restriction of activity, support and resistance exercises to surgical reconstruction depending on the extent and duration of symptoms.

Osgood-Schlatter's disease is a self-limited inflammation of the patellar tendon insertion into the tibial tubercle, or an "epiphysitis." It is intermittently painful and occasionally causes a prominence at the tibial tubercle. Symptoms usually subside with the termination of growth. Treatment for the occasional acute episode consists of lowering the activity level until the child is asymptomatic.

Dislocations and Separations

Dislocation is the end-result of complete ligament rupture. The shoulder is the most frequent major joint to be dislocated, the humeral head dislocating anteriorly in 98% of cases. The relatively weak ligamentous support allowing the great mobility accounts for the high-frequency of dislocation. The mechanism of injury initially may be direct trauma which tears the anterior ligaments and capsule. Subsequent dislocations result from the arm being forced into the abducted, externally-rotated position as in swimming, cocking the arm back in throwing, or arm-tackling in football. In this position, the large humeral head is levered anteriorly out of the shallow glenoid socket. Once dislocated, especially in the young adult, the incidence of recurrent dislocations is very high, even if the initial dislocation was promptly reduced and immobilized. Reduction is usually best accomplished by direct traction, or by hanging a weight or bucket of water over the suspended forearm of the prone patient. Immobilization of the acute dislocation should be for three to four weeks. After several recurrences, which usually do not respond to a conservative muscle strengthening physiotherapy program, surgical intervention is necessary. Surgery may limit external rotation of the shoulder or reconstruct the anterior supporting structures.

Shoulder dislocation should be distinguished from shoulder separation which is in reality a sprain of the acromioclavicular joint. The mechanism of injury is usually a fall on the point of the shoulder which injures the ligaments spanning the acromioclavicular joint in the mild to moderate sprains. As the force continues, the stronger coraco-clavicular ligaments are ruptured resulting in a third degree sprain where the clavicle rides upward causing a prominence of the outer end of the shoulder. Although the clavicle can be pushed down into place, maintenance of the reduction is difficult. Fortunately, however, little disability other than the cosmetic bump results from this injury, and although opinion is divided, surgery for the acute injury is often not justified. A short period of immobilization followed by intensive rehabilitation to regain motion and strength usually gives a good functional result. Should pain, weakness or limitation of motion due to traumatic arthritis develop, surgery is usually quite successful in the chronic case.

Ankle Sprains

The most common ligament sprain of a major joint involves the ankle, the mechanism of injury being plantar flexion, internal rotation and inversion. The sprains are classified as first, second and third degree depending on the severity as demonstrated by stress testing with an anterior drawer maneuver and inversion instability. Osteochondral fractures may occur on the articular surfaces of the tibia and talus and result in loose bodies and detached or semi-attached fragments.

With the inversion stress, the anterior talo-fibular ligament is torn. As the force continues, the calcaneo-fibular or middle ligament is involved, thus resulting in a double ligament tear. If there is a third degree sprain or rupture of both ligaments, an unstable ankle joint results, and in the chronic case accounts for the so-called "weak ankle" or frequent "giving out" syndrome especially on uneven ground. In extreme cases, the posterior talo-fibular ligament is injured.

Most ankle sprains are of the first and second degree, with only a partial tear of the ligaments and respond to a short period of immobilization followed by strengthening exercises concentrating especially on the peroneal muscles and proprioceptive feedback response techniques. Third degree sprains, as demonstrated by positive inversion stress x-rays and a positive anterior drawer sign, should be treated with six weeks of cast immobilization followed by intensive rehabilitation, although there are orthopaedic surgeons who would opt for primary surgical repair of the ruptured ligaments. The chronically unstable ankle not responsive to conservative measures in an athletic individual does well with surgery which entails reconstructing a lateral ligament out of the peroneus brevis tendon.

Muscle and Tendon Strains

Strains are defined as injuries to the muscle-tendon unit. Mild (first degree), moderate (second degree) and severe or complete rupture (third degree) are analogous to the grading of ligament injuries. In general, muscle strains heal with conservative treatment, due to the good vascularity. Tendon ruptures, however, often require surgical repair, as the ends of the ruptured tissue retract and a gap develops. The patella and quadriceps tendon in the lower extremity as well as the rotator cuff, biceps tendon and pectoralis major tendon in the upper extremity are examples of tendon ruptures occurring in athletes which require surgical repair.

Tennis Leg

Strains of the posterior calf musculature frequently relate to overuse of the gastrocnemius muscle. Most of these injuries occur in sports involving short, sharp, side-to-side and forward movements as tennis, racquetball and squash. The injury is thought to occur when the plantar-flexed foot is suddenly dorsiflexed with the knee in extension. Contributory factors are muscle fatigue and degenerative changes of the muscles and tendons in middle-aged players.

The typical history is one of sudden, sharp calf pain that occurs while running. The patient typically feels as if hit in the back of the calf with a ball or racket. Tenderness over the medial head or mid-belly of the gastrocnemius may be associated with swelling and ecchymosis and occasionally a palpable defect. Dorsiflexion of the foot is painful and often restricted. The so-called plantaris tendon rupture is more likely a rupture of the medial head of the gastrocnemius muscle. Treatment for the acute injury is similar to all acute musculoskeletal injuries, i.e., Rest, Ice, Compression, Elevation and Support (crutches or cane). A 3/4" heel lift is then worn for three to six weeks followed by rehabilitation to strengthen the calf muscles. In general, stretching of the calf muscles, hamstrings, quadriceps and hip adductor muscles should precede athletic activities, especially running sports in advanced-age athletes.

Achilles Tendon Rupture

The actual pathogenesis of Achilles tendon rupture is debatable. The tendon usually ruptures 2.0 to 6.0 cm. proximal to its calcaneal insertion with a sudden muscular contraction or a direct blow to the tendon. A diminished blood supply has been demonstrated in this area. Biopsy specimens of acute ruptures show pathologic evidence of acute and chronic cellular reaction and microtears. Thus, the repetitive trauma of athletic participation again seems to cause inflammation in an area of decreased vascularity.

A healthy Achilles tendon does not generally rupture through its substance unless trauma is great, and a normal tendon withstands tremendous tensile forces during activity. The larger the microscopic tears or the more advanced the state of degeneration, the less the insult needed to cause complete rupture. Rupture primarily affects men in their third to fifth decade; they are often poorly conditioned, athletically aggressive men who engage in intermittent sports activities.

The classic findings of an Achilles rupture are a palpable gap in the back of the ankle, calf swelling, ecchymosis and a positive Thompson test. This is performed with the patient prone and the feet hanging over the edge of the examining table. The calf muscle is then squeezed. The normal reaction is plantar flexion of the foot. When there is no plantar movement, the test is positive.

There are several pitfalls in the diagnosis of Achilles tendon rupture. Foot flexion in the affected extremity is often preserved by action of the deeper muscles. Diffuse swelling and edema with negative x-rays may suggest the diagnosis of ankle sprain or gastrocnemius rupture, but the Thompson test is diagnostic.

Non-surgical treatment of ruptured Achilles tendon consists of applying a short leg equinus (plantar flexed) cast for eight weeks, followed by a 1" heel lift for four weeks. Surgical treatment consists of operative repair possibly with fascia or plantaris reinforcement of the ruptured tendon. A cast is worn for 8–10 weeks following surgery, after which an elevated heel lift is worn for three months followed by a course of resistance exercises to strengthen the triceps mechanism. Surgical functional results are reportedly superior, with improved strength and endurance compared to those treated non-surgically. Surgery should certainly be recommended for more active patients.

Prevention consists primarily of appropriate conditioning, strengthening and stretching exercises. This is especially important when racket sports players also engage in distance running, as this latter activity may predispose to Achilles tendinitis and secondary degeneration in younger age groups than one would generally expect.

Overuse Syndromes in Running

The constant repetitive act of long-distance running in which each foot strikes the ground 1,000 times per mile has brought about a spectrum of overload syndromes to the lower extremities ranging from shin splints to stress fractures. Shin splints are believed to be a periostitis or inflammation, and micro-tears of the posterior tibial muscle attachment to the tibia resulting from repetitive contraction of the muscle at its bony attachment. If this type of overuse syndrome is thought of as a continuum, the other end of the spectrum is the stress fracture where the bone eventually fatigues under additive stress and microfractures become more complete. Stress fractures occur most commonly in the tibia, fibula and metatarsals. If they are allowed to progress by continuing activity, a complete bi-cortical fracture can develop. Although it may be difficult for a long-distance runner to stop running to allow a stress fracture to heal, it is essential to do so, and if necessary for cardiovascular fitness or psychological purposes, to substitute swimming, bicycling or other non-impact sports until there is x-ray evidence of healing. If the initial set of x-rays of a clinically-suspected stress fracture are negative, a bone scan will be a more accurate test especially in a competitive athlete. For the recreational athlete, two to three weeks of rest and repeat x-rays if there is no improvement in symptoms might be more feasible and cost-effective.

Knee problems including chondromalacia and anterior knee pain syndrome are common. Achilles tendinitis is not infrequent, as is iliotibial tract tendinitis. The latter is a localized tendon inflammation as it abuts on the lateral femoral condyle during repetitive flexion and extension of the knee in running. Malalignment problems and poor muscle development also predispose to knee problems in runners. Treatment depends on the area involved but must take into consideration the entire individual, including flexibility, muscle tone, and foot and leg alignment. Generalizations of treatment of overuse-injuries to the lower extremities in runners include flexibility exercises especially to the calf and hamstrings, muscle-strengthening exercises especially to the quadriceps, change in training methods by decreasing mileage and alternating the distance and speed of the run on consecutive days, with frequent rest days. Occasionally orthotics are beneficial in a poorly-aligned foot or lower extremity. Change in footwear and running terrain may similarly improve a patient with this type of syndrome.

SUGGESTED READINGS

Berson, L.B., McGinness, G.H. Common Tennis Injuries. *Hospital Med.* p. 122, April 1983.

Hawkins, R.T., Kennedy, J.C. The Impingement Syndrome in Athletes. *Am. J. Sports Med.* 8:151, 1980.

Inglis, A.E., Scott, W.N., Scolco, D.P., Patterson, A.H. Ruptures of the Tendo-Achilles: An Objective Assessment of Surgical and Non-Surgical Treatment. *J. Bone and Joint Surg.* 48A:990, 1976.

Millar, A.P. Strains of the Posterior Calf Musculature: Tennis Leg. *Am. J. Sports Med.* 7:173, 1979.

Nirschl, R.P., Sobel, J. Conservative Treatment of Tennis Elbow. *Phys. Sports Med.* 9:42, 1981.

Noyes, et. al. The Symptomatic Anterior Cruciate Deficient Knee, Parts I and II. *J. Bone and Joint Surg.* 65A: 154–174, Feb. 1983.

O'Donoghue, D.H. *Treatment of Injuries to Athletes*. W.B. Saunders Co., Phila., 1976, pp. 82–84.

O'Connor, R. *Arthroscopy*. J.B. Lippincott, Phila., 1977.

CHAPTER 12

INFECTIOUS ARTHRITIS

Leland Abbey, M.D.

JOINT INFECTIONS

Arthritis, or inflammation of joints, is part of many diseases. Some of these such as rheumatoid arthritis and osteoarthritis, gout, scleroderma, polymyositis, and hyperparathyroidism are covered in other chapters. This chapter will review arthritis associated with infectious processes, rheumatic fever, and sarcoidosis.

An acute suppurative arthritis represents a rheumatologic emergency. If left untreated, it may cause the rapid destruction of a joint with resultant loss of function. If recognized and treated appropriately, it can often be cured with little or no ultimate loss of joint function. The overall incidence of septic arthritis has remained relatively constant but there have been changes in the spectrum of responsible organisms. A wide variety of organisms may be involved including pyogenic bacteria, mycobacteria, viruses, and fungi. This discussion will deal mainly with the first three.

Bacteria enter joints in one of three fashions:

1) direct penetration

2) extension from an adjacent focus

3) hematogenous spread.

Direct penetration of a joint may be either accidental or iatrogenic. Penetrating trauma, with the resulting contamination of the joint, may cause a septic arthritis. The injection of contaminated materials, failure of sterile technique, or implantation during surgery may also result in an infected joint. An abscess, an infected bursa, or an osteomyelitis adjacent to a joint may extend into that joint. However, hematogenous dissemination from a distant site is most common. Thus infections elsewhere can often give one clue as to the organism and suggest treatment while awaiting bacteriological confirmation.

Although anyone can have a septic arthritis, certain people are more likely to be affected. People who have chronic debilitating diseases such as diabetes mellitus, cancer, chronic renal disease, cirrhosis, alcoholism, or rheumatoid arthritis are more prone to developing joint infections. Any pre-existent joint disease or former arthrotomy is also a predisposing factor.

Many drugs depress the immune system. Medicines, such as corticosteroids and chemotherapeutic agents, used to treat cancer, or immunosuppressive agents (azathioprine and cyclophosphamide) may make the patient more susceptible to infections. The previous administration of antimicrobial agents may select organisms that are resistant to those of antibiotics. Drug abusers, who use non-sterile materials, often inject bacteria and other organisms directly into the blood stream leading to many infectious complications including septic arthritis. Patients on renal dialysis are also at higher risk because of inadequate immune competence and the frequent invasion of the vascular system or peritoneal cavity that is necessary to accomplish hemodialysis or peritoneal dialysis. Patients with rheumatoid arthritis present a special and often not appreciated problem. They may be more susceptible because of the debilitating nature of severe rheumatoid arthritis, the presence of pre-existing joint disease, and medications (especially corticosteroids and immunosuppressive agents) that are sometimes necessary for their treatment. Because such patients already have joint inflammation, one often does not recognize when a joint is infected. It is necessary to be especially vigilant.

Once bacteria gain entrance to the synovial space, they begin to multiply and call forth an inflammatory reaction, resulting in accumulation of synovial fluid. Proteolytic enzymes released into the synovial fluid degrade the cartilage matrix; first proteoglycan, then collagen. Chondrocytes are unable to replace the collagen infra-structure of cartilage. Eventually the chondrocytes themselves are damaged or destroyed. If still untreated, the infection may progress to involve the underlying bone causing osteomyelitis. Even if bone is not involved, the loss of cartilage can result in severe long term problems. Since the joint surfaces will no longer be congruent, the abnormal biomechanics may lead to secondary osteoarthritis. The end result of a septic arthritis may even be the obliteration of the joint space and eventual fusion of the joint with complete loss of function.

Proper diagnosis and treatment requires a complete history and physical examination. Several areas should be emphasized. The history should highlight the mode of onset of the arthritis and differentiate between arthritis and arthralgia. Arthritis is inflammation of joints with its attendant signs of heat, swelling, tenderness, redness, and pain on motion. Arthralgia is the feeling of pain in a joint without demonstrable inflammation. Initially with infection, one may have arthralgias, but eventually arthritis develops. Although infection frequently involves only one joint, this is by no means the rule. Some organisms, such as gonococcus, may cause migratory arthralgias, tenosynovitis, and arthritis involving only one or several joints. With other organisms, tenosynovitis may not be prominent. Most patients report fever (sometimes chills), pain, redness, heat, and swelling of the involved joints. There is pain on motion and the joints are tender. A history of recent illness, medication, invasive procedures (e.g.

cystoscopy, dental work, barium enema), drug abuse, or alcoholism should be sought. Signs of recent or concurrent infection may suggest a causative organism. A careful sexual history is very important. One should also ask if there has been any trauma since this may precede the development of a septic arthritis.

The general physical examination should include a search for the signs of infection at other sites, such as the eyes, lungs, genitourinary tract and skin. One should carefully examine the skin and note any lesions that suggest gonococcal disease or the urticarial type rash sometimes seen in the prodrome of hepatitis B virus infection. One can then note swelling, tenderness, redness, and heat in the affected joints. One should look for the occurrence of an effusion. Although motion may be difficult or impossible because of pain, one should attempt to record both active and passive ranges of motion. Active motion will generally be less because of the greater stress on the joint. Tenosynovitis, which may be a prominent part of gonococcal arthritis, should be noted.

If an effusion is present, the joint should be aspirated. The volume of fluid, the color, turbidity, and viscosity should be recorded. A cell count and differential; glucose and protein; and gram stain, culture, and sensitivity tests should be performed. Normal synovial fluid is clear and pale yellow in color. As synovial fluid becomes inflammatory, it becomes turbid due to the accumulation of white blood cells. Septic arthritis usually yields synovial fluids with greater than 50,000 cells/mm^3. Although there are reports of infected joint fluids with low WBC counts (5,000 or 10,000 cells/mm^3), the higher the WBC count and the nearer to 100,000 cells/mm^3, the more likely one is dealing with a septic arthritis. The differential count reveals a predominance of polymorphonuclear leukocytes (often 90% or more) as opposed to the normal mononuclear cell predominance.

The viscosity of synovial fluid is caused by hyaluronic acid. The white blood cells contain hyaluronidase, an enzyme which degrades hyaluronic acid. This causes a decrease in the viscosity, as can be demonstrated by an absent "string sign." Normally synovial fluid will "string out" before separating from the syringe. If the hyaluronic acid has been degraded, this is no longer the case. A similar phenomenon is revealed by doing a mucin clot test. When glacial acetic acid is added to synovial fluid, a clot is formed which remains solid upon shaking. If the hyaluronic acid has been degraded, this clot will break up into little pieces upon shaking the tube.

Measurement of synovial fluid glucose is most helpful. Normally it is 1/2 to 2/3 the serum glucose level. If one is dealing with septic arthritis, it will be below 1/2 the level of a simultaneous serum glucose. This may not be true for the patient with hyperglycemia. Other exceptions to this rule are rare. A low synovial fluid glucose alone should be adequate evidence to treat for a septic arthritis while awaiting bacterial confirmation. Synovial fluid should not be allowed to stand a long time without processing. Because synovial fluid glucose may be artifactually lowered by the metabolic activity of white blood cells, they should be separated promptly.

Gram stain, culture, and sensitivity are vital in directing therapy. One may see either gram positive or gram negative cocci or gram negative bacilli in the synovial fluid. (Gram positive bacilli would be a rare finding.) Culture and sensitivity testing will confirm the exact organism and its antibiotic sensitivity.

Newer techniques have also been used in evaluating synovial and other body fluids. Counter-immunoelectrophoresis has been used to detect *N. meningitidis* and *H. influenza* antigens. Elevated levels of synovial fluid lactic acid may be an indicator of infection. The utility of these and other experimental tests has not been determined.

Lastly, one should examine the synovial fluid for crystals (most commonly urate and calcium pyrophosphate dihydrate) using compensated polarized light microscopy. Clinically, acute crystal induced arthritis may resemble septic arthritis. It is important to remember that septic arthritis can occur simultaneously with a crystal induced arthritis. In this case a positive gram stain or a low synovial fluid glucose should suggest the diagnosis and appropriate therapy should be instituted. It is unusual to find a low synovial fluid glucose in an uncomplicated crystal induced arthritis.

Radiologic evaluation of the involved joints should be done. Initially, one may see only soft tissue swelling or evidence of a synovial effusion. Within the first seven days juxta-articular osteopenia, a non-specific finding, appears. If left untreated, one then sees loss of the joint space. This represents the destruction of the articular cartilage. Later there is subcortical bone resorption and periosteal reaction. Gas forming organisms may cause lucencies because of gas in the surrounding tissues or joint space. Late complications may be osteomyelitis, osteoarthritis, fusion of the joint, or the appearance of calcifications in the periarticular tissues.

Any organism may be responsible for a septic arthritis. However, the majority of cases can be accounted for by a relatively small number of bacteria. *Neisseria gonorrhea* is responsible for 35–50% of septic arthritis in multiple series. It should always be considered in the otherwise healthy patient and appropriate cultures performed, including urethra, cervix, rectum, and throat. Infection with *Neisseria gonorrhea* has been reported in both the young and the elderly. An association exists between disseminated gonococcal disease and menses or pregnancy.

The presentation of gonococcal disease is considered to occur in two phases which may often overlap. The first is the appearance of fever, skin rash, and arthralgia. This represents the bacteremic phase of the disease. Organisms may be cultured from the blood and rarely from skin lesions. More frequently, they may be seen on gram stain of the skin lesion. The rash is usually vesicular, pustular, or hemorrhagic papules or bullae. They show a leukocytoclastic angiitis on biopsy. In the next phase, a tenosynovitis or septic arthritis develops in one or several joints. Although any joint may be involved, involvement of the knees, wrists, or ankles is most frequent. The synovial fluid is typically inflammatory. Gram negative cocci may or may not be seen on gram stain. The culture is positive in less than 50% of cases, leading some to suggest that the arthritis may, in part, be due to immune complex or other hypersensitivity reactions. Meningococcal disease may mimic gonococcal disease. They may sometimes be differentiated by the lack of tenosynovitis in the former. In meningococcal disease, the joint effusions are frequently sterile, suggesting an immune complex etiology. The disease may also appear as the meningitis is improving. Part of the poor yield on culture of these bacteria may be due to inadequate handling. They are fragile organisms that must not be allowed to cool. As soon as the culture is taken, it should be put in a carbon dioxide enriched atmosphere.

Of the gram positive cocci, *Staphylococcus aureus* accounts for most cases. Streptococci and pneumococci account for a smaller number. Staphylococci and streptococci may have originated in distant sites of infection such as the skin or an abscess. Pneumococci may have caused a previous pneumonia and are also a common cause of otitis media in the adult.

When dealing with gram negative bacilli, the spectrum of disease appears to be changing. In previous series, less than 5% of cases of septic arthritis were caused by gram negative bacilli. More recently, this has risen to 11–22%. This probably represents the increased survival of patients with cancer, diabetes, cirrhosis, and the more aggressive use of chemotherapeutic agents. Any gram negative bacillus may be involved, although *Escherichia coli, Pseudomonas aeruginosa, Proteus spp., Serratia marcescens* are common. In children, gram negative bacilli cause infection in the perinatal period. *Hemophilus influenza* is usually a disease of the young (<4 yrs.) and the very old. Patients with sickle cell disease are said to be particularly susceptible to salmonella infections.

As already alluded to, the patient with rheumatoid arthritis presents a special problem. So often an inflamed joint is said to be the result of a flare in the rheumatoid disease. When one joint is inflamed out of proportion to the underlying disease activity or the arthritis does not fit the previous patterns of the patients disease, it is imperative to suspect a septic arthritis.

Treatment of a septic arthritis involves both general and specific measures. One must splint the involved joints in a position of function during the acute stage of inflammation. This prevents contractures and preserves function of the extremity. For example, the position of function of the knee is fully extended. For the wrist, one positions the hand in neutral or slight dorsiflexion to preserve grip. Splinting will also rest the joint. As the acute inflammation resolves, the patient is begun on a program of passive range of motion. Then, as tolerated, active motion is begun. The goals are to reestablish joint function as fully as possible, and restore muscle strength which is rapidly lost during an acute arthritis.

A septic joint is a closed space infection and behaves like an abscess. Therefore, the joint must be drained. Unless the fluid is very viscous or has become loculated within the joint, needle aspiration is usually adequate. Aspiration removes harmful enzymes which may degrade the cartilage and relieves pain by decreasing the distension of the inflamed joint capsule. This should be done daily or even twice a day if necessary. The changes in the synovial fluid are useful in following the resolution of the infection. The culture should become sterile; organisms should disappear from the synovial fluid; the glucose should rise; and the white blood cell count should decline. The fluid can also be used to verify that bacteriocidal levels of antibiotics have been achieved. When necessary, surgical drainage, which can often be done through the arthroscope, should be performed. Except in two situations, open surgical drainage is not usually required. If there is failure to respond in four to five days, one should perform open surgical drainage. Infection of the hip joint, particularly in children, should lead to early surgical intervention. It is difficult to perform repeated needle aspiration of this joint. In general, morbidity is less in the patient who responds to medical therapy. Recovery of joint function is usually more complete and the need for prolonged physical therapy less.

The choice of antibiotics will depend on the clinical state and age of the patient, the result of the gram stain, and the culture result if available. If the gram stain shows gram positive cocci, one should treat for *Staphylococcus Aureus* with a semisynthetic penicillin, such as nafcillin. Until culture results are available, this should be adequate coverage for gram positive cocci. If the gram stain shows gram negative bacilli, one should treat with a regimen that will at least cover pseudomonads and *E. Coli,* taking into account resistance patterns in the community and hospital. If the gram stain is negative and the patient otherwise healthy, one should treat for *N. gonorrhea.* If the patient has predisposing factors, as previously outlined, one must provide antibiotics effective against *Staphylococcus aureus* and gram negative bacilli. If one sees gram negative cocci, one is most likely dealing with *N. gonorrhea* or *N. meningitidis.* One should treat the patient with high dose intravenous penicillin. In a child, one must consider *H. influenza.* The use of ampicillin with or without chloramphenicol (depending upon resistance patterns) would be appropriate. With a negative gram stain in a child, therapy will vary with age. Neonates need coverage for *S. aureus* and gram negative bacilli. Older children need coverage for *S. aureus* and *H. influenza.*

The prognosis depends upon both the patient and the organism. Patients who have severe underlying diseases and/or infection with gram negative bacilli may have a poor outcome. Patients with rheumatoid arthritis do particularly poorly, with increased loss of joint function and even occasionally death. Delay in therapy will invariably lead to a poor outcome. Gram positive bacilli have a better outlook if treated promptly. However, not all patients recover rapidly. Often, there is a lingering chronic synovitis and recurrent effusions. These are sterile and synovial biopsy reveals only chronic inflammation. The time needed for resolution varies. The rate of recovery can often be predicted by the degree of purulence of the synovial fluid. If the WBC count is low, recovery is usually rapid. As the WBC count rises, recovery is slower with increasing likelihood of persistent synovitis.

Tuberculosis of bones and joints accounts for approximately 1% of tuberculosis in the United States. Although any joint may be involved, tuberculosis commonly involves the spine (Pott's disease), hip, knee, and ankle. Delay in diagnosis is often long and the arthritis indolent and destructive. As opposed to infection with pyogenic bacteria, the joint is often swollen and only slightly warm. There is usually marked muscle atrophy about the joint. The chest film is normal in about 50% of patients and the PPD test is positive in 95% of patients. The synovial fluid reveals elevated protein. The white cell count may vary from 1000–100,000 cells/mm^3, and there is a predominance of polymorphonuclear leukocytes. Glucose is usually low and in one series was less than 50% mg in the majority of cases. Ziehl-Neelsen stain of the synovial fluid is positive only in 19% of cases. Although it takes six weeks, the synovial fluid will frequently grow the organism. The best diagnostic technique is synovial biopsy, yielding a high number of positive histologies and organism growth in 95% of cases. Treatment is controversial, but should include at least two antituberculous drugs for a minimum of 18 months. When there is a sequestrum or severe joint destruction, surgical debridement is necessary. If the spine is involved, the surgeon may have to drain the paravertebral abscess and stabilize the spine with a fusion.

Many viruses can cause arthritis. Hepatitis, rubella (natural and vaccine), and mumps are commonly involved. Smallpox is also capable of causing an arthritis. Recently Human Immunodeficiency Virus (HIV) has been associated with arthritis. Other viruses rarely cause arthritis or are not seen in the United States.

Mumps causes arthritis in about 1% of cases. It usually involves small joints and resolves within 60 days. Both natural rubella infection and rubella vaccine have been associated with arthritis in incidences of up to 35% for natural infection and 10% for vaccine. There is usually symmetrical involvement of the knees, wrists, and proximal interphalangeal joints. Usually, it resolves within 30 days. In vaccine associated cases, monarticular knee involvement occurs and recurrences are common. In up to 30% of patients with hepatitis B infection, there is a prodrome, usually lasting two weeks but sometimes up to six weeks.

It consists of fever, urticarial rash, and migratory arthritis or arthralgias. The joint may be acutely inflamed with a large effusion only to become normal in a few days and to be replaced by another inflamed joint. The synovial fluid is inflammatory. Hepatitis B surface antigen is usually detectable in the serum and synovial fluid. Synovial fluid complement is low suggesting an immune complex etiology. When clinical hepatitis evolves and the liver function becomes abnormal, the prodrome disappears.

Acquired immunodeficiency syndrome (AIDS) is caused by a retro human immunodeficiency virus (HIV). Recently, there have been reports of the occurrence of Reiter's syndrome (urethritis, conjunctivitis, and arthritis) in patients with AIDS. The two may appear simultaneously or either may occur first. In one series nine of thirteen patients were HLA-B27 positive. Psoriasis has also been observed in this setting and may get worse with the development of severe AIDS. Several reports have emphasized that methotrexate or other immunosuppressive therapy is contraindicated in these patients because of the development of fulminant AIDS.

Lyme Disease

Lyme disease is caused by *Borrelia burgdorferi*, a previously unknown spirochete, and transmitted by the tick *Ixodes dammini* (*I. pacificus* on the west coast). Over the last few years, the incidence of Lyme disease has been increasing, creating a public health problem in endemic areas. Interestingly, manifestations, now known to be part of Lyme disease, had been described in Europe many years ago. Lyme disease may result in an arthritis and other systemic involvement. The clinical spectrum of disease was originally described in Lyme, Connecticut. It is endemic on the east and west coasts and also in the north midwest. Exposure to the spirochete can be detected serologically. The disease is characterized by a large spreading rash with a clearing center, which develops at the site of the tick bite. The rash is called *erythema chronicum migrans*. Unfortunately, only about 60% of patients remember the tick bite and the rash is not always present. The arthritis commonly involves the knees, but may also involve other joints. Recurrences of the arthritis are common. Also cardiac and neurological disease may be associated with Lyme disease. Early treatment with tetracycline at the onset of the rash is likely to prevent the other manifestations of the disease. When the arthritis or other systemic involvement has already occurred, high dose intravenous penicillin for at least ten days, and as long as 21 days, is the therapy of choice. Ceftriaxone has also been used successfully. The best treatment is prevention. One can avoid exposure by covering the skin and using insect repellents when in or near forested endemic areas. Since the tick lives on deer and white footed mice, this is especially important if these animals live in the area. If bitten, the tick should be removed as soon as possible. The incidence of infection is often correlated with the length of time the tick is attached.

RHEUMATIC FEVER

Rheumatic fever is an inflammatory disease of heart, brain, joints, and skin, which is associated with a streptococcal infection. Although rheumatic fever has been commonly found in the Third World, there have been reports of an increasing incidence of rheumatic fever in middle class populations in several areas of the United States. These reports are associated with the reappearance of a specific type of streptococcus which had been uncommon until recently and which has been associated with past outbreaks. It has been estimated that 1–3% of children develop rheumatic fever after a streptococcal infection. The infection may only be mildly symptomatic.

The diagnosis of rheumatic fever is best accomplished using the major and minor criteria of the Modified Jones Criteria in conjunction with the whole clinical picture. The Jones Criteria consist of the following. The major criteria are: 1) carditis, 2) arthritis, 3) chorea (Sydenham's Chorea), 4) erythema marginatum, and 5) subcutaneous nodules. The minor criteria are fever, a prolonged p-r interval on the electrocardiogram, increased erythrocyte sedimentation rate, elevated C-reactive protein, increased white blood cell count, arthralgias, and previous rheumatic fever or rheumatic heart disease. The presence of two major criteria or one major and two or more minor criteria along with the demonstration of a preceding beta hemolytic streptococcal infection is consistent with a diagnosis of rheumatic fever. The streptococcal infection may be shown by culture or by the use of various antibody tests. These criteria are not perfect and should be used as a guide. For example, up to 25% of children with chronic juvenile polyarthritis have evidence of a preceding streptococcal infection and would fulfill the Jones Criteria for rheumatic fever. A helpful clinical point is that the arthritis of rheumatic fever rarely lasts longer than six months. In adults, subcutaneous nodules and rash are rare. Chorea does not occur in adults.

Carditis is the major problem because it can cause permanent heart disease. It can be manifested by the murmur of valvular heart disease, pericarditis, congestive heart failure, or tachycardia. Chorea (rapid, jerky, purposeless movements) is a late manifestation, sometimes occurring months after the streptococcal infection. Occurring in 10%–15% of patients, it is more common in females and rarely occurs after puberty. Subcutaneous nodules occur in 5% of patients and are found over bony prominences. Erythema marginatum is also a rare finding. It consists of an erythematous rash with well defined darker edges.

Arthritis, although often a prominent feature, resolves without sequelae. It usually involves large joints, but can affect any joint. Characteristically, it is migratory and lasts one week to one month. Typically, there is swelling, redness, and pain. The synovial fluid is inflammatory. Occasionally, in patients who have had rheumatic fever, Jacoud's arthritis has been reported to occur years later. These patients have ulnar deviation and swan neck deformities which are reducible. It is the result of chronic inflammation, fibrosis, and laxity of the supporting capsular and ligamentous structures. Erosions are not seen on radiographs. Rheumatic fever is most common in children but may occur in adults. Carditis and arthritis are the main manifestations in adults. Erythema marginatum and subcutaneous nodules are rare and chorea (caused by rheumatic fever) never occurs in adults. Proper treatment requires the administration of penicillin to eliminate the original streptococcal infection. Then, one gives prophylaxis with penicillin to prevent a recurrence. In penicillin sensitive patients, other antibiotics, such as erythromycin, are appropriate. High dose aspirin is the drug of choice to suppress the acute manifestations of the disease. One tries to achieve a salicylate level of 20–25 mg. In patients with severe disease and major cardiac complications, corticosteroids may play a role in treatment.

SARCOIDOSIS

Sarcoidosis is a multisystem disease (affecting heart, brain, lung, liver, skin, eyes and lymphatics) characterized by granulomatous inflammation. A granuloma contains epithelioid and giant cells (derived from macrophages), lymphocytes, and plasma cells. Although the etiology is unknown, there is some evidence for an unidentified transmissible agent. An immune etiology is suggested by multiple abnormalities such as hypergammaglobulinemia, rheumatoid factor (1/3 of patients), anti-nuclear and thyroid antibodies, anergy, circulating immune complexes, and elevated complement levels with evidence for complement activation.

About 25% of patients develop one of two types of joint disease. The first is characterized by bilateral hilar adenopathy, erythema nodosum, and a systemic polyarthritis (Lofgren's triad). The ankles, knees, wrists, and small joints of the hands are commonly involved. Arthritis is usually limited to only a few joints at a time. Rather than actual arthritis, the disease involves mainly the periarticular structures. Tenosynovitis may occur. The arthritis usually resolves without residua in four to six weeks. It is often responsive to indomethacin. Colchicine may be helpful.

Other patients develop a chronic recurring polyarthritis which is usually symmetric, involving the hands, knees, wrists, and ankles. They may have sarcoid granulomas in their skin but do not develop erythema nodosum. These patients develop joint space narrowing on x-ray films, joint deformities, and bone cysts (lace-like bone). Non-steroidal anti-inflammatory drugs may be helpful. If there is other serious systemic involvement, the use of corticosteroids may be necessary.

Arthritis associated with infectious agents may be caused by a wide variety of organisms from bacteria to viruses. Some organisms have been identified only recently. In addition, some forms of arthritis such as rheumatic fever and sarcoidosis may result from the immunologic consequences of infection.

SUGGESTED READINGS

INFECTIOUS ARTHRITIS

Espinoza, A., Ed. Infections in the Rheumatic Diseases. Grune & Stratton, New York, 1988.

Goldberg, D.L., et. al. Acute Infectious Arthritis: a Review of Patients with non-gonococcal Joint Infections (with Emphasis on Therapy and Prognosis), *Am. J. Med.* 60:369–377, 1976.

Lochshin, M.D., et. al. Infectious Arthritis in *Disease-a-Month,* 28(4), 1982.

Manshady, B., et. al. Septic Arthritis in a general Hospital 1966–1977, *J. of Rheumatol.* 7:523–530, 1980.

Schmid, F.R. (ed.). Infectious Arthritis in *Clin. Rheum. Dis.* 4:(1), 1978.

McCarty, D.J., Ed. Arthritis and Allied Conditions, Lea & Febiger, Philadelphia. 11th edition, 1989. Sec. 11 Infectious Arthritis.

HIV AND ARTHRITIS

Duvic M., et. al. Acquired immunodeficiency syndrome-associated psoriasis and Reiter's syndrome, *Arch. Dermatol.* 123(12):1622–1632, 1987.

Lambert, R.E. and Kaye, B.R. Methotrexate and the acquired immunodeficiency syndrome, *Ann. Intern. Med.* 106(5):773, 1987.

Lin, R.Y. Reiter's syndrome and human immunodeficiency virus infection, *Dermatologica* 176(1):39–42, 1988.

Winchester, R., et. al. The co-occurrence of Reiter's syndrome and acquired immunodeficiency, *Ann. Intern Med.* 106(1):19–26, 1987.

Withrington, R.H., et. al. Isolation of human immunodeficiency virus from synovial fluid of a patient with reactive arthritis, *Br. Med. J.* 294(6570):484, 1987.

LYME DISEASE

Dattwyler, R.J., et. al. Ceftriaxone as effective therapy in refractory Lyme disease, *J. Infect. Dis.* 155(6):1322–1325, 1987.

Dattwyler, R.J., et. al. Treatment of late Lyme Borreliosis—Randomized comparison of Ceftriaxone and Penicillin, *Lancet* 1(8596):1191–1194, 1988.

Steere, A.C., et. al. Successful parenteral penicillin therapy of established Lyme arthritis, *NEJM* 312(14)869–874, 1985.

Steere, A.C., et. al. The clinical evolution of Lyme arthritis, *Ann. Intern. Med.* 107(5):725–731, 1987.

RHEUMATIC FEVER

Ad Hoc Committee to Revise the Jones Criteria (Modified) of the Council on Rheumatic Fever and Congenital Heart Disease of the American Heart Association. Jones criteria (revised) for guidance in diagnosis of rheumatic fever, *Circulation* 32:664–668, 1965.

Feinstein, A.R. The natural histories of acute rheumatic fever, *Bull. Rheum. Dis.* 17(3):423–428, 1966.

Stollerman, G.H. *Rheumatic Fever and Streptococcal Infection.* Grune & Stratton, 1975.

Tadzynski, L.A., et. al. Diagnosis of rheumatic fever. A guide to the criteria and manifestations, *Postgrad. Med.* 79(4)295–300, 1986.

SARCOIDOSIS

Grigor, R.R., et. al. Chronic sarcoid arthritis, *Br. Med. J.* 2(6043):1044, 1976.

James, D.G., et. al. Bone and Joint Sarcoidosis, *Semin. Arthritis and Rheum.* 6(1):53–81, 1976.

Keary, P.J., et. al. Benign self-limiting sarcoidosis with skin and joint involvement, *New Zealand Med. J.* 83(560):197–199, 1976.

Perruquet, J.L., et. al. Sarcoid arthritis in a North American Caucasian population, *J. of Rheumatol.* 11(4):521–525, 1984.

Rosenberg, A.M., et. al. Arthritis in childhood sarcoidosis, *J. of Rheumatol.* 10(6):987–990, 1983.

Spilberg, I., et. al. The Arthritis of Sarcoidosis, *Arthritis Rheum.* 12(2):126–137, 1969.

Uddenfeldt, P., et. al. Musculo-skeletal symptoms in early sarcoidosis. Twenty-four newly diagnosed patients and a two-year follow-up, *Acta. Med. Scand.* 214(4):279–284, 1983.

TABLE 12-1
MAJOR ORGANISMS CAUSING SEPTIC ARTHRITIS
(Modified From Kelly, p. 1565, 2nd ed.)

Gram Stain	*Organism*
Gram Negative Coccus	N. gonorrhea N. meningiditis
Gram Positive Coccus	S. aureus
Gram Negative Bacillus	Pseudomas spp. E. coli
Gram Negative Coccobacillus in a child	H. influenza
Gram Stain Negative	
Healthy Adult	N. gonorrhea
Underlying disease or medication	S. aureus +/- gram negative bacillus
Child	
Neonate	Gram negative bacillus +/- S. aureus
>1 Month	H. influenza S. aureus

III THERAPEUTICS

"...it follows obviously, that a diseased condition once established, in any part of the body, cannot be made to disappear by the chemical action of a remedy. A limit may be put by a remedy to an abnormal process of transformation; that process may be accelerated or retarded; but this alone does not restore the normal (healthy) condition."

Animal Chemistry by J. Liebig, M.D., 1st American Edition, Cambridge, Mass., 1842, p. 252.

CHAPTER 13

THE DIAGNOSTIC PROCESS

Harry Spiera, M.D.

Proper treatment of any medical condition depends on correct diagnosis. A diagnosis places a patient into a defined category thereby excluding other considerations. It also predicts what may be expected to occur and what treatments are more likely to succeed. Patients presenting with the same type of complaint may have completely different diagnoses. For example, a patient who presents with an acute painful swelling of his knee could have, among other conditions, an acute infection, gout, or intra-articular bleeding. The infection would be treated with antibiotics, but if left untreated could totally destroy the joint. The gouty joint would respond quite well to anti-inflammatory medicines, while the joint which is swollen because of bleeding may only need to have the blood evacuated to restore comfort and function to that joint.

The traditional basis for proper diagnosis is first the taking of a careful history. This includes the chief complaint, the events bringing the patient to medical attention and past medical history. Other historical information such as past or concurrent illnesses, previous episodes of the same nature, medication the patient may be taking, certain social and environmental factors as well as possible hereditary factors should be elicited. Relative importance of these factors will differ from case to case. Thus if the patient who has been well, trips down the stairs and strikes his shoulder and then has severe shoulder pain it is most likely that the pain in the shoulder is due to the trauma sustained. On the other hand, if a patient becomes ill with fever, pain and discomfort in many joints he may have a more complex situation. Hence a more careful and detailed history may be necessary.

After the history is obtained, a physical examination is performed. Not only is the part of the body which is painful or inflamed examined, but often a full physical examination is necessary. Thus the diagnostic clue suggesting gout in a patient with a swollen elbow, may be the finding of a tophus (a deposition of uric acid in the ear lobe or about the finger). Another example is a patient with a swollen foot who may have psoriatic arthritis. Here the finding of stippling of his fingernails may be important. There are many other such examples.

After the physical examination is done, the physician will then formulate what is referred to as a differential diagnosis. This is a consideration of those illnesses that are most likely to explain the complaints and physical abnormalities. This is not necessarily formally written down, but in the physician's mind a certain set of circumstances will lead to one or a number of different possibilities. Sometimes a diagnosis will be obvious and apparent after the history and physical examination and no further diagnostic testing may be required. However, in many instances further testing will be necessary. This could include a number of blood tests, urinalysis and other chemical determinations. It may often involve aspiration of the joint for examination of the synovial fluid. X-Ray studies are often extremely important. Sometimes more sophisticated imaging techniques such as computed axial tomography (CAT) or magnetic resonance imaging (MRI) are necessary. Radio-opaque dyes may be injected into a joint before X-Ray to outline internal structure. This technique is called arthrography, which is often helpful in diagnosing various cartilage injuries. Coming into more extensive use recently is the technique of arthroscopy, where an orthopedic surgeon using an instrument called an arthroscope looks into the joint and examines the internal structures. At times actual surgical exploration of various areas is done and tissue removed for analysis. Oftentimes pathological examination of involved tissues is essential for correct diagnosis. This is particularly true where a patient has a single joint involved and possibility of a joint tumor or chronic infection is considered.

It should be clear from the foregoing that the diagnosis of various rheumatic diseases involve history and physical examination done by a physician who is acquainted with the many possibilities that can cause problems. At times the diagnosis will be obvious to the general practitioner or internist. At other times consultation with a rheumatologist or an orthopedist is required. Sometimes consultations with various other specialists are necessary, for example neurologists and psychiatrists. In some extremely complicated problems, many different medical specialists are involved in an attempt to arrive at the correct diagnosis.

Sometimes the most thorough work-up fails to yield a clear diagnosis. This is particularly true early in the course of some of the diffuse rheumatic diseases wherein the diagnosis may not become immediately apparent. In that situation a physician may take a "wait-and-see" attitude treating the patient empirically until enough time has passed for a more clear-cut picture to evolve. Understandably, this may be terribly frustrating for the patient who has undergone an extensive medical investigation. It is important for the health professional to explain to the patient that our knowledge is limited and only with time will the correct diagnosis become apparent. This type of understanding and sympathetic communication on the part of the health professional may be most important. There are many instances where patients develop illnesses of the musculoskeletal system which seem to be self-limited and do not fall into any clearly definable category. These patients may get better and the problem resolves without a diagnosis being made.

In some instances no diagnosis can be made despite intensive study and yet the patient is too ill to assume a "wait-and-see" attitude. In that situation the physician may make a presumptive diagnosis and treat accordingly and observe the patient for what then occurs.

Probably the best means of diagnosing a condition is if one can know the cause. A typical example of this is infectious arthritis wherein a microorganism causes the disease in question. Therefore eradication of the infection gives the best chance of achieving a good outcome. Indeed, infectious arthritis is one of the few examples of arthritis being "cured." Unfortunately infection, as far as we know, is responsible for only a small percentage of the musculoskeletal disease that is seen in everyday practice. If it turns out that rheumatoid arthritis is an infectious disease, as suspected by some, the previous statement may have to be modified.

Another way of categorizing a disease is on the basis of certain structural and pathological changes. Thus, osteoarthritis is defined as a disease in which there is a wearing away and loss of the articular cartilage with secondary reactivity of the surrounding bone. There may be a number of causes for this type of change but the disease is still referred to as osteoarthritis.

Some diseases may be defined on the basis of characteristic microscopic appearance. That is, they have certain histological changes in cells and tissue which define the disease. Thus, amyloidosis which results from the deposition of a certain type of protein into the tissues is recognized on the basis of a characteristic appearance both on standard and polarized microscopy.

Still other diseases may be defined on the basis of a metabolic abnormality and accumulation of certain metabolic products. The classic example of this would be gout where, as the result of a number of biochemical disturbances there is an accumulation of uric acid in the blood. The uric acid may precipitate in the joint and so trigger the acute gouty attack.

In some inflammatory diseases of the joints and connective tissue such as rheumatoid arthritis, systemic lupus erythematosus and polymyositis, there has been an attempt to define the disease by the presence of certain immunological abnormalities. Some investigators believe that the presence of antibody to double-stranded DNA defines the disease as being lupus and an antibody to an extractable nuclear antigen (ENA) defines it as a "mixed connective tissue disease" (MCTD). Most investigators, however, do not feel that these autoantibodies are specific enough to define these diseases.

The majority of the inflammatory diseases of the joints are of unknown cause and thus there is no etiological basis for classification. Furthermore, the histopathological findings are usually too non-specific to make a clear-cut diagnosis. The serological findings are also too non-specific in the opinion of most investigators to establish the diagnosis. As a result, the diagnoses of the various diffuse connective tissue diseases are made on the basis of a group of findings including clinical observation, and laboratory and histopathological abnormalities. Examples of this can be seen in the appendix of this book. Criteria have been developed for the diagnosis of rheumatoid arthritis, systemic lupus and scleroderma. For the most part patients can be categorized as having one or another disease; however, many patients do not clearly fit into one category.

Rheumatoid arthritis is a prime example of a disease of unknown cause in which there is no absolutely specific laboratory or pathological finding. It is diagnosed on the basis of a patient having inflamed joints lasting for a certain period of time in which other diseases capable of causing the same type of signs and symptoms can be excluded. It can thus be seen that rheumatoid arthritis may indeed be a diagnosis of exclusion, and what we call rheumatoid arthritis may be a group of different diseases of different causes. Illnesses such as ankylosing spondylitis, psoriatic arthritis and Reiter's syndrome can be considered as variants of rheumatoid arthritis. However, on the basis of clinical, laboratory and genetic differences, they have been clearly differentiated. Further understanding of the various rheumatic diseases and their intelligent classification will depend on the progress that is made in understanding their etiology and pathogenesis.

The question is with a disease of unknown etiology and pathogenesis, why it is necessary to establish different diagnostic categories. That is, what does a diagnosis mean in those circumstances. It would seem that there are three reasons.

1. If it makes for a difference in treatment.
2. If there is a difference in prognosis.
3. If some fundamental biological difference can be distinguished among the groups.

An excellent example of this approach is ankylosing spondylitis. It was formerly called rheumatoid spondylitis and considered to be a variant of rheumatoid arthritis. On the basis of clinical considerations, it was clearly distinguished from rheumatoid arthritis. Some of the major differences are: Rheumatoid arthritis is predominantly a disease of women in a 2–3:1 ratio, while ankylosing spondylitis is overwhelmingly a male disease. Whereas ankylosing spondylitis involves the axial skeleton and only in about a quarter of cases is there peripheral joint involvement, rheumatoid arthritis is a disease of the peripheral joints in which the axial skeleton is only rarely involved. Furthermore, about 70% of patients with rheumatoid arthritis have rheumatoid factor in their serum as opposed to ankylosing spondylitis where rheumatoid factor is found in no higher frequency than in the general population.

The treatment of ankylosing spondylitis differs in many ways from that of rheumatoid arthritis in that the main agents used are the non-steroidal antiinflammatory drugs such as indomethacin which is particularly effective in ankylosing spondylitis but only moderately effective in rheumatoid arthritis. Moreover, disease-modifying agents such as gold, penicillamine and antimalarials are often effective in rheumatoid arthritis but have no place in the management of ankylosing spondylitis. The prognosis of the two diseases is quite different. Although rheumatoid arthritis may be a remitting disease, many patients develop a chronic deforming disease. On the other hand, most patients with ankylosing spondylitis eventually remit, and though left with a rigid axial skeleton continue to function at a relatively good level. Of greatest importance, however, is the biological difference that has been found. In the study of the immunogenetics of disease, 80–90% of patients with ankylosing spondylitis are HLA-B27 positive in contrast to 8% of the general population; whereas in rheumatoid arthritis, there is no increase in the incidence of HLA-B27 positivity. It is only because AS was clinically distinguished from RA that the association between HLA-B27 and AS was established. This discovery was proved to be the cornerstone of modern immunogenetic diseases in the rheumatic diseases.

It is extremely important for every health care professional to know that many diagnostic categories are often merely a shorthand means of communication. Thus these differentiations, on the basis of experience, have given us a better idea of prognosis, and of treatments likely to be effective in one situation or another. Furthermore, if a disease can be separated from another on clinical grounds, in the future we may be able to define that disease on the basis of specific biological features.

In summary, the proper diagnosis of rheumatic diseases is essential for proper treatment. The diagnosis is based on a thorough history and physical examination and the appropriate use of laboratory testing, imaging techniques and histopathological findings. Even in diseases of unknown etiology and pathogenesis, this type of approach has led to more rational and effective treatment of many of the diseases with which we deal.

GENERAL REFERENCES

Katz, W.A., Ed. "Diagnosis and Management of Rheumatic Diseases," JB Lippincott Co., Philadelphia, 2nd ed. 1988.

Kelley, W.N., Harris, E.D. Jr., Ruddy, S. and Sledge, C.B. (Eds.) "Textbook of Rheumatology," (2 vol.) W.B. Saunders Co., Philadelphia, 3rd ed. 1989.

McCarthy, D.J. (Ed.) "Arthritis and Allied Conditions." Lea & Febiger Co., Philadelphia, 11th ed. 1989.

Schumacher, H.J. Jr. (Ed.) "Primer on the Rheumatic Diseases," Arthritis Foundation, Atlanta, 9th ed. 1988.

CHAPTER 14

DRUGS

Thomas G. Kantor, M.D.

Personnel involved in patient care often find their arthritis patients on some sort of drug therapy. It must be understood that only in the case of infected joints can a cure be effected and that all other conditions ordinarily treated by rheumatologists are incurable. In some instances, disease remission can be established by drugs but only very rarely is this lasting. Totally controllable conditions, such as gout, may require life-long treatment, and this is addressed in another chapter of this book.

However, the pain and inflammation associated with arthritic conditions can frequently be controlled by drugs, allowing the patient to function within his socio-economic milieu and partake in physical medicine procedures which preserve joint function. In some of the more devastating connective tissue syndromes, drugs can be life-saving.

Since drug therapy is not curative and merely reduces symptoms in the face of ongoing disease, drugs often must be taken over long periods of time. This creates special problems in drug development and regulation. Drugs must not only be effective and stay that way, but must be safe over periods of months or years.

This section will consider the drugs used in this field of medicine—not in pharmacological detail—but in order of effectiveness, from least to most, and with consideration of the disease to be treated. This will be followed by a section on ancillary drugs.

FIRST LINE DRUGS

The non-steroidal anti-inflammatory drugs (NSAIDs), including aspirin and other salicylates, are the first line drugs for many arthritic and some connective tissue syndromes. Aspirin was introduced at the turn of the 20th century as an analgetic drug, its anti-inflammatory properties only widely recognized after 1964. Paradoxically, the non-steroidals were introduced as anti-inflammatory drugs and only recognized as all-purpose analgetics after 1964, too. It is now apparent that all NSAIDs, including the salicylates, can be used for either indication with perhaps a lower dose conferring only analgetic effect.

All NSAIDs perform both effects in the periphery where pain is most often associated with inflammation. Reduction of fever, a characteristic of all these drugs, is a central nervous system effect that depends only on the ability of the drug to cross the blood-brain barrier.

At the present time, it is felt that the effectiveness of NSAIDs depend on their ability to inhibit the enzyme cyclo-oxygenase which produces from arachidonic acid, endoperoxides and prostaglandin end products such as thromboxane, prostacyclin (PGI_2) and PGE_2. All of these have profound physiological effects, with the endoperoxides apparently being one of the mediators of inflammation. Further metabolism of endoperoxides result in production of PGI_2 and PGE_2 which sensitize peripheral pain receptor sites to the further action of histamine and bradykinin, which in turn triggers the pain signal.

Thus, both anti-inflammatory and analgetic effects are interdependent. Other inflammation mediators, such as bradykinin, histamine and complement fragment C5, are not directly affected by the NSAIDs to any consistently measurable extent.

Table 14-1 lists some NSAIDs by chemical class and approximate elimination half-lives. These lists include the NSAIDs available to the American public as of this writing, but approximately twenty more are available in other parts of the world. The reason for this profusion will be discussed later. It is pharmacologically unusual to have so many chemicals, all capable of inhibiting one enzyme.

Pharmacologists have recognized certain chemical functions which are common to the entire group, and from this information have deduced the chemical configuration of the enzyme itself. By its donation of an acetyl group to cyclo-oxygenase, aspirin destroys this enzyme which then needs to be reconstituted by the body. The other NSAIDs temporarily inhibit the enzyme, but when the drugs are metabolized and excreted, the enzyme is as good as new.

Many investigators are dissatisfied with ascribing all of the effects of these drugs to the inhibition of the one enzyme, cyclo-oxygenase. For one thing, it does not explain the effect of non-acetylated salicylates, such as sodium salicylate and other inorganic salts of salicylic acid, which do not inhibit the enzyme in-vitro, nor does it explain the effect of organic salts, such as salsalate (Disalcid) and choline-magnesium salicylate (Trilisate), which do not contain an acetyl group.

The effect of aspirin is quite different on the cyclo-oxygenase of the blood platelet, an organelle incapable of manufacturing any cell constituents on its own after it has broken away from its parent cell, the megakaryocyte. Thus, functions of the platelets that are dependent on prostaglandin production, such as the ability to aggregate and thereby initiate blood clotting, are totally absent during the week-long residence of platelets in the blood.

With the other NSAIDs, however, the enzyme may continue to function when the drug has been metabolized and/or eliminated, and the effect on clotting is only temporary. Aspirin should be stopped in patients who already have a coagulation defect, whether it is disease (hemophilia, certain cases of rheumatoid arthritis, or lupus), or drug-induced (coumarin derivatives and heparin). It should also be stopped a week prior to elective surgery unless the surgeon wishes to take advantage of the protection against thrombophlebitis which the prolongation of bleeding time by aspirin produces. Other NSAIDs may be given up to the time of surgery, dependent on their half-lives in the circulation (Table 14-1).

It should be explained that the elimination half-life of most of these drugs, when multiplied by a factor of six or seven, is the total residence time of the drug in the body. Thus, tolmetin (Tolectin) is only present in the body for at most seven hours after a single dose, while piroxicam (Feldene) is present for almost two weeks (Table 14-1). In addition to the platelet effect, residence time in the body profoundly affects dosage schedules and the duration of adverse effects. For example, a long half-life drug (over 10 hours) requires only a twice-a-day or once-a-day dose. This has a distinct advantage in patient compliance as compared to short half-life drugs which require three or four times-a-day dosage.

However, in patients with hepatic or renal insufficiency, or in the elderly, a long half-life drug may pile up in the body and cause serious toxicity. All of these drugs are metabolized by the liver and excreted by the kidney and some have enterohepatic circulations. In the latter situation, a drug or its metabolites may be excreted in the bile but then reabsorbed from the intestine. Essentially, the choice of drug may depend upon the pocket-book of the patient, his trustworthiness on dosage schedules, his age, his use of other drugs, and the possibility of other diseases.

The NSAIDs bind to albumin and in doing so may replace other drugs which also bind to this plasma protein. A drug bound to protein is in equilibrium with unbound drugs in the plasma, and an unbound drug is the pharmacologically active form of the drug. Therefore, a drug displaced by an NSAID may be in a more active form which in fact happens when other drugs, such as oral hypoglycemics and coumarin derivatives, are given. NSAIDs may be contraindicated with such drugs or doses may need to be modified.

As noted above, there are some questions as to the exact mechanism of anti-inflammatory effect for the NSAIDs. There is, however, little question about the mechanism of their side-effects which are much the same among them all. The inhibition of prostaglandin synthesis is the cause of the important side-effects. Prostaglandins are extremely active physiological substances and are ubiquitous in their location in the body. They control salt and water metabolism in the kidney by modulating the efforts of angiotensin and renin. They control much of the physiology of the gastric mucosa by decreasing free stomach acid production, and increasing mucous and mucosal blood flow.

Inhibition of the production of prostaglandins leads to retention of salt and water by the kidney with consequent edema, hypertension and reversal of the effect of anti-hypertensive agents. Patients with active peptic ulcer should never receive any of these drugs and those with a history of ulcer should receive them only with great caution. The stomach effect causes gastric irritation and peptic ulcer.

Prostaglandins are also involved in the physiology of the uterus, and NSAIDs are superb drugs for the control of dysmenorrhea which is due to excess of prostaglandins in the uterine cavity. At the same time, prostaglandins are also involved with the events of parturition and NSAIDs may prolong the delivery process and, by their platelet effect, lead to excessive bleeding during delivery.

Hepatic and renal toxicity have occasionally been reported for all of these drugs but serious difficulties are rare. The renal problems may have some basis in the reduction of prostaglandin synthesis but the causes of hepatic toxicity are unknown. Despite the rarity of these difficulties, frequent monitoring of hepatic and renal function should be performed since even the most serious of these adverse effects are usually reversible on stopping the drug. There may be differences among NSAIDs with respect to renal toxicity.

A rare group of patients is truly allergic to aspirin in that they get hives and asthma. Such patients are also allergic to all the other NSAIDs and should be precluded from treatment with this group of drugs. The mechanism of this allergic process may be a shunting of arachidonic acid metabolism from the cyclo-oxygenase pathway to the lip-oxygenase leading to the production of leukotrienes C, D and E, which can cause bronchial constriction.

A familiar feature of NSAID therapy, well-known to clinicians, is the unpredictability of their therapeutic effect. It is not possible to predict which patients will develop unacceptable adverse effects. The commonest of the latter, by far, is gastrointestinal intolerance. Poor compliance due to this adverse reaction probably accounts for a considerable percent of the failures in effectiveness. In addition, there are unaccountable failures in effectiveness in patients who are compliant. These non-responders do not pharmacologically handle the drug any differently from responders, and these apparent idiosyncratic differences between patients in effectiveness are as yet unexplained. It would seem that there is a target population for any number of these drugs which accounts for their profusion in Europe and for the many awaiting FDA approval in this country.

There are a few, but only a few, rheumatological conditions where there seems to be some specificity for any of the NSAIDs. Most rheumatologists agree that indomethacin and phenylbutazone have greater effectiveness than other

NSAIDs in the spondyloarthropathies, such as ankylosing spondylitis, Reiter's syndrome, and the spinal component of juvenile arthritis. The two drugs, however, are not infrequently troublesome with adverse effects unique to them. These include psychotomimetic problems and bone marrow toxicity.

In summary, the NSAIDs have unique, non-curative, symptom-lessening properties in almost all arthropathies, including osteoarthritis. Choosing the right one for an individual patient depends on pharmacological and clinical knowledge, but effectiveness and potential for adverse effects are unpredictable in any given patient. However, choice need not be capricious.

SECOND LINE DRUGS

In inflammatory arthridities or connective tissue diseases not responding satisfactorily to NSAIDs, second line drugs are often used. They are sometimes called SARDs (slow anti-rheumatic drugs) or DMARDs (disease modifying anti-rheumatic drugs), and are characterized by the fact that complete remissions may be associated with their use and that weeks or months are required to note significant clinical effect. They are frequently used in conjunction with the more rapidly acting NSAIDs or even with small doses of corticosteroids.

There are three groups of drugs in this category: gold, penicillamine, and the antimalarials. All were discovered to have disease modifying activity by serendipity or faulty reasoning.

Gold

Inorganic gold salts were used at the turn of the 20th century as antibiotic agents. Forestier, a French physician, reasoned that rheumatoid arthritis was an infectious disease and successfully treated some rheumatoid patients with gold. Now that we are uncertain that a conventional infectious agent is the cause of the disease, there is no rationale for the proven success of this treatment.

The most important development, after the initial concept, was the shift to organic salts of gold which are much less toxic (thio-gluconates and thiomalates). At present, these must be injected. Myochrysine is a water clear solution of gold thio-malate and Solganal is a colloid suspension in oil of aurothioglucose. The latter seems less likely to cause some of the toxic reactions caused by this treatment.

Conveniently, a total dose of 1,000 mg of gold is given by weekly intramuscular doses of 50 mg each, after smaller test doses are given. If there is no demonstrable beneficial effect after 1,000 mg have been given, the trial is abandoned. This occurs with some 20% of patients. In another 60% or so, some beneficial effect is noted. The remaining 10–15% may achieve close to a complete remission.

While this treatment has been used primarily in rheumatoid arthritis, some patients with juvenile arthritis and psoriatic arthritis seem also to be improved, and the author has used it with seeming success in Reiter's syndrome. Gold it not recommended for any of the connective tissue diseases.

Gold treatment of about twenty weekly injections is cumbersome and potentially dangerous; this, in a setting of diseases which are rarely morbid. Toxicity includes serious reduction of any or all bone marrow elements (particularly platelets), renal insufficiency, nephrosis, skin rashes which may be severe, and glossitis. Neuropathies and gastrointestinal toxic effects are rare. Skin rashes mostly affect the trunk and may be intensely pruritic, occurring in an incidence of 20–25%. This is usually reversible on stopping the drug, and treatment may then be resumed using smaller doses. The other toxic effects are grounds for permanent termination of treatment.

Patients receiving gold should be closely monitored as most toxic effects are usually reversible. A convenient monitoring schedule is to obtain urinalysis and a blood count, including a platelet count, on alternate weeks.

Auranofin

An oral gold preparation, auranofin is now available. This drug also has a thiol group in its formulation. In an oral dose of six to nine mg daily, it has about the same time of onset of effect and perhaps slightly less total effectiveness as injected gold formulations. Side effects are also quite similar with the addition of about a 10–15% incidence of diarrhea which is clearly dose-related and sometimes unacceptable.

Despite these similarities, there are some biologic and pharmacologic differences between oral and injected gold. For example, oral gold seems to have a greater effect on inflammation, chemotaxis, aggregation and oxygen production by leukocytes to a greater degree than the injected form. Many practitioners are now using oral gold in preference to the intramuscular injectable preparation.

d-Penicillamine

Penicillamine was introduced by Jaffe in 1963 as a means for reducing serum titers of rheumatoid factor which, in complex with immunoglobulin G, is considered to be pathogenic in the joint inflammation of rheumatoid disease. Therapy at first employed a mixture of the d & 1 isomers of the drug which gave a high incidence of gastrointestinal toxicity. When the two isomers were separated, the d form was found to be less toxic and more effective. This is the form now used as an oral preparation. Ironically, the drug contains a thiol group similar to that found in the gold salts noted above and previously discounted as the efficacious component. Trials of other thiol compounds are now being undertaken in Europe.

As treatment schedules have become better defined, it is apparent that doses of d-penicillamine which are relatively safe and effective do not achieve the concentrations in plasma necessary to reliably reduce the rheumatoid factor titer. Thus, again we have no viable concept of how this drug works, although effects on cell traffic and immunological function are suspected. Jaffe's dictum, "go low, go slow," is established as a safe method of giving the drug with doses starting as low as 125 mg daily, and progressing by doubling to 1,000 mg daily over a six to twelve month period.

Toxicity is surprisingly similar to that of gold toxicity. (Perhaps not so surprising if the thiol moiety is taken into account.) In addition, there have been reports of initiation of other auto-immune disease such as lupus, polymyositis and myasthenia gravis. Monitoring by frequent urinalyses and blood counts is a must.

The drug is certainly useful for rheumatoid arthritis, probably useful for juvenile arthritis, and uncertain for the other arthridities. It is not recommended for connective tissue diseases nor for osteoarthritis.

Antimalarials

A legend concerning the use of anti-malarials in the rheumatic diseases tells us that when the British in World War II were pressed for manpower in their armed services, they switched able-bodied colonial administrators for disabled personnel at home. Since many of the colonies were in malarial zones, and prophylaxis with quinacrine (Atabrine) was then routine, some of the disabled new colonial administrators who had rheumatoid arthritis were placed on quinacrine and their arthritis forthwith improved.

A brief trial was performed in London and later a more formal trial of a second generation anti-malarial, chloroquine, was done in Canada on rheumatoid patients. Both trials were favorable and chloroquine, which everyone assumed was a very safe drug, was suggested for rheumatoid arthritis, in doses ten to twenty-fold higher than the anti-malarial dose. Some patients subsequently became totally and permanently blind and chloroquine was temporarily withdrawn from use as an anti-rheumatic drug. Only later was it appreciated that the very long half-life (five to seven days) led to an insupportable accumulation of the drug, especially in retinal tissues.

More recently, rheumatologists have become less timorous concerning the use of these drugs because of more sophisticated ophthalmological testing which can predict retinal damage long before it becomes clinically apparent, and because of reduced dose schedules. Additionally, new drugs of the 4-aminoquinoline chemical class seem less toxic to the eye.

Drugs utilized today are hydroxychloroquine (Plaquenil), quinacrine, and comolquin (Amodiaquin). Quinacrine, because it stains the skin yellow, is infrequently used, and the dose of comoquin is still uncertain. Hydroxychloroquine is most often used in adults in a 200–400 mg daily dose, although doses as low as 200 mg/three times-a-week sometimes seem successful.

Besides skin rashes and gastrointestinal upset, there are few side effects but the clinician is well-advised to have the patient get a preliminary ophthalmologic examination performed, and then again at three-to-six month intervals during therapy.

These drugs have weak anti-rheumatic effect on the average but seem to be helpful in some connective tissue syndromes, especially discoid lupus. Ankylosing spondylitis and osteoarthritis do not seem to benefit from any of the second line drugs.

THIRD LINE DRUGS

Immunosuppressives

If the second line drugs have failed or toxic effects preclude their use, then anti-metabolic or "immunosuppressive" drugs may be tried. The rationale for the use of these drugs is again somewhat speculative. They are all commonly used in the treatment of lymphoma and solid malignant tumor, the lymphocyte being particularly sensitive to their anti-metabolic effects. Since lymphocytes in T & B cell forms have much to do with humoral and cellular immunological events, and since these are precisely the events considered to be awry in the arthritis and connective tissue disorders, drugs which electively interfere with or kill certain lymphocyte populations might modify these diseases.

Some authors talk of immunomodulation or regulation as if a radio were being tuned. However, such precision eludes us still and these drugs act pretty much in shotgun fashion, disturbing both "good" and "bad" lymphocytes and monocytes. More telling is the fact that when these drugs have a clinical effect, there may be no measurable effect on any immunological function. It is possible that these drugs may affect mononuclear cell traffic and polymorphonuclear function as a more likely explanation for their efficacy.

The drugs most often used in this category are selected primarily because they can be given orally. They are methotrexate, azathioprine (Imuran), cyclophosphamide (Cytoxan), and chlorambucil. All of these are effective in rheumatoid arthritis and the connective tissue diseases, although in inflammatory arthritis conditions, excepting rheumatoid arthritis or psoriatic arthritis, we have only anecdotal experience to draw upon.

It must be discussed with the patient and made clear that these drugs have serious acute effects and ongoing potential for even more devastating problems. For example, some of these may cause permanent sterility through a toxic effect on the ovaries and testes. If a female patient happens to be unknowingly pregnant, there may be serious consequences for the fetus since these drugs are protoplasmic poisons. There is some evidence that lymphomas and solid malignant tumors may be induced with these drugs, particularly with cyclophosphamide. Cyclophosphamide, in particular, may also be associated with permanent hair loss. Since these drugs are most often used in diseases which have a female predominance, the physician must be quite open and frank with the patient in terms of options and potential adverse effects which may be particularly devastating to women.

While toxic bone marrow effects are common to all the drugs and are potentially permanent, methotrexate at least has a possible "rescue" feature that the others do not. Folic acid is a specific antidote for methotrexate in that the drug apparently works by competitively inhibiting the physiological effect of folic acid on cell growth and maintenance. Methotrexate, however, is the most hepatotoxic of this group, particularly so in patients who drink to excess. Chronic hepatitis and cirrhosis may occur.

In actual controlled trials, cyclophosphamide works more rapidly (often within several weeks) than the others, but its bone marrow, hair follicle, and sex organ effects are greater in incidence. Azathioprine works more slowly, and in the case of rheumatoid arthritis and renal lupus, more unreliably. Methotrexate has been used in psoriatic arthritis and rheumatoid arthritis and safer courses of treatment with methotrexate have been recently established. There is very little literature on chlorambucil. Cyclophosphamide works very well, to the extent that it is the drug of choice in Wegener's granulomatosis.

Both cyclophosphamide and azathioprine interact with allopurinol, a drug used in gout. Since increased blood levels of uric acid occur in treatment with all of these drugs due to the cellular damage caused, physicians are often tempted to treat this situation with allopurinol. In the case of cyclophosphamide, allopurinol has been found to increase the half-life of the drug, possibly increasing its already toxic effect on bone marrow. Cyclophosphamide is toxic to cells because it is an alkylating agent related to the nitrogen mustards.

The first metabolite of azathioprine is 6-mercaptopurine (6-MP), another potent cytotoxic agent which interferes with the synthesis of adenine and guanine, and therefore the further synthesis of DNA. 6-MP is further metabolized to inactive compounds by the enzyme xanthine oxidase. Allopurinol competitively inhibits xanthine oxidase and may produce toxic levels of 6-MP.

If both azathioprine and allopurinol must be given together, reduction of the azathioprine dose to 25% of its usual dose seems safe.

While these drugs are usually given in doses expressed as milligrams per kilogram in oncological patients, little attention is paid to this by rheumatologists who commonly give doses up to 150 mg/daily of azathioprine and cyclophosphamide to patients of average size. While the dose schedule of methotrexate is still somewhat unsettled, one to two consecutive days of 2.5 mg oral or intramuscular doses are usually well-tolerated and can be raised to as much as two consecutive days per week of 15 mg per day, with care. Frequent blood counts must be obtained with all these drugs.

In summary, cyclophosphamide and azathioprine are effective enough to warrant their use in extremely aggressive and destructive rheumatoid arthritis or progressive renal disease in lupus. Methotrexate is more commonly used in rheumatoid or psoriatic arthritis. None of these drugs are effective in osteoarthritis.

Corticosteroids

The steroids have been left for last in this discussion because they have very specialized uses. Possibly their most common use among rheumatologists at the present time is in the form of local injections, with systemic use a distant second. Corticosteroids have extraordinarily powerful anti-inflammatory effects, much greater than the NSAIDs. The mechanism by which this is accomplished is complex.

Steroids sequester mononuclear cells, especially T cells and monocytes, out of the circulation and into reticulo-endothelial depots and the bone marrow. The same effect diminishes eosinophiles and basophiles in the circulation. Steroids also stabilize membranes, thus repairing or preventing the leakage of plasma components and cells of the capillaries. There are profound effects on cell function with cortisone-like drugs easily entering into the cell to bind to constituents in the cytosol which promote the manufacture of certain substances at the expense of others.

Membrane stabilization also prevents arachidonic acid from being formed, therefore inhibiting production of prostaglandin products of both the cyclo-oxygenase and lipoxygenase pathways. However, these powerful effects are also associated with a variety of side effects, and worse, are subject to tachyphylaxis, a term describing the necessity for constantly increasing the dose of a drug to maintain the same effect.

Adverse effects include hypertension, salt and water retention, hyperglycemia, osteoporosis, and reduction of resistance to infection. There is some controversy as to whether or not peptic ulcer is produced by steroids or if they protect against it. In high doses, they can certainly cause stress ulcers along the greater curvature of the stomach. Because of the changes in cell metabolism induced, steroids cause myopathy, a weakening of the muscular support structure of joints which is disastrous in arthritis. Prednisone does this less so than other steroid preparations and is, therefore, preferable in long-term therapy.

Forms of steroids used in rheumatology are oral tablets of prednisone, the drug most used, and the very potent halogenated compounds such as triamcinolone and dexamethasone. All of these are synthetic derivatives of the natural adrenal hormone, cortisone. In vivo, cortisone release is triggered by hormones supplied by the pituitary. The giving of corticosteroid therapy will lead to the eventual suppression of the pituitary adrenal axis with actual atrophy of the adrenal cortex. This atrophy occurs within a few weeks after the onset of therapy and may not be fully repaired until a year after cessation of therapy.

The stress of surgical procedures, trauma or systemic infection should be treated with corticosteroid doses for at least a year following therapy. Patients under stress require cortisone to mobilize body defenses, and if it is missing, may go into shock and die.

Methyl prednisolone and cortisol are soluble corticosteroid products capable of intravenous or intramuscular administration. Intraarticular injectable forms are often suspension of methyl prednisolone or triamcinolone.

Corticosteroids have very little acute toxicity and may be used in very large parenteral doses when the situation warrants. The more serious side effects become apparent with continuing use beyond a few weeks and are dose dependent. In such conditions as lupus crisis, polyarteritis and dermatomyositis, high dose therapy may be life-saving. In the arthridities, such as rheumatoid arthritis, they are occasionally used as a rapidly acting bridge while the delayed effect of a SARD or DMARD is building up. When this occurs, steroids should be discarded by tapering.

ANCILLARY DRUG THERAPIES

Patients faced with chronic pain and the uncertainties of incurable disease often become anxious and depressed. Clinicians frequently treat their patients with anxiolytic agents such as diazepams (Librium, Valium, etc.), or potent narcotics such as the oxycodeinone combinations (Percodan, Percocet). Except in extraordinary circumstances, this is inappropriate therapy. At best, anxiolytic agents only further depress and the tolerance produced by strong narcotics will eventually preclude their usefulness and only complicate the course of the disease with the production of habituation.

A sound relationship between patient, physician and other health personnel is of paramount importance in maintaining the morale and cooperation in what is often a continuing uphill battle. In the case of drugs, mild analgesics such as acetaminophen (Tylenol) are helpful alone or in combination with the less potent narcotics, codeine and propoxyphene. These can be given over prolonged periods with little or no tolerance as long as their use is carefully explained to the patient and monitored.

More recently, as our understanding of the neuro-transmission and central nervous system pathways of pain increases, uses can be made of what is already known. The anti-depressive drugs amitriptyline (Elavil) and doxepin (Sinequan) have serotonin augmenting properties. Serotonin is a neurotransmitter of a brain initiated neural pathway which descends to modulate incoming pain sensation at the spinal cord level. This pathway seems to become exhausted in the face of chronic pain and the patients become very sensitive to serotonergic and anti-cholinergic effects of these drugs. Therefore, they should be used in very small doses, given only at bedtime, with the dose increased very cautiously. A proper dose seems to normalize the sleep pattern and to eventually modify the overall degree of pain.

SUMMARY

Drug therapy in the rheumatic diseases is only one of the modalities available to medicine in total therapy, but it is an important one. Except for antibiotic treatment of infected joints, there are no drugs that cure nor reliably contain the progression of these diseases. However, in their ability to alleviate pain, aid in preservation of function and maintain quality of life, they are very useful adjuncts, and the understanding of their pharmacological characteristics is necessary for their proper use.

SUGGESTED READINGS

"Oral Gold in Therapy in Rheumatoid Arthritis: Auranofin." Proceedings of a Symposium. *Amer. J. Med.*, Suppl., Dec. 1983.

Gottlieb N: "Gold Compounds." *Textbook of Rheumatology*. Second Edition, Vol. 1, Ch. 52. Eds. Kelly W, Harris E, Ruddy S and Sledge C, WJ Saunders & Co., Phila., 1985.

Huskisson EC: "Anti-Rheumatic Drugs." *Clinical Pharmacology and Therapeutics Series*. Vol. 3. East Sussex, Great Britain, and New York City: Praeger Publishers, 1983.

Jaffe IA: "D-Penicillamine." *Bull. Rheum. Dis.*, 28:948–52, series 1977–78.

Kantor TG: "Salicylates in the 80's." *Clin. Rheum. in Practice,* 1:151–72, 1983.

Kantor TG: "Selecting the Appropriate NSAID." *Drug Therapy,* 14:59–66, Feb. 1984.

Kantor TG: "Ketoprofen: A Review of its Pharmacologic and Clinical Properties." *Pharmacology,* 6(3):93–103, 1986.

Kelley, W.N., et al. Ed. Textbook of Rheumatology. WB Saunders, Phila. 3rd ed. 1989. Ch. 50, Methotrexate, Weinblatt, N.E.

TABLE 14-1
NSAIDs USED IN CLINICAL PRACTICE*

Class	*Compound*	*Trade Name*	*Half-Life (H)*
Pyrazoles	Oxyphenbutazone	Oxalid, Tandearil	72–96
	Phenylbutazone		84–96
Indole acetic acids	Indomethacin	Indocin	3.4–.5
	Sulindac	Clinoril	13 (active metabolite)
	Tolmetin	Tolectin	1
Phenylalkanoic acids	Fenoprofen	Nalfon	3
	Ibuprofen	Motrin, Rufen	2–3
	Naproxen	Naprosyn	13
	Naproxen sodium	Anaprox	
	Ketoprofin	Orudis	
Fenamic Acids	Meclofenamate	Meclomen	2–5
	Mefenamic acid	Ponstel	2–5
Oxicams	Piroxicam	Feldene	44–50
Salicylates	Aspirin		3–16
	Choline magnesium trisalicylate	Trilisate	7–18
	Diflunisal	Dolobid	8
	Magnesium salicylate		2–2.5
	Salsalate	Arcylate, Disalcid	8

*Other NSAIDs introduced more recently into clinical use include flurbiprofen (Ansaid) and diclofenac (Voltaran), (eds.).

CHAPTER 15

SURGERY

Roger Levy, M.D.

INTRODUCTION

One of the brightest chapters in the history of orthopaedic surgery has been the remarkable advances in the surgical treatment of arthritis made possible by the startling technological advances of the past 15 years. The advent of joint replacement implant arthroplasty has entirely revolutionized the surgical approach to arthritic joints. In a predictable way, patients with severe arthritic problems involving the hip and knee, can be routinely evaluated for surgery with high expectation of success. Patients with involvement of other joints such as the shoulder also can be benefited very greatly. Patients with problems involving the elbow, wrist and hand, and the ankle and foot joints can be treated by a judicious combination of new and old procedures.

The startling successes of the joint replacement experience has lead to this same technology being utilized for a variety of other problems such as primary and secondary tumors of bone. The orthopaedic treatment of many childhood joint difficulties has likewise been altered by the success in adult life of joint replacement to direct therapy so that an abnormal joint in early childhood can be made at least good enough for later reconstructive surgery as an adult.

It is in the face of all this success that the problems inherent in substituting a mechanical replacement for an original biological part must be considered. One can state that any artificial joint will ultimately mechanically fail if it is subjected to enough stress for a sufficient period of time. This is to say that if artificial joint implants are of necessity placed in patients whose anticipated lifespan and use of that joint will be sufficient then ultimately revision surgery may be required to replace the worn or loosened artificial joint. It does not diminish the value of these procedures to recognize this most important fact. It therefore becomes an important philosophical aspect for the patient and other health professionals to appreciate that these joints must be regarded as a great luxury, to be appreciated and protected, but never abused.

Any indication for surgical treatment of an arthritic joint always presumes that the patient has had an ample, well designed, and thorough trial of non-surgical treatment. Non-surgical treatment includes as its mainstay, rest and relief from mechanical stress on the joint. This often necessitates weight reduction or the temporary or permanent use of external walking aids such as walkers, crutches and canes. Splints to temporarily immobilize an inflamed joint in a position of function are still valuable adjuncts to treatment. Careful, and thoughtful programs of physical therapy are extremely important but must not be followed in a routinized manner since there is so much variation between patients. Unless medical contraindications exist, a thorough trial of non-steroidal anti-inflammatory drugs as well as analgesics should be attempted. Joint replacement surgery is rarely an emergency and timing can be arranged to best fit the patient's life.

It is important for all members of the health care team to recognize the fact that the patient must be regarded as a fellow human being rather than as a collection of painful and anatomically imperfect joints.

In this chapter an attempt will be made to cover the key points of surgery for arthritis. It will be impossible to cover in detail every aspect of the technique of surgery or of every possible new development currently on the horizon. It is the philosophy of arthritis surgery that is intended to be transmitted. No form of medical treatment can be relied upon to achieve uniformly perfect results without possibility of disabling or life-threatening complications. The arthritis surgery discussed in this chapter is no exception to this rule. The choice of the best possible alternative for a given patient is a burden to be shared by the physician, other members of the health care team, the patient and the patient's family. Well performed and properly indicated surgical procedures can be complicated by myriad problems of damage to bones, blood vessels, nerves, and virtually any tissue of the body as well as reactions to drugs or blood products. Fortunately, these problems are uncommon, indeed.

GOALS OF SURGERY

The decision to proceed to a surgical procedure in the arthritic patient is a complex step in decision making. Numerous factors must be analyzed and separately considered for the individual patient and then synthesized into an appropriate decision model for the individual patient. The decision to perform a surgical procedure must be regarded as one step in a series of steps involved in the care of the total patient. Numerous factors are called into consideration. These factors include but are not limited, to the following;

1. Age of the patient
2. The future use of the joint
3. Unilateral or bilateral

4. One extremity or several
5. The general medical status of the patient
6. The psychological status of the patient
7. The cost and benefits of surgery at the present time
8. The consequences of not operating at that time

Whenever possible, objective score systems should be utilized. Numerous systems exist for the evaluation of individual joint problems such as those at the hip or at the knee. An example of hip evaluation score systems would be the modified D'Aubigne-Postel system that was popularized by Sir John Charnley, the innovator of total hip replacement, or the equally popular Harris Hip Scale. A variety of knee evaluation systems likewise are in utilization ordinarily depending upon a one hundred point scale. The author has utilized the Charnley modified D'Aubigne-Postel system for many years and finds it to be a most suitable method for evaluation of preoperative function and post-operative improvement.

This system utilizes a one to six score for the separate categories of pain, walking ability, and total range of motion. The system proceeds from severe to normal from one to six. A normal individual without pain in the hips, walking normal distances, and enjoying an average range of motion at the hip joint would have an evaluation of 6-6-6. A prefix letter A, B, or C is also utilized. A indicates a unilateral hip involvement; B indicates a bilateral hip involvement; and C indicates another factor present which would tend to minimize the patient's anticipated lifespan. This system points out many of the factors inherent in the evaluation of a patient for surgery including the important factor of long-term durability, which, of course would be related to the patient's anticipated lifespan from the time of joint replacement as well as the relative use to which the joint would be subjected. A typical patient undergoing hip replacement surgery would ordinarily have a score that had dropped from the normal six down to a score at the three levels in the various categories. Post-operatively, most patients after hip replacement, will once again regain a score at the six level for relief of pain and frequently at the six level for walking ability and range of motion as well.

The author has utilized a one hundred point knee evaluation score. On this score system an individual with normal knee function will typically get a score of one hundred points. This is to indicate that one need not be an olympic performer to obtain one hundred points. Patients who undergo knee replacement surgery will typically have scores of less than fifty points. Post-operatively, patients will usually regain eighty-five out of one hundred points. Many patients will regain scores in the high nineties but, in general, one should anticipate a postoperative score in the mid eighties.

None of these individual score systems are reliable for evaluating the total function of the individual human being who presents with the problem in a given joint or several joints, as the case may be. It is important to recognize the fact that the patient is not a given joint but is a human being operating under adverse circumstances in a world of obstacles and difficulties. The goal of surgery can be simply stated as an attempt to help the patient regain independence. If one analyzes that statement you realize that this means that surgery is directed toward the relief of pain from a given joint, toward the restoration of lost functions relative to that joint and to achieving those goals in the simplest and most expeditious way for that patient, exposing him/her to the least amount of risk. It is the sum of these parts that leads to either the maintenance or restoration of independent function as a human being.

The technological advances of the past one and one-half decades have brought an extraordinary change in the surgeons ability to help the arthritic patient to achieve improved function and pain relief. The beneficial value of joint replacement surgery is now extremely well established. Hundreds of thousands of afflicted individuals have been helped toward a restoration of more normal life by total hip replacement, total knee replacement, as well as replacement of other joints. In general, these procedures have had a very high success rate. However, their success has also brought along a new set of problems related to the late mechanical failure of these individual parts. We should assume as a working hypothesis that any artificial joint, no matter how well designed in terms of its engineering concepts and no matter how well implanted in that given patient by excellence of meticulous surgical technique, will ultimately wear out if used hard enough and long enough. All of the attempts to improve the function of joint implants has been directed toward improving the durability factor of these implants in the body.

It is appropriate at this point to spend some time on the shortcomings of joint replacement surgery since much of the remainder of this chapter will deal with the benefits to be expected from such surgery. Total hip replacement consists of a metal femoral prosthesis and a high density polyethylene plastic acetabular component, each one fastened to its respective bone with polymethylmethacrylate acrylic bone cement. At the time of inception of total hip replacement, it was thought that it would be the plastic acetabular socket which would be the weak point of the system. It was anticipated that the metal ball would ultimately bore through the plastic acetabulum. This was believed to be the case because John Charnley's original work utilizing a metal femoral component with a plastic acetabular component of a different fabrication resulted in premature wearing of the plastic components. High density polyethylene has proved to be a relatively durable component in the body, at least in the hip. The weak point of the system would appear to be at the prosthesis-cement-bone interface. Late mechanical loosening of the component tends to occur at this point in a small percentage of patients. This tendency can be reduced by strict attention to technical details at the time of surgery, by improved utilization of the cement substance and very significantly by careful selection of patients to avoid when possible, relatively young, relatively hyperactive individuals who will tend to abuse the implant. Research is currently proceeding toward the possibility of either improved forms of cement or else eliminating the need for cement completely by means of bony ingrowth into a porous surface on the given implant. It is not known whether this will result in improved durability of such components but it is anticipated that the use of such components may make later revision surgery easier if it should be necessary.

The age of the patient is an important factor, therefore, in evaluating a patient for surgery in arthritis, if the patient is old enough then one can anticipate the long term durability of a joint replacement being secure enough so that later revision surgery would probably not be required. On the other hand, if the patient is young enough the potential for joint replacement surgery requiring revision at a later date may be so great that one would clearly elect to do some other procedure first in hopes of "buying time" until the patient's age would be more appropriate for joint replacement.

The use to which the joint will be put is very much a parallel issue. Even in an older individual, one would be relatively loathe to recommend joint replacement surgery to an individual who has only one joint involved and who wishes to return to active athletics following successful surgery. Under these circumstances one might anticipate that the greatly increased load bearing under conditions of running as compared to conditions of walking (3–4 times greater) might be too great for reasonable durability of the given joint. On the other hand, one might be more inclined to recommend joint replacement surgery to an even younger patient with polyarthritis whose other ailments would necessitate that the patient would never be a very long distance walker under any circumstance.

Whether a condition is unilateral or bilateral is also of consequence as is the related issue of whether or not the upper and lower extremities are also involved. In selecting a procedure for a patient with monoarticular arthritis choices are more clear cut because the patient's return to function is much more predictable. In the patient with polyarthritis, the presence of other areas of joint involvement creates special problems of patient selection. The author has adopted the phrase "rehabilitate to the next joint" as the philosophical guideline for patients with several joints involved, such as the large population of patients with rheumatoid arthritis. In these, and in other patients, one joint may appear to be the most prominently involved joint. The left hip may be extremely painful in a patient who also has bilateral knee involvement. The patient may be less aware of the knee involvement because the extreme limitations placed on weight bearing by the very symptomatic left hip may prevent that individual from ever walking for enough steps to ever begin to stress the already damaged knee joints. The patient, surgeon, and other members of the health care team must be alert to the fact that following successful rehabilitation of that left hip the patient will no doubt once again be able to walk enough distance to begin to put stress on the already involved knee joints. Planning should proceed at the initial time of surgery for a reasonable program for the knees. For example, an exercise program, bracing, or consideration for reconstructive surgery on the knees may all have to be considered prior to doing the first operation. Timing of procedures is likewise important. A patient with rheumatoid arthritis with involvement of various joints in the upper extremities as well as in the lower extremities, may have great difficulty in resuming walking activities following an otherwise successful lower extremity joint reconstructive procedure because the patient's difficulties in using external walking aids have not been properly considered as part of the rehabilitation program. Patients may need to have a procedure selected for them so that they can perform various activities of daily living which may be difficult with either bilateral lower extremity involvement or the combination of both upper and lower extremity involvement. The early participation of the occupational therapist is a must in such situations.

The patient's general medical condition must be carefully evaluated. It is understood that no patient would ever be operated upon unless they are in an appropriate medical condition to tolerate the given procedure.

In a more general sense the patient's medical condition needs to be evaluated in terms of the change that the joint reconstruction will make in her life. In today's world of advanced technology, it is by no means unusual for the orthopaedic arthritis surgeon to perform joint replacement procedures on patients who have had vascular reconstructions in the lower extremities for the release of peripheral vascular obstruction as well as coronary bypass procedures for the relief of myocardial ischemia. Patients with artificial joint replacements may also have artificial heart valves. The problem of evaluating the patient's general medical status becomes more acute in facing the reconstruction of the severely crippled polyarthritic. There exist within the population of patients with rheumatoid arthritis those with the most severe form of the disease and who may be completely crippled by bilateral involvement of many joints in the lower and upper extremities. Sometimes these patients can be operated upon in the course of one long hospitalization in which several joints will be reconstructed. At times, simultaneous bilateral joint reconstruction can be performed by either one or two teams of surgeons at the hips and knees or alternatively, a hip and knee replacement can be performed in the same lower extremity in the course of the same anesthesia. We ordinarily prefer to wait three weeks between procedures in the rheumatoid patient who is typically on steroid medications as well as immunosuppressive drugs. At times the reconstructive program must be halted because the patient's general physical reserve is not sufficient to allow the patient to continue without a relief period of several months to regain her strength. The reconstructive orthopaedist must be physician as well as surgeon in his judgment in these instances.

The patient's emotional status must also be considered. Many patients with involvement of a single joint may feel suddenly isolated from the rest of their peer group or suddenly "made old" by the advent of the arthritis. It is important for these patients to help them to distinguish between their individual identity and worth as a human being and their particular joint problem. Likewise, the patient with multiple joint involvement does not have the liberty of looking upon a single joint reconstruction as a renaissance and an alleviation of all vestiges of the rheumatoid process from her body. Some patients with polyarthritis will suffer from chronic depression and often exist in a long term family support system which, at times, tends to encourage them not to relinquish their disability. Here too, gentle handling of the patient is required so that she can gradually begin to appreciate the difference in her lifestyle that improvement in a given joint or joints may enable them to accomplish.

One must stress the care with which post-operative physical therapy must be administered. The reconstructive surgery sets the stage for improvement of the patient and it is therefore important and obvious to all that the patient will benefit from a gradual program of physical and occupational therapy designed to restore muscle tone and range of motion and coordinated use of the extremities. In general, however, patients do not lack for efforts in this regard and the usual error is one of excess rather than one of too little therapy. It is especially in the rheumatoid patient where an extremely small margin for error exists. The patient and therapist try to pursue as active a program as possible to improve power in muscles made weak by long months or years of disuse and disability as well as to try to restore motion to joints that previously were either stiff or unstable. The rheumatoid patient frequently will be made symptomatically worse for long periods of time by brief excesses of effort in physical therapy. The author usually does not recommend passive assisted motion of the involved joint. Motion should be active with very little assistance on the part of the therapist. The rule of thumb with the rheumatoid patient should be to err on the side of conservatism.

REGIONAL CONSIDERATIONS

The Hip

It was the advent of total hip replacement arthroplasty which ushered in a new era of arthritis surgery. The hip remains the area of leading advance of implant technology with regard to reconstructive surgery. Total hip replacement arthroplasty has changed in subtle but significant ways since it was first described. Seemingly modest changes in the conformation of the design of the femoral stem as well as the potential for metal encasement of the high density polyethylene acetabular components have led to improved performance characteristics of current day implant components as compared to those used in the earlier years of this procedure. Similarly, the development of ultra-high strength metals has increased the strength of these components without unduly increasing the cross sectional area so that an individualized test fit of component to bone can be achieved for a given patient with very little potential for fatigue failure of the metal component itself. The relatively few cases of high-density polyethylene failure have largely been attributed to errors in component design and those characteristics are no longer incorporated in current day implants. This again points to the weak point of any hip implant system being at the juncture of the implant and the bone whether that takes place through the medium of polymethylmethacrylate cement to stabilize the components in the bone or else via porous ingrowth surfaces for potential direct bony attachment. Current day techniques of cement utilization involve the use of low viscosity cement so that the best possible interdigitation of the cement into the bone can be obtained. Additional pressurization is performed to maximize the mechanical interdigitation and interlocking of the cement into the bone which is the means by which the relative surface area is increased and thus stabilizes the component. The bearing surface of the metal against the high density polyethylene provides for a relatively low friction interface while the maximum interdigitation of cement into bone provides for an extremely high frictional resistance to movement. The same type of interlock is hoped for by developers of porous ingrowth mechanisms. A variety of these porous ingrowth mechanisms are at use at the present time, including rough surfaced ceramic or metal surfaces, but they are still in a developmental stage. The reproducibility of surgical technique in case after case has been an extremely important feature in the success of total hip replacement surgery as well. The closer the surgeon can approximate the idealized engineering situation, theoretically the greater the possibility for long term durability.

The ideal patient for a hip replacement would be a patient in the 60's or older with relatively good quality bone stock. The younger the patient and the greater the degree of osteoporosis, the greater the potentials for long term mechanical loosening of the components.

The average patient undergoing a hip replacement procedure is one who has had a thorough trial of conservative treatment including rest, the use of an external walking aid such as a cane, and a sufficient trial of non-steroidal oral antiinflammatory agents and analgesics. Human beings differ markedly in their perception of pain and in their ability to tolerate it. Pain occurring at rest and which regularly wakes the patient from sleep generally can be regarded as a symptom of intractable pain which will require surgical treatment. The typical patient undergoing hip replacement can expect a relatively complete relief of pain at the hip and consequent upon that, a restoration of walking ability to the extent that the remainder of the patient's physical being can permit. That is to say that if the patient does not have other musculoskeletal areas of involvement nor any cardiorespiratory or vascular problems which would serve to limit walking ability then unlimited walking can be expected. This may prove to be several blocks or several miles. The use of a cane as a permanent requirement for walking should not be anticipated although in many geriatric patients who have used a cane previously an impaired sense of balance can be very well compensated for with the light but judicious use of a cane. Range of motion is usually ample after hip replacement surgery. A considerable degree of effort has been directed toward developing hip replacement components which will have relatively wide ranges of motion on engineering bench testing. Our own experience, however, confirms to us the clinical fact that the amount of motion that will occur in the operated hip is predetermined by the amount of motion present in the opposite normal hip. Patients will usually get within 5–10 degrees the amount of motion present in the contralateral hip after hip surgery. This is because the way one sits, stands and conducts various activities is determined by that fact. Early motion may exceed this but with full healing it is rare for patients to have more motion in the operated hip than on the normal opposite one. An exception to this rule is the presence of very limited motion in the contralateral hip. The average patient after hip replacement surgery can expect to be able to reach their foot for foot care or putting on shoes and stockings. This is not universally present and can be a problem particularly in obese individuals.

Post-operative care usually involves protected weight bearing. Surgeons disagree as to the need for how much and how long this is to be used. It is our general procedure to insist upon double support for fully six weeks after surgery. This can be accomplished with the use of a walker, forearm crutches, or conventional crutches. A second six weeks of the use of a single cane in the opposite hand is likewise recommended. Many surgeons will prefer a shorter period of external support. Our rationale for insisting upon the described program is to allow for as much bone healing at the cement bone interface as can possibly occur without imposing excessive weight bearing pressures during the early phase. A thin line of necrosis is always present at the area of cement bone or porous implant bone interface and needs to be protected so that healing can occur in the early phases.

Relatively simple exercise routines are likewise initiated in the early postoperative period. It is our routine to have patients out of bed on the day immediately after surgery. Patients can stand or sit in a chair with the hip joint not bent beyond 90° and with the knees apart so that the hip remains abducted. Early activity following surgery probably does not improve hip function in the long run but it would appear to have a beneficial effect in reducing the incidence of undesirable complications such as phlebitis, pulmonary embolus, pulmonary atelectasis, skin breakdown, and possibly, confusion. The patient's hip will ordinarily tolerate the early activity and allow for the beneficial effects described. Hip exercises can be relatively simple and should be designed to improve the power of flexion, abduction, and extension, at the hip. We usually demonstrate simple hip flexion, abduction and extension exercises to the patient in the standing position since they are able to do it relatively easily that way and are encouraged by the early efforts. Patients are instructed in appropriate protective weight bearing but should immediately begin a normal heel-toe gait to avoid the incorporation of maladapted walking patterns. As the weeks progress patients will gradually increase the number of repetitions and intensity of the exercises. Alternative forms of exercise can be incorporated to maintain the interest of the patient. We frequently recommend swimming as a beneficial therapeutic exercise at approximately six weeks post-operative for those patients for whom swimming would come easily and to whom access to a pool is convenient. This is also of value to initiate these patients into swimming as a permanent form of aerobic activity for their general benefit in the future since other types of endurance exercise would tend to be possibly contraindicated.

Infection after total hip replacement surgery is a rarity both in the early or late stages. Isolated cases will occur but are few and far between. The use of "clean room technology" has been of great value in reducing the apparent incidence of infection. Late infections appear to be of hematogenous spread and for this reason patients with any joint replacement are advised to take prophylactic antibiotics at the time of any procedure that might cause a transient bacteremia such as dental procedures or urinary tract manipulations.

Alternative procedures at the hip

Alternative procedures need to be considered for those patients who are too young or too active to logically benefit from total hip replacement surgery. These patients are typically young people with single joint involvement although not necessarily limited to this group. Prior to the advent of total hip replacement surgery patients with arthritis of the hip were treated by a variety of techniques. The results in terms of frequency of success, tended to be about 80% successful as compared to the 95% success rate usually quoted for hip replacement. In addition, the quality of pain relief and restoration of function tended to approximate but not equal that enjoyed by patients undergoing hip replacement. Nevertheless, if the patient would logically be too young then alternative procedures must be considered. At the present time, these alternative operations would be either an osteotomy at the hip or else a hip fusion.

An osteotomy means cutting across the bone. At the hip this would be performed either below the ball (femoral osteotomy) or above the socket (pelvic osteotomy). In either instance after the bone is cut it is manipulated into an improved mechanical position and held in place with a metal fixation device until the bone has healed. A hip fusion is performed by denuding the joint surfaces. The exposed raw bone edges are pressed together and held firmly with a metal fixation device. This sends the same signal to the body as does a broken bone. Bone grows across the surfaces to heal the fracture and the joint becomes solidified by bone. A variation on a total hip replacement, surface replacement at the hip was introduced in the late 1970's. This procedure preserved the bone stock of the femoral head but reshaped it.

A metal cap was cemented onto the femoral head with a thin walled plastic acetabular component cemented into the acetabulum. It was the hope that this procedure would prove to be more suitable for the younger patient and likewise conserve bone stock. Unfortunately, an extremely high incidence of revision surgery was required in this group and for the most part its use has been discontinued except at a few centers where its potential value is still being explored in long term studies. At the time of this writing, surface replacement is reserved for those centers.

Osteotomy at the hip can be either of the femur or of the pelvis. Certain young patients, possibly even up to the early twenties, can be considered for a pelvic osteotomy designed to improve coaptation of the femoral head and acetabulum and to provide broader surface areas of contact and thereby improve weight transmission across the hip joint and hopefully preserve the joint for many years, while at the same time providing a potential anatomical joint of improved characteristics for later reconstructive surgery. More commonly, femoral osteotomies are employed. These are usually in the subtrochanteric or intertrochanteric area and are designed to tilt the femoral head into an improved weight bearing position of better congruency with the acetabulum. This procedure likewise improves weight transmission across the hip joint and probably also serves to temporarily decompress the inflamed capsular and ligamentous structures and may also alter the hemodynamics of the hip joint. All of these factors together can result in pain relief. Appropriate radiographic studies are done preoperatively to determine if the hip can be improved by this procedure. Patients must have an ample range of motion preoperatively to allow for this procedure to be performed. Relative stiffening of the hip appears too frequently if there is less than 70° of flexion preoperatively.

These procedures can be worthwhile and result in considerable pain relief for many years. Patients often limp as a consequence of these procedures if a varus osteotomy is performed or may have some malalignment of the knee joint if a valgus osteotomy is performed. The patient must understand that these procedures are elected in order to delay the ultimate need for hip replacement surgery in a young patient in their 30's or 40's. Hip fusion or arthrodesis of the hip is a time honored procedure that needs to be considered for the young patient with monoarticular hip involvement. This procedure will completely eliminate all motion at the hip by creating bone growth across the hip joint. It will also result in a painless hip capable of very hard use and so can be considered as a procedure of choice, perhaps, in a young patient who is going to pursue an extremely active lifestyle with regard to occupation or recreation. Late problems after hip fusion tend to involve excess weight bearing strains in the low back area as the lumbar spine will make up for the motion in the anterior-posterior plane that is lost by the hip fusion. In addition, the contralateral hip and the ipsilateral knee will likewise tend to suffer excessive wear to make up for some of the rotational motion that was lost by the hip fusion. It is possible to consider doing a hip fusion in a young patient with conversion to a hip replacement, possibly twenty years later. Considering the marked advances that have taken place in the technology of implant surgery in the past ten to fifteen years it is difficult to project what the technology of twenty years hence will provide.

For those patients who have early osteonecrosis of the hip where a prompt diagnosis can be made, it is possible that many of them can be salvaged by the procedure of core decompression of the femoral head. Early studies suggest that not only is pain relieved, but that the process is arrested provided the procedure can be done in the extremely early stages.

Paramount in the surgical treatment of arthritis at the hip, must be the intelligent understanding on the part of the patient that modification in lifestyle is a necessity following any procedure in order to enhance the ultimate durability of the result.

The Knee

Patients with pain and disability related to the knee must be evaluated in a similar fashion for surgical procedures. As a prerequisite to any surgical indication it is understood that the patient must have had a thorough trial of non-surgical treatment. This would include the need for rest, modification of activities, the use of nonsteroidal antiinflammatory drugs and analgesics and possibly the use of a brace and a cane. Bracing for the knee can be a problem. The use of a long leg double upright brace extending from the foot to the ischium is what is truly required to stabilize the knee and relieve weight bearing pressures from it. Few patients would be able to tolerate this type of heavy and cumbersome orthosis. The use of lightweight knee cages can be helpful for selected patients. Problems can exist in obtaining proper fit of these relatively light braces in patients who have an obese thigh with its typical inverted pyramidal shape. With regard to the knee, the patient's age and the use to which the joint will be put are likewise extremely important factors.

Total knee replacement arthroplasty needs to be approached even more critically than hip replacement arthroplasty. The past ten years have seen the progressive development of a wide range of knee implants. Many of these implant systems are reported by the originators to have extremely low incidences of complications and extremely high success rates. It is then somewhat surprising to see these extremely salutary reports followed by the introduction of another version of that implant designed to improve upon its function and to eliminate complications which reportedly occur so seldom. At the present time, considerable improvement does exist in knee replacement systems. Improved design allows for abnormal weight bearing forces to be minimized on the implant. The development of latest generation instrumentation likewise helps the surgeon to be able to insert the implants in a reproducible manner in case after case so that the implant in the patient can more closely approximate the idealized engineering testing of that implant. The durability of knee replacement implants is at the present time more suspect than in the hip and consequently, a considerable degree of conservatism needs to be employed in selecting patients for these procedures. On the other hand, porous surfaced implants designed to help eliminate or at least minimize the amount of cement to be utilized at the time of surgery seems somewhat more advanced than in the hip so that later revision surgeries may not provide as many problems in the future as they have in the past.

The selection of a patient for total knee replacement arthroplasty must take into account the patient's age and level of activity. In the case of patients with monoarticular knee arthritis and no other restraining factors, knee replacement needs to be restricted to the geriatric age group, in the opinion of the author. However, there are many clinical situations where judgment must rule and where the surgeon and patient may agree that knee replacement is the best possible of all alternatives even though the patient does not meet the idealized situation. In the case of patients with rheumatoid arthritis with multiple joint involvement, knee replacement is frequently indicated in the much younger patient because of their greatly reduced level of activity and also because no other procedure can provide the patient with a return to independence. It is in the case of the young patient or middle aged patient with monoarticular involvement that the most caution needs to be observed.

A variety of knee replacement systems exist which allows the surgeon to be able to meet most clinical situations and restore to a painful and stiff or unstable knee, relatively painless function with relatively good stability and a serviceable range of motion. The typical patient undergoing knee replacement will have extremely limited walking ability due to pain in the knee as well as pain which interferes with most other activities. Motion is ordinarily limited except in the case of rheumatoid arthritis where very abnormal motion with instability may be present. Post-operatively, the average patient after knee replacement surgery will achieve painless to relatively painless function of the knee. Stability is usually good for every day activities and walking ability is usually good although excessive walking should not be encouraged. Whereas the patient with a total hip replacement can walk for miles, this probably should be discouraged in the patient with a total knee replacement, in my opinion. Range of motion ordinarily is at least 0–90° of flexion. This would appear to be the amount required for life in society in the United States although additional degrees of motion can be useful. Occasionally, as the patient develops increasing motion beyond 90°, she may also develop increasing ligamentous instability at the knee.

Post-operatively, patients are usually out of bed the day following surgery. Two different types of post-operative routines are followed. In the classic post-op routine the patient's knee is usually kept immobilized in a splint or cast for a number of days after surgery before motion is instituted. This may be for as short as a few days and as long as seven to ten days. Once exercises are begun, the desired range of 0–90° is encouraged. For those patients who fall short of 90° with their own efforts and the assistance of a therapist, manipulation of the knee may occasionally be required under an anesthetic.

Standing can be permitted very soon after surgery as soon as symptoms permit and weight bearing with protection shortly thereafter. Once motion is begun weight bearing is ordinarily permitted with external protection which can gradually be eliminated between six and twelve weeks after surgery.

A recent innovation is the use of continuous passive motion devices; motorized splints, to slowly move the knee through a gradually increasing range of motion. Use of these machines is begun in the recovery room and usually used on a 24 hour a day basis for approximately one week. Pain appears to be minimized and motion possibly improved with this device but controlled studies are needed to confirm this.

For patients with bilateral knee involvement, the contralateral knee must be considered very carefully at the time of surgery on the more painful side. If there is a marked flexion contracture present in the relatively good knee, or very limited range of motion in that knee, it will be exceedingly difficult to maintain full extension or a suitable range of motion in the operated knee. Again, similar to the hip, the way in which a person sits or stands or conducts her various activities is usually determined by the less mobile joint. While this is seldom a problem at the hip it can lead to a somewhat more aggressive approach to surgery on the opposite knee in persons with bilateral knee involvement.

Mechanical failure with loosening of the components and subsequent pain in the knee is gradually becoming a much less frequent problem as component design and instrumentation have improved. Nevertheless patient selection and voluntary restriction on the part of the patient remains an important factor in this regard. While late infection after hip replacement is quite rare, it does not appear to be nearly so rare after knee replacement. For reasons that are not entirely clear, patients with knee replacements seem more likely to develop late hematogenous infections from other sources than do patients with other joint replacements.

Alternative procedures

Knee fusion was once considered as the procedure of choice for many patients with monoarticular arthritis of the knee. While this may still be true for the young vigorous patient with only one knee involved, its use is currently largely as a salvage procedure for failed total knee replacements, usually as a consequence of irretrievable infection. Some infections after total knee replacement can be successfully treated by debridement of the joint and reimplantation of a prosthesis with a decreasing incidence of success as compared to primary procedures. Many of these procedures unfortunately fail and patients with infected total knee replacements can then profit from removal of the components, debridement of the knee, and a secondary knee fusion. This procedure provides a stable and painless knee. It has the problem of completely eliminating motion at the knee so that difficulty can be encountered in reaching the foot for hygiene or putting on shoes and stockings without additional aids. A patient with a knee fusion will be able to walk unlimited distance with a cane which is a great asset. It is sometimes quite difficult to obtain a solid bony union of the knee after a total knee replacement had previously been performed because of loss of adequate bone stock as the debridement will include not only the infected components but also those areas of bone which are infected with impregnated cement. Possibly the use of bony ingrowth knee replacements may minimize some of these problems should failure occur in the future. In order to obtain knee fusion, many months of immobilization are frequently required as well as more than one surgical procedure. Various types of additional internal fixation may be used such as a long femoral-tibial intramedullary rod, bone plates and screws for stable fixation, or the frequent use of external fixation devices derived from fracture treatment. Secondary bone graft procedures may be required and in certain instances the possible adjunct value of direct electrical or external electromagnetic pulsed stimulation may be of value in helping to achieve union. In addition, there is the feeling that many of these patients do quite well in a functional sense even if they do not achieve a bony ankylosis but have only a reasonably stable fibrous ankylosis and use an external orthosis to stabilize the knee. If this route is taken for the more disabled patient, then it greatly simplifies the many months of care that would otherwise be required.

Osteotomy of the knee remains an important procedure for many patients up to and including middle age with arthritis of the knee. For the patient with the commonly found degenerative joint disease involving primarily the inner half of the knee, proximal tibial osteotomy can have an extremely beneficial effect in relieving pain and restoring function. In this procedure an appropriately dimensioned wedge of bone is removed from the proximal tibial area below the joint surface and above the tibial tubercle so that the limb is realigned from a varus or "bowleg" position to a slight valgus "knock knee" position. This will accomplish improved weight bearing distribution across the joint. In the typical varus knee, approximately 75% of the weight bearing is transmitted through the medial compartment which is already substantially damaged. After appropriate realignment of the knee, weight bearing tends to be more equally distributed between the two compartments. It is never completely relieved from the medial compartment. Post-operatively patients will typically wear a cast for approximately six to eight weeks during which time they will be weight bearing. Certain techniques allow for internal or external fixation to be utilized and the cast to be eliminated. This permits for earlier institution of motion but a range of motion of from 0–90° is to be anticipated by either technique and frequently more degrees can occur. Patients can be assured, in the successful cases, of pain relief in substantial degree lasting for upwards of a decade. The goal of such surgery is to delay the time for ultimate knee replacement surgery to be performed in a patient who would be too young or too vigorous to otherwise be a candidate for knee replacement surgery.

For those patients with a valgus deformity of the knee and who have primarily lateral compartment degenerative disease, a proximal tibial osteotomy will not only not relieve their problem but it will frequently tend to make it worse because for a variety of anatomical and biomechanical reasons, it tends to result in an increased malalignment of the joint surfaces relative to the weight bearing line. For these patients who are usually women, a varus supracondylar osteotomy can be performed in the supracondylar portion of the femur just above the knee. An internal fixation device will be utilized with this to obtain secure fixation of the bone and the patient will usually wear some type of cast brace orthosis in the post-operative period to allow for range of motion of the knee while the femoral osteotomy is healing. This procedure in carefully selected patients can yield results quite similar to that seen in proximal tibial osteotomy.

Double osteotomy of the knee is an operation that was described by Benjamin in England in the mid 1960's. This procedure utilized an osteotomy in the proximal tibial area as well as one in the distal femoral area. The patient's limb was then manipulated into a relatively straight position and a cast applied. Very early weight bearing was initiated with a cast which was subsequently removed at approximately six to eight weeks and range of motion exercises begun. In our own experience with this procedure, it does not offer any advantages in the patient with osteoarthritis of the knee over the conventional proximal tibial osteotomy. We have found it to be uniquely useful for a very small percentage of the rheumatoid population who possess a knee that is relatively well aligned but has early articular involvement with considerable synovitis. This type knee is usually not suitable for synovectomy because of the articular involvement but if the patient is physically and emotionally capable of beginning extremely early weight bearing following this procedure, it is a very helpful adjunct to treatment of the rheumatoid knee in this very select group.

Synovectomy of the knee is of value in the rheumatoid patient who has persistent synovitis despite good medical control of the disease in other areas for a period of three to six months. If the articular surfaces remain intact, then synovectomy of the rheumatoid synovium will usually have a very beneficial effect with regard to pain relief. Many years ago it was felt that this procedure would protect the knee from the further ravages of the disease. On an empiric basis, this appears true in many patients in whom this procedure has been performed, but studies of the synovial fluid reveal that rheumatoid characteristics tend to be reestablished in the joint within a period of months after the surgery. Synovectomy remains useful for a small group of rheumatoid patients.

Synovectomy previously had a substantial trial in patients with osteoarthritis and was shown ultimately to be of no value. At the present time with the development of arthroscopic surgical techniques, synovectomy and debridement on a limited scale of a variety of arthritic joints is again being done. It is much too soon to evaluate the results of these procedures. There is considerable enthusiasm at the present time for their benefit but if one looks at the history of surgery of arthritis of the knee, a more conservative approach should be considered until long term results of these procedures can be evaluated.

A special circumstance sometimes seen in the rheumatoid knee is that of a giant popliteal cyst associated with synovitis of the knee. These cysts can assume massive size and extend from the popliteal crease completely down the calf and can sometimes be misdiagnosed as a thrombophlebitis. Synovectomy anteriorly is required as well as the removal of the posterior cyst in order to prevent recurrence of this problem.

The Foot and Ankle

The foot and ankle should be considered together since the ankle joint and the subtalar joints together are often considered in biomechanical terms as a universal joint. Many patients with arthritis of the ankle joint can be treated for very long periods of time conservatively especially with the use of below knee orthoses. They can usually help stabilize the ankle so that relief of pain for as long as one year can be obtained in terms of delaying surgery. Joint replacement at the ankle has been attempted with mixed results. It is a procedure that is still being developed at several centers but the revision rate after a total ankle replacement appears to be unduly high at present to recommend it uniformly to patients.

Ankle fusion is an operation that has stood the test of time. A variety of surgical approaches to accomplish this exist and all seem to work well with a high incidence of fusion occurring. Cast immobilization is invariably required after surgery and some form of either internal fixation in the form of screws or external fixation in the form of an external immobilizing device are often utilized. Following successful ankle fusion, the subtalar joints will tend to develop compensatory motions simulating the tibial-tarsal joint. For this reason it is important to be certain that the subtalar joints are not arthritic prior to performing ankle fusion. While this is not typically the case in the post traumatic osteoarthritis it very often is the case in the patient with rheumatoid arthritis and needs to be considered. Post-operatively the use of shoes with a metatarsal rocker bar and beveled heel will often help to provide for some of the lost motion obtained by the ankle fusion. Patients with ankle fusions often function extremely well for many years.

The subtalar joint often is afflicted in rheumatoid arthritis. It can also be a source of post traumatic degenerative arthritis following calcaneal or other fractures in the hindfoot. If conservative care in the form of shoe modifications and orthotic arch supports do not suffice then triple arthrodesis involving fusion of the talo-calcaneal, talo-navicular, and calcaneal cuboid joints can be performed which usually leads to a very excellent relief of the symptoms. Many patients with rheumatoid arthritis who have marked hindfoot (subtalar) involvement will usually develop a marked valgus position of the heel. Such patients should be carefully questioned for the presence of burning pain in the soles of their feet. If present, this can strongly suggest posterior tibial nerve compression on the medial side of the ankle as it traverses the tarsal tunnel. The tarsal tunnel syndrome can then be further confirmed by appropriate electromyographic and nerve conduction studies. If present an attempt at conservative treatment in the form of local injections can be attempted but if this does not relieve the burning paresthesias then surgical release of the tarsal tunnel may be required. Unfortunately many rheumatoid patients with this problem may also have an associated vasculitis and neuropathy so that their symptoms are not always relieved by the mechanical release of the relatively tight ligamentous tunnel.

Metatarsalgia with arthritic metatarsal phalangeal joints are very common and probably does not belong in the purview of a chapter dealing with surgery for arthritis except that in the rheumatoid patient who cannot be relieved with full conservative treatment including the use of molded shoes then forefoot resection in the form of surgical removal of the arthritic metatarsal phalangeal joints can be very helpful to enable the patient to resume painless function with appropriate shoe modifications. It is possible in selected situations with the use of silastic joint implants that more improved function may result.

SURGERY OF THE UPPER EXTREMITY

The Shoulder

Degenerative joint disease and rheumatoid involvement of the glenohumeral joint is not rare but patients can often function remarkably well for many years in the face of such involvement. Surgery is seldom required for these problems considering the large pool of patients with these afflictions but when properly indicated, it can result in a very gratifying relief of pain and improvement of function. Conservative treatment should include rest, a full trial of modalities of physical therapy, restoration of range of motion, nonsteroidal oral antiinflammatory drugs and analgesics, as well as the occasional intraarticular steroid injection. These latter should be kept to a minimum.

Partial debridement of the glenohumeral joint to include partial acromionectomy can sometimes be of value in selected cases. Total shoulder replacement for those patients with advanced rheumatoid involvement, osteonecrosis of the humeral head, or advanced degenerative joint disease can lead to extremely gratifying results, quite comparable to those seen in total hip replacement. It remains unclear whether simple humeral head replacement alone or humeral head replacement along with a polyethylene glenoid replacement is required. Results seem somewhat comparable. Post-operatively these patients will require early institution of range of motion and exercises designed to regain strength in the weakened shoulder mechanism.

The Elbow

Arthritis at the elbow seldom requires surgical treatment. For many years, arthritic elbow joints of either post traumatic or rheumatoid source have been treated relatively successfully by the rather conservative procedure of synovectomy, debridement, and radial head resection. The procedure will usually result in substantial relief of pain and relatively good motion. Post-operatively patients are usually immobilized in a posterior plaster splint and relatively early motion begun within a week. Guided and guarded motion is usually continued for several weeks with the goal of obtaining sufficient elbow flexion to bring the hand to the face and sufficient elbow extension to be able to reach for objects.

If the above procedure fails then total elbow replacement may be indicated. Current elbow replacements possess the unfortunate characteristic of being relatively constrained, i.e. the humeral and ulnar components are frequently joined together. This leads to an inability to dissipate rotary torque forces through the elbow joint which are instead transmitted through the axes of the component prosthetic stems to ultimately create prosthetic loosening at the cement bone junction. Those patients who use that extremity as an assistive rather than a dominant one, this procedure has proved to be quite useful. Considerable care is required in patient selection to avoid those patients who will overuse this rather delicate component.

The Wrist and Hand

Arthritic involvement at the wrist is ordinarily either a post traumatic degenerative osteoarthritis or else is a consequence of rheumatoid arthritis or its variants. Many patients with arthritic wrist problems have difficulties consequent upon associated involvement of the hand. This is most frequently the case in rheumatoid disease.

Post traumatic arthritis at the wrist is ordinarily a consequence of malunions of prior fractures in this area. In many instances simple conservative treatment will suffice. The use of protective wrist splints can be most helpful in this regard. For patients with post traumatic problems that are not responsive to conservative treatment, the resection of the distal ulna (Darrach procedure) can sometimes be of value to relieve the pain of the deranged radio-ulnar joint. This operation is rarely required after malunion following distal radial fracture but can sometimes be helpful to relieve local pain and even occasionally assist in restoration of rotatory motion of the forearm.

More advanced problems of arthritis tend to more typically be a consequence of carpal fractures or dislocations. Wrist fusion can be relied upon to secure a painless and stable wrist which will serve as the solid base for good hand function. The extent of the radialcarpal fusion can sometimes be limited to permit some intercarpal motion. Motion at the wrist is a mixture of motion taking place at both the radial carpal joint as well as between the carpal bones themselves.

Patients with rheumatoid arthritis can develop complex problems involving the wrist and hand. The wrist will frequently develop a radial deviation and will often sublux dorsally. In these patients simple resection of the distal ulna can sometimes lead to increased instability of the wrist. Depending upon available bone stock and the presence of adequate muscle power to balance the wrist, wrist fusion or possibly implant selection at the radialcarpal joint can be chosen. Wrist fusion has stood the test of time and has a documented history of relief of pain and restoration of stability. Wrist implants have been utilized for a number of years and are essentially of two types. A silicone implant for the distal radius can be helpful in many instances in restoring length and providing a smooth surface for future motion at the wrist. Alternatively, a total wrist replacement component can be inserted. There is considerably more experience with the use of the silicone distal radial implant and results are generally satisfactory. The total wrist prostheses remain in a developmental stage but reports from those centers who have devoted themselves to the development of these are somewhat encouraging.

Surgery of the arthritic hand is largely that of rheumatoid disease and as an isolated subject would be much too complex for a detailed inclusion in this chapter. The typical rheumatoid deformity is that of radial deviation at the wrist and ulnar deviation at the metacarpal phalangeal joints. Associated "swan's neck" deformity or "mallet finger" deformities may also be present. Surgery for the rheumatoid hand is designed to realign abnormal muscle and tendon pulls, to release contracted capsular structures and to reinforce weakened ones. Silicone metacarpal phalangeal joint implants can be utilized to help restore alignment and balance to the finger. The silicone implants have had a spotty history in terms of long term durability. Surgery of the rheumatoid hand and wrist needs very careful timing as to the staging of procedures and complete involvement of physical therapy and occupational therapy departments with both preoperative and post-operative dynamic splinting. Frequently overlooked in the patient with multiple wrist and hand arthritic abnormalities may be the presence of median nerve compression at the wrist. The carpal tunnel syndrome should be thought of, looked for, and confirmed with appropriate electrical testing. Early release of the volar carpal ligament will usually produce a gratifying result in terms of relief of painful burning paresthesias in the palm of the hand and restoration of hand function.

The Spine

Arthritic abnormalities of the spine can be present at any area of the cervical, dorsal, or lumbar spine. Like the hand, a detailed exposition of the various problems associated with the arthritic spine is well beyond the scope of this chapter.

Cervical spine instability is commonplace in the rheumatoid patient particularly at the C_1-C_2 interspace. This should be considered in any rheumatoid patient undergoing anesthesia as the intubation during anesthesia might prove to be possibly dangerous for a patient with instability of the spine. Conservative treatment in the form of cervical collars will usually suffice but occasionally cervical spine fusion may be required for patients whose cervical spine symptoms of pain are so intractable or who develop a radiculopathy consequent upon this.

Spinal stenosis is an important topic to touch upon briefly. Often confused with vascular insufficiency in the lower extremities, the pain in the lower extremities due to arthritic narrowing of the lumbar spinal canal is typically present with walking and relieved with rest. Symptoms may be unilateral or bilateral. Careful physical examination will usually confirm the presence of adequate vascular supply. Conventional radiographic examination may reveal the telltale signs of greatly enlarged facet joints on the anterior posterior film. Computerized axial tomography of the involved areas will reveal the classic narrowing of the internal diameter of the lumbar spinal canal or possibly only bony encroachment from arthritic facet joints causing narrowed lateral recesses. Either one of these anatomic problems can lead to compression upon nerve roots with subsequent radicular pain with activity.

Conservative treatment will suffice for many patients and this should include rest, weight reduction, the possible use of an appropriately designed lumbosacral corset or brace, and the use of non steroidal oral antiinflammatory drugs. For those patients whose symptoms remain intractable despite adequate conservative treatment surgical decompression is indicated and will usually produce a substantial relief of symptom.

SUGGESTED READINGS

American Acaedmy of Orthopaedic Surgeons, National Institute of Arthritis, Metabolism and Digestive Diseases of the National Institute of Health, and The Orthopaedic Research Society: Mechanical failure of total joint replacement, Workshop, Atlanta, 1978.

Charnley, J. Acrylic Cement in Orthopaedic Surgery, Baltimore, 1970, Williams and Wilkens, Co.

Charnley, J. and Cupic, Z. The nine and ten year results of low friction arthroplasty of the hip, Clinical Orthopaedics and Related Research, 95:9, 1973.

Katz, W.A., Ed. Diagnosis and Management of Rheumatic Disease. 2nd ed. 1988. JB Lippincott, Philadelphia. Ch. 88 Arthritis Surgery.

Kelley, W.N. et al (Eds.) Textbook of Rheumatology. WB Saunders, Philadalphia. 3rd ed. 1989. Sec. 23 Rheumatic Diseases.

Levy, R. Total Hip Replacement. The Mount Sinai Approach, Orthopaedic Profiles, 1984.

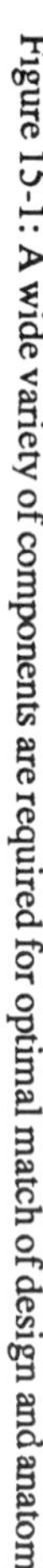

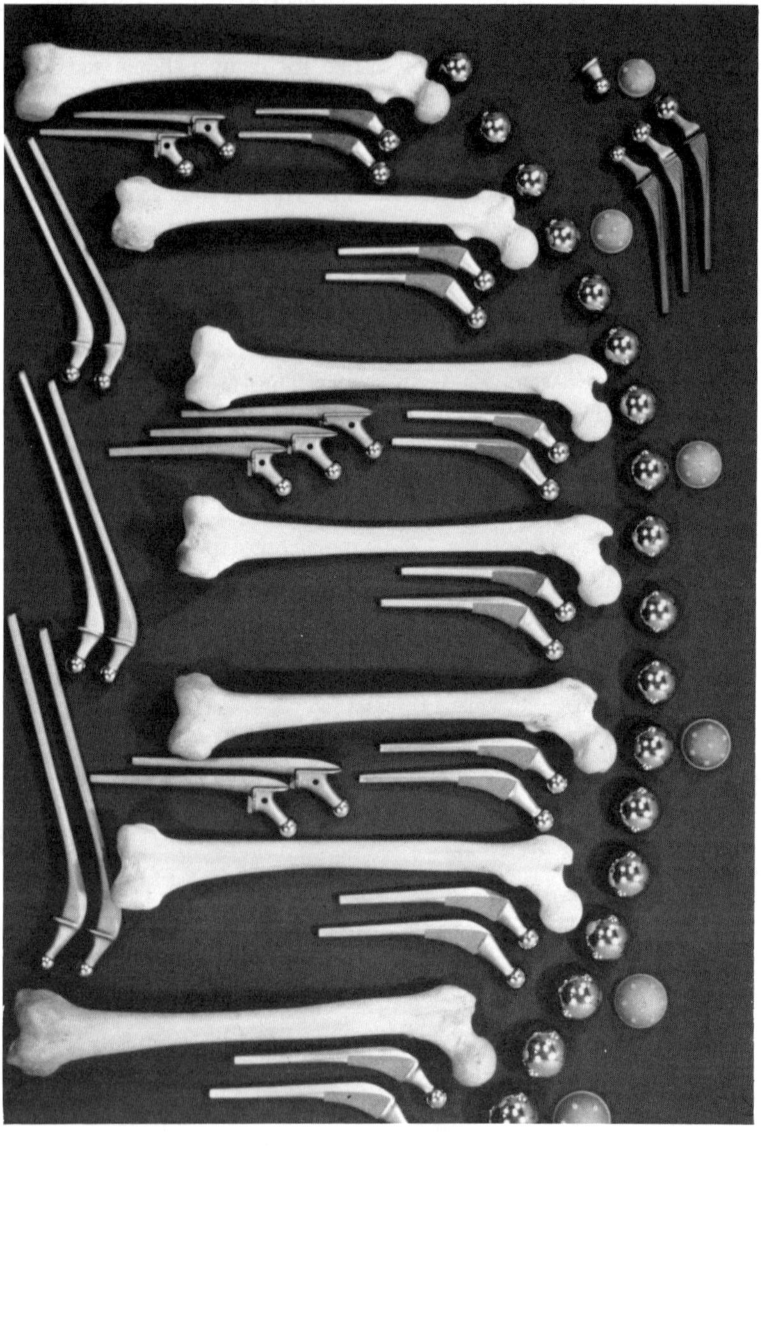

Figure 15-1: A wide variety of components are required for optimal match of design and anatomy.

CHAPTER 16

REHABILITATION MEDICINE

Ramon Vallarino, M.D.

BASIC CONCEPTS

Rehabilitation medicine, also called physical medicine and rehabilitation, is a medical discipline whose goal is maintenance and restoration of the patient's optimal level of function—physically, psychologically, vocationally and socially.

The rheumatic disorders are disabling conditions and may cause the patient to suffer a number of losses, such as:

Loss of the feeling of well-being due to the systemic character of the illness or the burden of persistent pain.

Loss of mobility caused by joint pain, deformity, stiffness or weakness.

Loss of income caused by inadequate fitness to continue practicing his or her established occupation.

Loss of social life because of lack of stamina to participate in activities or to venture out in public.

Loss of sexual activity because of the discomfort encountered

Loss of self-esteem.

All of these losses affect the functioning of the person as a whole. When they accumulate, when they are severe, or when the person fails to react to them in a positive manner, he/she becomes in varying degrees disabled.

Assessing the disabled patient by pointing out their losses and finding their origin is the diagnostic component of Rehabilitation Medicine. Treating the disability from its origin to its end-result is the therapeutic part of the specialty.

Physiatrist and Therapist

The physiatrist is a physician specializing in rehabilitation medicine. The general public and even many physicians sometimes fail to identify this medical specialty.

A number of factors explain this lack of awareness, such as: insufficient discussion in medical school of the problems of the disabled, little chance for the medical student to meet physiatrists and see them in action, relatively small number of physiatrists in the community (only 2,000 in the entire country). In addition, and probably as a result, it is unusual for a patient to be referred to a physiatrist by his or her doctor, who, more often, will refer patients to physical therapists, who are the better known rehabilitation professionals in the field.

In the United States, the physician who wishes to become a physiatrist must after graduating from medical school and completing an internship, enter a three or more year training program in an approved residency in physical medicine and rehabilitation.

During this training the resident studies the etiology, pathogenesis and physio-psychopathology of many disabling conditions. The resident must review neurology, rheumatology, cardiology, pulmonology, angiology, orthopedics and endocrinology. Frequently, the disabled individual is an elderly person, therefore, the resident must be at ease with the core of geriatrics and gerontology. A physiatrist will often take care of children affected by cerebral palsy, congenital deformities or metabolic disorders. The resident in rehabilitation medicine must, therefore, review the principles and practices of pediatrics. The physiatrist is called to lead and supervise the work of physical, occupational and speech therapists. It is necessary for the resident to master the principles and techniques of those specialties, such as the use of physiotherapy equipment, physical modalities, therapeutic exercises, functional activities, activities of daily living, kinesiology, orthotics and prosthetics, speech disorders and swallowing impairments. The physiatrist must be able to lead a team that will include activities and recreational therapists, psychologists, vocational counselors and social workers. Thus, the resident must learn the basics of all those disciplines and become knowledgeable about supportive services for the disabled. He/she must also become fluent in choosing disposition options, i.e., long-term care facilities, supervised residential settings, health-related facilities, nursing homes and home care services.

Upon completion of this extensive and intensive training, and after a prescribed period of time has elapsed in the practice of this specialty, the physiatrist becomes Board Eligible. To be certified by the American Board of Physical Medicine and Rehabilitation, the physiatrist must pass a written test and a comprehensive oral examination. Because of their vocational aptitude, and the training in the management of the disabled, the physiatrist is the natural leader of a sound rehabilitation effort.

In that capacity, the physiatrist:

Evaluates the disabled or potentially disabled individual, analyzing to its ultimate details, the etiology and pathogenesis of the condition.

Estimates a prognosis for the prospective functional capabilities of the whole person.

Establishes the goals of the therapeutic program, both for each discipline participating and for the entire program as a comprehensive effort.

Prescribes specific orders to be followed by the therapists.

Assembles a therapeutic team, i.e., physical and occupational therapists, nurses, social workers and the patient's spouse.

Assigns specific roles for each member of the therapeutic team, and supervises their work.

Keeps an on-going consultation with the members of the team and is ready to modify the prescribed program if the results of this consultation suggest a beneficial change for the patient.

Maintains a record of the progression toward the goals and is ready to alter these goals if the patient's condition requires it.

Plans and implements, with the help of the team, long-term therapeutic and supportive actions, i.e., home care, individualized programs of exercises for the patient to do on their own, timely follow-up visits with a therapist, in order to prevent the recurrence of the handicap.

Physical, occupational and speech therapists are non-physician health professionals trained in the management of specific problems in the area of rehabilitation. Their role, while essential, is different from the physiatrist. A way to try to describe this difference would be to say that the physiatrist tries to cure a human being with specific losses, while the therapist tries to cure the losses of a human being. This is not a semantic difference but an expression of the different broadness of the formation, knowledge and skills of one professional to another.

In that more concise role, the therapist at the physician's request:

Evaluates focal problems, such as pain, weakness, stiffness, deformity, and in general, any malfunction analyzing its direct mechanical basis and its immediate origin.

Establishes immediate goals and charts the course to take in order to execute the physician's prescription in the most efficient and efficacious manner.

Attempts to correct the malfunction or teaches the patient how to compensate for an incorrectable one by using, within the framework of the physician's prescription, the modalities and techniques at their disposition.

Establishes early rapport with the patient through direct frequent contact. Uses such rapport to motivate the patient towards making the best effort to achieve set goals.

Learns, first hand, the way the patient reacts physically and psychologically to the program, and shares this information with the team, assisting the physician to reprogram and adjust the goals where necessary.

Provides the patient with practical advice for his or her daily activities and/or exercises to enhance and facilitate the recovery of the patient and to prevent or minimize the possibility of recurrence of the disorder.

A question frequently asked, particularly at a time when cost containment is a major preoccupation in the minds of health professionals, health facility administrators and legislators is, ("When shall one use a physiatrist and when shall one use a therapist?") In our view, the answer is quite simple; use a physiatrist when the person is disabled or suffering with a condition that imposes a serious threat to the patient's ability to function. Call a physiatrist, too, for in-depth diagnostic assessment of the mechanisms affecting the patient's function. The patient may be referred directly to a therapist if: (the patient is not disabled; there is no serious or immediate threat to the patient's ability to function; and, the therapist will treat a local malfunction of which the attending physician has a clear diagnosis and a reasonable knowledge.)

Some examples should clarify our point of view. A rheumatologist wants to prevent losses in range of motion in a newly diagnosed case of rheumatoid arthritis in a vigorous individual with a sound emotional state. A physical therapist can handle this care perfectly well on the rheumatologist's referral. If this same patient, however, suddenly starts calling in sick and missing days at work due to this condition, a physiatrist would probably be in a better position to identify the problem and know how to resolve it.

An orthopedic surgeon has operated on a deranged knee and wants to have the patient regain range of motion and strength; a therapist will implement the right program. This patient has a history of a cerebrovascular accident a few years ago and has been walking with a cane since that time. A physiatrist is most likely the right choice.

A gastroenterologist's patient develops pain and loss of range of motion in a shoulder and a definitive diagnosis cannot be established. It would be wrong to send this patient to a therapist. The patient should see a rheumatologist, or an orthopedic surgeon or a physiatrist then, once the etiological diagnosis is made, is referred to the therapist.

THE REHABILITATION PROGRAM

The concept of rehabilitation has always been in the core of the management of the rheumatic patient. "Rest and exercise" are words that classically share the same paragraph with "salicylates" in every rheumatology treatise. These words were forgotten by many at the beginning of the steroids era with serious consequences for patients that saw their function lost while undergoing an illusion of state of pain-free well-being. At present, every physician knows that pain relievers and hormonal or non-hormonal anti-inflammatories are insufficient to protect the overall functional state of a patient.

Rehabilitation does not alter the histologic progression of the disease but can significantly influence the functional outcome, making the difference between being able or disabled.

Rehabilitation programs are based on the following scheme:

Assessment of the patient

Establishment of therapeutic goals

Implementation and coordination of the therapeutic program

Evaluation of the results

Assessment of the Patient

The purpose of this step is to determine the patient's current and premorbid level of functioning, and to estimate future functional outcome. To assess the patient, the physiatrist must, review the history, do a physical examination and review laboratory and X-Ray findings. The examination must focus on the patient's ability to function and must include evaluation of:

The functioning of the body, particularly of the musculoskeletal system: Detecting and recording the presence of pain, deformity, swelling and measuring the strength and range of motion.

The functioning of the patient's mental state: Cognitive status, affect and motivation.

The patient's stamina: Staying power resulting from corporal and mental strengths.

The functioning of the person as a whole and their performance of activities of daily living: Transfers, ambulation, toileting, rooming, bathing, dressing, going to work, taking public transport, etc. Obviously, the list of these activities is very long, and varies from person to person, depending on variables such as age, occupation, interest, responsibilities, level of education and socio-economic status.

This type of assessment reveals how the patient's body and mind function at present and how they functioned prior to the illness. Throughout the entire process, the physiatrist looks for the mechanisms causing a detected impediment, going beyond the etiology of the illness by analyzing the physio-psychopathology of the impediment. For example, if a shoulder shows limited range of motion, one should not be satisfied with a simplistic explanation such as, "This is due to some form of arthritis," and not even with a more precise, "This is due to osteoarthritis." We have to try to understand which specific component of osteoarthritis caused the limitation, differentiating pain, stiffness, mechanical derangement, or capsular contracture. Furthermore, we must bear in mind the possibility that, in spite of the presence of osteoarthritis, the shoulder limitation may have nothing to do with it, and maybe secondary to another process, i.e., acute trauma. Finally, it also may be possible that the patient is simply faking a limitation to obtain a secondary gain.

Another example would be the case of a patient who has stopped attending work. We will have to determine if this is due to physical problems, such as malaise or poor mobility, socio-economic problems, such as insufficient funds to pay for a more expensive form of transportation, or emotional problems, i.e., embarrassment in showing disabilities to peers. On the other hand, we must not fail to recognize the occasional case of the arthritic patient that stops going to work to make himself eligible for disability or compensation payments. This diagnostic effort may be tedious and time consuming, but it must be done if one really wants to understand the mechanisms that render a patient disabled, and to establish a sound program of therapy.

The concept of projection into the future, the prognosis, must be present throughout the assessment process. This means that one has to predict forthcoming disabilities, not present at the time of the assessment, but that are likely to occur in the natural course of rheumatic disease.

Establishment of Therapeutic Goals

In rehabilitation, the goals may be focal, i.e., for a joint or limb, or in general for the person as a whole. Goals are also short-term and/or long-term. Goals have to be realistic but they must also be as optimistic as possible. Experience teaches us the almost limitless capabilities of the disabled as long as they have a clear mind and a strong motivation. The best way to establish adequate goals is to look carefully at what the patient was doing just prior to the current illness. We will often make incredible discoveries, like finding that a feeble looking patient was driving his car a couple of weeks prior to entering the nursing home or that a severely deformed arthritic patient has been independent in daily living activities in spite of many years of pain and joint deformity.

Most of the time, the goals may be to regain the premorbid state. When this is no longer feasible because there have been permanent losses, the goal will be to approach the premorbid level and as closely as possible, working around the permanent loss, i.e., developing new skills, using assistive devices, modifying the patient's environment, changing the patient's needs. Goals must be flexible to adjust to the changing pattern of the rheumatic illness. The rehabilitation professional has to maintain a vigilant attitude to detect changes in the course of the illness and to react promptly with changes in therapy and in goals as they may be needed. Some examples will clarify this concept.

Wheelchair mobility may be the initial stated goal for a seriously ill patient with SLE. However, perhaps a few days later, as a result of successful medication, the goal may be changed to that of achieving fully independent ambulation. On the other hand, one may be giving ambulation training to a lupus patient who lost their ability to walk because of pain in the knees, and suddenly finds that this goal is no longer possible because the patient has entered into a phase of severe cardiac failure.

In still another case, the therapist may intend treating the pain, loss or range of motion and muscle weakness in a patient with rheumatoid arthritis but finds that the patient's vigor has decreased to a point that no longer allows an involved session of therapy. In this case, the therapist may have to defer some goals and determine which ones are still feasible under the new conditions.

Therapists and all other health professionals involved in the rehabilitation process must immediately inform the primary physician or the physiatrist about the changes they perceive in order to adjust the goals as needed. Goals should be frequently recalled to insure that the right course of therapeutic effort is maintained. Probably, the most frequent cause of failure of a rehabilitation program is losing sight of the goals. When this happens the therapeutic effort becomes an aimless routine.

As with every other team, the rehabilitation team follows two basic rules:

There must be a leader, i.e., the physician in this case.

The members of the team must work together. This assures that they communicate effectively with each other.

Small teams include just the doctor, a therapist, the patient and relatives. Large teams add other health professionals, i.e., different kinds of therapists, social workers, discharge planners, vocational counselors, psychologists, nurses, pastoral care representatives, etc. The composition of the team depends on the needs of the patient and the setting in which it works, namely an acute hospital, a longer term institution or the community. The team may or may not have formal meetings. However, small or large, with or without meetings, the team must communicate! The members of a rehabilitation team communicate by means of two basic instruments:

The prescription and the progress report

The doctor is expected to write a prescription. Aside from their questionable legality, verbal prescriptions, as often suboptimal and undetailed. A written prescription is a document to which one can return to recollect the goals. It is also a record of the starting point. The prescription must include the diagnosis, in a detailed and comprehensive form, the doctor's goals, specific warnings and limitation, the requested services or modalities, the number and sequence of services, when applicable, and the time when a report or follow-up is expected.

The therapist must not accept, as a prescription, from a doctor a casual statement such as, "Take care of doing some rehab, or see if you can give some heat or exercise." Some therapists seem to like this kind of referral, apparently because it gives them total freedom and feeling of self-sufficiency. However, competent and experienced therapists reject them because they know that a serious interplay of professionals demand that each one assumes their role fully and responsibly.

An adequate prescription in a hospital would read as follows:

Patient Name:	John Doe, Age 66
Diagnosis:	Osteoarthritis of both knees Cardiac arrhythmia Loss of efficiency in transfers and ambulation
Goals:	To regain lost functions, probably using a gait aid
Warnings:	Cardiac precautions
Physical Therapy:	Hot packs to both knees Strengthening exercises to both quadriceps Transfer training Progressive ambulation. Use a walker initially, then proceed as adequate. Teach patient a home program of therapy Treat five times per week for the first two weeks, then as adequate Patient must see me after six weeks of therapy

Therapists and other health professionals can play a very important role in improving the level of care by teaching physicians to write this kind of prescription.

Choosing a modality in physical or occupational therapy is as important as choosing a medication. If the doctor requests specific modalities, it is the duty of the therapist to faithfully follow this request, using the best of their science and art to apply such means of therapy, with the most perfect technique.

If we take, for example, our prescription model, the therapist is expected to provide:

> Hot packs to the knees: It will be the therapists choice to determine how to position the patient, what the patient could be doing through the length of time of the treatment, i.e., isometrics or relaxation, how to assure that the heat is maintained and how to ascertain the patient's safety.
>
> Strengthening to quadriceps: The therapist will decide whether to give resistance with hands, ankle weights, weight boots or machines. He/she will also establish the number of repetitions and the sequence of the muscle contraction.
>
> Transfer training: The therapist must choose whether to challenge the patient asking him or her to stand from a low seat or rather facilitate and encourage the patient by elevating the seat.
>
> Progressive ambulation: The therapist decides how far, how fast, whether

or not to put obstacles in the patient's way, when to progress to a cane after starting, as prescribed, with a walker, when to try stair climbing.

Teaching the patient a home program: This is an outstanding opportunity for the therapist to bring up all talent to help the patient, choosing from a wide number of options for the implementation of such a program.

As one can see, there is always enough leeway for a therapist to be independent and creative while faithfully following a doctor's order. Proper use of that independence and that creativity is what determines whether a service is mediocre or excellent.

Doctors are shocked and legitimately so when they find that their patients have gone from one day to another, from heat to cold, to massage and to electricity or that they have ended having a corset or a brace that they had not requested; or when they find that, while they were preparing to send their patient home after hospitalization, the social workers had prepared everything for discharge to a nursing home.

The therapist and every other member of the team is expected to write a progress note, indicating his or her own observations, the services provided and the results that are being achieved. The frequency of such reports varies as the result of rules, regulations and practices in a given setting.

Good care implies writing a note every time it is relevant to do so. When there is an observation to bring to the teams' attention, when the condition shows significant change, when the patient is not responding after a prudent number of sessions, when a new sign or symptom occurs, or when the treatment has been successful and becomes unnecessary.

Recalling our previous example of a patient with osteoarthritis of the knees, one could expect the following to be an adequate physical therapy program note, written after a few paragraphs of general information about the patient and the program delivered:

"Patient is now able to stand without assistance from regular chairs. He walks with a walker with supervision for one hundred feet before knees become quite painful. Progress to cane deferred for the time-being. Program will continue daily. Notice: Patient has 15 degree flexion contracture on both knees. Kindly give clearance for use of ultrasound on knees plus active assistive range of motion with stretching."

This kind of communication, brief and relevant and similar ones between other members of the team, are the core of the sound practice of rehabilitation. They maintain the team effort and assure the best quality of care.

Evaluation of Results

All health services, including programs of rehabilitation, must be evaluated on the basis of their achievements. It is surprising to observe how many audits and reviews are limited to monitoring compliance with regulation, such as promptness of services, documentation and sequence of visits. Quality assurance efforts often serve just to collect data that tells us nothing about the excellence or mediocrity of the services rendered. Unfortunately, we find a tendency to measure what we do instead of assessing what we achieve. The sad consequence is that by doing so, we fool ourselves, our peers and our patients into believing that we are good simply because we do a lot even if we achieve nothing. In rehabilitation, the proper way to evaluate a program is to check its results against pre-established goals. Evaluating the results should mean monitoring the changes in the patient's condition as a result of our services. Each health discipline has many systems to measure functional changes. These instruments are intended to describe, often by means of numerical score, parameters such as joint function, muscle strength, overall performance endurance, proficiency in activities of daily living, patients' satisfaction and psycho-emotional adjustment. These tests are enumerable and offer the health professional a broad choice of possibilities to fit his particular preference.

Following the same principles enunciated when we described the assessment process, we like to see the patient's progress evaluated from a "local" and a "general" point of view. We are referring again to the function of the musculoskeletal system and to the function of the person as a whole. Therapists should, therefore, choose systems that measure changes in each of these spheres.

Whatever system is used, one has to be attentive to avoid involuntary misrepresentations and misinterpretations. The following example should illustrate this statement: Let us imagine an arthritic patient who has become bedridden as a result of deconditioning and whose realistic goal is to regain independent ambulation. After a week of therapy, the patient becomes able to walk with assistance. The patient's score has improved dramatically. We get the impression that this is a successful program. We may be wrong. First of all, the goal has not yet been achieved, since the patient is not independent. Secondly, we have to spell out what assistance means. Assistance may equally mean light contact guarding or dragging the patient while we carry all his or her weight.

In addition, therapists, because of their professional skills, have much less difficulty than other people in assisting a patient in performing a task. For example, it may be a minor effort for the therapist to assist in the transferring of a severely crippled arthritic from wheelchair to bed. Assisting in the same task may require a lot of effort from a relative. These biases may result in erroneous reports of "little assistance required," when in actuality, the skilled therapist gave a tremendous amount of assistance in a very efficient and knowledgeable manner. The required amount of assistance should, therefore, refer to the one delivered by a lay person, not a skilled health professional. The therapists should take this fact into consideration when reporting the amount of assistance required for a task.

To conclude the case of our imaginary patient, we may learn that after many weeks of therapy, the patient has become "independent" in ambulation with "just supervision." This is a fallacy because no activity that requires supervision should be called "independent." We will have to accept that the program has not reached the goal, or that the goal was unrealistic. Perhaps the right goal should have been, "unassisted but supervised ambulation." Or maybe we are over protecting the patient and under estimating his or her actual capabilities.

Rehabilitation is a powerful tool that can change the quality of life of a patient. Physiatry can operate almost "magical" changes in the patient's well-being and outlook. Physiatry can also be a waste and result in frustration. The outcome depends, in significant measure, on our skills, our good judgement, our creativity and our devotion.

SUGGESTED READINGS

Kelley, William; Harris, Jr., Edward; Ruddy, Shaun; Sledge, Clement. *Textbook of Rheumatology,* 3rd edition, W.B. Saunders Co., Philadelphia, 1989 (two volumes).

Kottke, Frederic J.; Stillwell, G. Keith; Lehmann, Justus F. *Krusen's Handbook of Physical Medicine and Rehabilitation,* 2nd edition, W.B. Saunders Co., Philadelphia, 1982.

McCarthy, Daniel J. *Arthritis and Allied Conditions: A Textbook of Rheumatology,* 11th edition, Lea and Febiger, Philadelphia, 1989.

Moskowitz, Roland W.; Howell, David S.; Goldberg, Victor M.; Mankin, Henry J. *Osteoarthritis: Diagnosis and Management,* W.B. Saunders Co., Philadelphia, 1984.

Riggs, Gail K. and Gall, Eric P. *Rheumatic Diseases: Rehabilitation and Management,* Butterworths, Stoneham, Mass., 1984.

Rusk, H.A. *Rehabilitation Medicine,* 3rd edition, The C.V. Mosby Company, 1971.

Ruskin, Asa P. *Current Therapy in Physiatry: Physical Medicine and Rehabilitation,* W.B. Saunders Co., New York, 1984.

CHAPTER 17

PHYSICAL THERAPY

Sandy Beth Gans, M.S., R.P.T.

INTRODUCTION

Physical therapists function in a wide variety of settings such as hospitals, rehabilitation centers, schools, sports medicine centers, geriatric treatment centers, motion analysis laboratories. They engage in private practice, home care, and they may perform biomechanical and ergonomic assessments in industrial settings.

Physical therapists evaluate patients with or without physician referral. In some states, they may treat without physician referral. Physical therapy is a major adjunct to rheumatology, but also plays a role in many other medical disciplines, e.g., orthopedics, neurology, surgery, pediatrics, geriatrics to name only some.

Physical therapists also act as consultants in all levels of governmental health planning activity. Finally, they are teachers and faculty members in the academic community participating in programs to prepare new physical therapists. In some settings they may instruct medical students or other health professionals.

Evaluation

Physical therapy management of rheumatic disease patients is a challenging task even for the most astute clinician. The importance of bedrest and therapeutic exercise has long been debated and continues to be controversial. This chapter looks at rest and exercise therapy in the treatment of rheumatic disease patients.

Physical therapy goals in the treatment of patients with rheumatic disease are four fold: (1) To prevent disability, (2) To restore function, (3) To relieve pain and, (4) To educate the patient. Before these goals can be achieved, a thorough physical therapy evaluation is performed which can include:

1. Functional Assessment
   A. Bed Mobility: Observing patient turning from supine to sidelying, sidelying to prone, supine to sitting.

B. Transfer Status: Observing patient transfer to and from various surfaces, i.e., bed, chair, toilet, car.

C. Gait Analysis:

1. Observational: Observing patient ambulate with or without assistive devices on level surfaces and stairs.
2. Instrumented: Using computerized video analysis, force plate analysis, foot switch stride analysis.

2. Range of Motion (ROM) assessment of all joints.

3. Muscle Evaluation:

A. Manual muscle test (MMT): Strength assessment of proximal/distal muscles, trunk and neck to determine weak musculature.

B. Instrumented biomechanical muscle test (IMBT): Isometric/Isokinetic objective strength measurement recorded for selected muscle groups.

4. Postural Assessment: Performed during standing, ambulation and functional activities.

5. Respiratory Status: Chest evaluation is performed consisting of: (1) Auscultation, (2) Chest expansion measurements and, (3) Inspirometry.

Once the physical therapy evaluation is performed, the clinician has a baseline for future comparison, and a basis for determining treatment goals. These specific goals are achieved through therapeutic exercise, rest, heat and cold modalities, ambulation training, biofeedback and electrical stimulation. But, perhaps the most important aspect of treatment is patient education. Because of the amount of daily contact between the patient and the therapist, the physical therapist is in an excellent position to monitor and insure patient understanding and compliance with rehabilitation programs.

Rationale for Therapeutic Exercise

In an exercise conscious society undergoing one fitness craze after another, the term "exercise" usually implies aerobic exercise, running, jogging, as well as weight lifting. Such exercise and therapeutic exercise are not synonymous.

According to Webster's Dictionary, "exercise is exertion made for the sake of training; a task or problem done to develop a skill." Therapeutic exercise on the other hand is a prescription of bodily movement for the purpose of preventing muscular atrophy, improving musculoskeletal function, increasing muscle strength, improving the efficiency of cardiovascular and pulmonary function, and maintaining a state of well-being. Therapeutic exercise may be limited to specific muscles or muscle groups, or expanded to include physical conditioning.

Therapeutic exercise used in the treatment of patients with rheumatic diseases are performed to: (1) prevent joint contractures, (2) strengthen weak muscles, (3) maintain or improve ROM and, (4) enhance respiratory efficiency through breathing exercises. The latter are important for the patient with ankylosing spondylitis.

Therapeutic Exercise

Therapeutic exercise helps to maintain overall physical and mental health. Following a thorough musculoskeletal evaluation, an individualized exercise program is designed to maintain joint motion, muscle strength and correct poor posture. Pain and/or swelling are often the limiting factors which contribute to loss or decrease of ROM concomitant with muscle wasting and functional impairment. Patients with rheumatic diseases need to perform the proper type of exercises. Too much exercise or exercise of the wrong type can do a great deal of harm and aggravate rather than relieve joint symptoms.

Therapeutic exercises used in the treatment of arthritic conditions are of the following types:

1. Range of Motion (ROM)—Excursion of a joint through available range of movement.
   - A. Passive Range of Motion (PROM)—Without active muscle contraction about the joint, the joint is moved through available ROM by another person, or the patient using slings, pulleys or opposite extremity.
   - B. Active Assisted Range of Motion (AAROM)—The patient performs ROM exercises with available muscle contraction with the assistance or another person, object or other extremity.
   - C. Active Range of Motion (AROM)—The patient performs ROM exercises without assistance.
   - D. Active Resisted Range of Motion (ARROM)—The patient performs ROM exercises with some form of resistance (Manual or mechanical resistance, elastic bands or weights). ARROM includes various forms of isotonic and isokinetic exercise.
2. Strengthening Exercises—Static or dynamic
   - A. Static—Isometric exercise in which the patient actively contracts or tightens the muscles around the joint without producing any joint motion.
   - B. Dynamic—Some form of resistance is used, either manually or with an externally applied load, i.e., weight.
3. Breathing Exercises—The patient performs inspiratory/expiratory exercises with or without assistive devices, i.e., inspirometer.
4. Relaxation Exercises—Specific exercises performed for muscle relaxation and stress reduction.

The specific type of exercise regime will depend entirely upon the acuteness of the disease process. Rheumatoid arthritis may occur in any one of three stages: acute, subacute and chronic. Osteoarthritis is usually seen in a static form and appropriate exercise therapy is similar to that which is used in the chronic stage of rheumatoid arthritis.

In determining what type of exercise is required, one must design the exercise program to minimize joint irritation and pain. The rule of thumb is that no exercise, strengthening or stretching should cause severe pain. The importance of modifying the exercise program depending on the patient's response throughout the course of treatment cannot be overstated.

During the acute stage, the aims of treatment are to control inflammation, to maintain ROM, and minimize loss of function. The inflamed joint is best safeguarded by application of appropriate splints, and proper positioning to prevent contractures. Gentle PROM, and AAROM is performed in this stage to maintain muscles at their proper length and maintain the integrity of the joints and periarticular structures. In the sub-acute stage, the aims of treatment are to improve ROM, maintain muscle strength and increase mobility. The patient goes through a transition period between recumbency (inactivity) and activity in which gentle movements, with gradual progressive weight-bearing and active exercise are performed. As the pain subsides, AROM is introduced to encourage voluntary movement. Isometric exercises are also begun during this stage to facilitate the strength and performance necessary to do the various activities of daily living.

In the chronic stage, ARROM (including isotonic and isokinetic exercises) can be performed to increase strength and endurance. It is not uncommon for patients with rheumatic diseases to exhibit poor aerobic function secondary to weakness, fatigue and inactivity. Preliminary research indicates that there may be a role for more vigorous conditioning exercises, during the chronic stage, specifically graded aerobic exercises concomitant with ROM and strengthening exercises (see Table 17-1). During all stages, patients learn very quickly to avoid painful or fatiguing motions during ADL, avoiding those movements required in therapeutic exercise to improve mobility and strength. It is not uncommon for the patient to complain of mild or diffuse aching during or after an exercise session.

The following precautions should accompany every exercise program that is prescribed for the patient:

1. Perform all movements slowly and smoothly, avoiding rapid, jerky movements.
2. Stop when you feel increased pain. If you have increased pain one–two hours after exercising, you have done too much and your program needs to be modified.
3. Change positions frequently.

4. Respect your pain and limitations.
5. Remember to move all your joints through their ROM at least twice a day.

Rationale for Rest

Rest is essential in the management of active inflammatory disease. Rest can be divided into three groups: systemic (body) rest, articular (joint) rest and emotional rest. Systemic rest helps to control fatigue and joint inflammation by resting the entire body. Articular rest lessens the harmful local effects of inflammation, deformity and pain during activities of daily living (ADL). Joint protection techniques, splinting, and assistive devices; ambulation aides; canes, crutches, or walkers are utilized to promote articular rest. Emotional rest is necessary to enable the patient to cope with the stress, pain and chronic disease process. Relaxation and stress reduction techniques are used to enhance emotional rest.

Exercise/Activity vs. Rest

The relative amount of rest versus activity is the subject of extensive debate. Immobilization through bed rest may result in contractures, muscle atrophy and osteoporosis. In rheumatoid arthritis, however, these effects may occur even without immobilization. The duration of bedrest, or articular rest, depends entirely on the time required for joint inflammation and systemic manifestations to subside. Exercise therapy in the past has been limited to ROM and non-stress muscle strengthening, with the goal of preserving joint motion and strength. There is evidence to indicate that both excessive rest and exercise can be detrimental in the treatment of arthritis. Atrophy, loss of motion, and postural deformities can result from rest/immobilization. Too much exercise or exercise of the wrong type can aggravate rather than relieve joint symptoms. Until controlled studies are performed to accurately determine the interaction between rest, exercise and disease status, this debate will continue.

Heat and Cold Modalities

Thermotherapy and cryotherapy have long been used in conjunction with therapeutic exercise in the treatment of rheumatic conditions. Neither heat nor cold modalities will change the disease process or repair a damaged joint. Heat and cold modalities provide temporary pain relief by raising the pain threshold, and should not be used as an alternative to arthritis medications prescribed to decrease inflammation or disease activity.

Heat may be applied to the surface of the body through changes in environmental temperature (convection), or by contact with warmed substances (conduction) or by radiating energy. Generally heat produces the following therapeutic effects: increased extensibility of collagen tissues, decreased joint stiffness, relief of muscle spasms, increased blood flow, and pain relief.

Heating modalities used in the treatment of rheumatic conditions can be divided into two categories, superficial and deep. Superficial heat includes: moist hot packs, electric and moist heating pads, whirlpool, therapeutic pool, and Hubbard tank, moist air machine, and fluidotherapy. Deep heating modalities include ultrasound, short wave diathermy and microwave diathermy.

General contra-indications for the use of heat are decreased sensation, inadequate vascular supply and heat hypersensitivity (see Table 17-2). Traditionally, most patients with rheumatic conditions prefer heat to cold, with the exception of post-surgical patients.

Cryotherapy produces marked vasoconstriction, lessens edema and inflammatory reaction and decreases pain sensitivity. Cold modalities include ice packs, frozen gel packs (cold packs), ice massage, immersion of limbs into iced water, and placement of limbs into a combination cold and intermittent pressure unit. General contra-indications for the use of cold are vasculities, Raynauds phenomenon, cryoglobulinemia, cold hypersensitivity, poor circulation and decreased sensation. Patients with cardiac and respiratory disease treated with these modalities should be closely supervised to ensure maximum safety. The physician should always be consulted.

It is imperative that the clinician be aware of the specific types of exercises and modalities utilized during the various stages of the disease process. There is no cookbook recipe for the treatment of rheumatic diseases, each patient needs to be evaluated and treated accordingly. In 1871, Trousseau said, "It behooves every practitioner to consider the form of treatment of each patient." He advocated rest and exercise as the two main therapeutic pillars in the management of arthritis. The proper balance between rest and exercise is the key for successful treatment.

SUGGESTED READINGS

Basmajiian, John V., ed. *Therapeutic Exercise.* Baltimore, Williams and Wilkins Co., 1984.

Ehrlich, George E., ed. *Rehabilitation Management of Rheumatic Conditions.* Baltimore, Williams and Wilkins Co., 1980.

Harkcom, T.M. et al. "Therapeutic Value of Graded Aerobic Exercise Training in Rheumatoid Arthritis." *Arthritis and Rheumatism* 28 (January 1985); 32–9.

Kottke, Frederic J., Stillwell, G., Keith, Lehamann, Justus F. *Krusen's Handbook of Physical Medicine and Rehabilitation.* Philadelphia, W.B. Saunders Co., 1982.

Lehmann, Justus F. *Therapeutic Heat and Cold.* Baltimore, Williams and Wilkins Co., 1982.

Lict, S., Kamenetz, H.L., eds. *Arthritis and Physical Medicine*. Baltimore, Waverly Press, 1969.

Simpson, C.F., Dickinson, G.R. "Adult Arthritis Exercise." *American Journal of Nursing* 83(2) (February 1983); 273–4.

Simpson, C.F. "Heat, Cold or Both?" *American Journal of Nursing* 83(2) (February 1983); 271.

Smith, R., Polley, H.F. "Rest Therapy for Rheumatoid Arthritis." *Mayo Clinic Proceedings* 53 (March 1985); 141–5.

TABLE 17-1
TREATMENT GOALS

Stages of Disease	*Treatment Goals*	*Exercise*
Acute	Control of Inflammation Maintain ROM Minimize Loss of Function	PROM AAROM
Sub-Acute	Increase ROM Maintain Strength	AROM ISOMETRIC
Chronic	Increase ROM Increase Strength Increase Endurance	AROM ARROM ISOKINETIC AEROBIC

TABLE 17-2
TREATMENT MODALITIES

Modality	*Specific Contraindications*
Superficial Heating	
1. Moist Hot Pack: Silica gel which absorbs and retains large amounts of water. Packs are placed in thermostatically controlled water at 175° F.	Open Wounds
2. Paraffin Wax: Liquid paraffin is heated and maintained at a temperature of 125° F, and can be applied in a variety of methods: (a) dip, (b) continuous immersion, (c) brush.	Open Wounds
3. Hydrotherapy: Whirlpool, therapeutic pool, Hubbard tank. Buoyant property of water permits motion with much of gravity eliminated. Movement is achieved with decreased strain on joints.	Rashes Open Wounds Incontinence Severe Cardiac Disease Severe Respiratory Disease
4. Moist Air Machine: A cabinet filled with heated moist air controlled thermostatically.	Infected Wounds
5. Fluidotherapy: Thermostatically controlled hot air blown through a pad of finely divided solids, e.g., glass beads.	Open Wounds Infected Wounds
Deep Heating	
1. Short Wave Diathermy: Application of high frequency currents with an induction coil, or condenser field.	Metal Implants Pregnancy Pacemaker
2. Microwave Diathermy: Electromagnetic wave radiation.	Metal Implants Pregnancy Pacemaker
3. Ultrasound: Acoustic vibration propagated along the axis of a beam with frequencies so high that it cannot be perceived by the human ear.	Pregnancy

CHAPTER 18

OCCUPATIONAL THERAPY

Judith Lannefield Klinger, M.A., O.T.R.

INTRODUCTION

Occupational therapy, as an important health profession in rehabilitation, is deeply concerned with the functional capabilities of the person with arthritis. These range from basic activities of daily living, i.e., self-care and mobility, to jobs, leisure time, sexuality, social and community relations. The role of the occupational therapist is three-fold:

1. To assess the health and rehabilitation needs of the client.
2. To identify and minimize the effects of the disease, and
3. To design and provide a therapeutic program to improve the patient's ability to function in self-care and life-role activities.

Occupational therapy contributes to both the physical and emotional independence of the individual with rheumatic disease, looking at him or her as a whole person with responsibilities and desires. From initial screening and assessment to discharge and follow-up, the ultimate goal of occupational therapy is to help the patient find a way to travel life's path, enjoying the process to its fullest.

The occupational therapist (OT) does not work alone. At the center of the multidisciplinary team is the patient, the raison d'etre. Guiding the treatment in occupational therapy and other disciplines, is the physician. Depending on the setting, the rehabilitation or home care nurse, the physical therapist, social worker and other professionals share in this process of rehabilitation.

As arthritis is a changing disease, with intermittent periods of exacerbation and remission, the treatment program in occupational therapy will vary. It may include, among other things:

a. Patient education in methods of joint protection, energy conservation and work simplification.
b. Hand and upper extremity intervention, focusing on increasing range of motion, strength and endurance as well as preventing deformities.
c. Provision of orthotic devices and splinting to allow complete rest,

decrease pain, prevent deformity, and protect joints and muscles following surgery.

d. Application of adaptive or self-help equipment and environmental modifications to increase function and decrease stress to affected joints and muscles.

e. Vocational and avocational modifications to allow fuller activity and decrease stress.

f. Family counseling to encourage and allow attainment of goals that the patient has set.

g. Transition to community, whether job, school, leisure-time or volunteer activities.

h. Follow-up to ascertain that the patient is functioning completely to his or her abilities, and to make modifications as necessary.

Occupational therapy for rheumatic disease continues to evolve and changes as new treatment methods are found valuable. The parameters of the occupational therapist's job varies from health care facility to facility, from hospital to home care. In some settings, the occupational therapist carries out only activities of daily living; in others, is responsible for all upper extremity treatment and training including orthotics. In home care settings, the occupational therapist may also do family counseling on a deeper level if a social worker is not available.

Occupational Therapy Assessment

Occupational therapy assessment refers to the process of determining the need for, nature of, and estimated time of treatment, determining the needed coordination with other health care professionals and persons involved, then documenting these findings.

The assessment may begin with *screening*, or review of the potential client's case to determine the need for treatment. This includes discussions with the other health care professionals. In some settings, such as home care, the screening may be done by the physician or hospital discharge service, with the therapist then receiving orders.

Patient-related consultation is ideally done as a case conference within the health care setting as it allows sharing of relevant information with other professionals in order to develop a full-treatment program. When this is not possible, a mini-conference with the assigned nurse or physician will help pinpoint the most important factors. In some instances, a review of the chart is the sole source of information before evaluation. During the consultation, the occupational therapist may give and receive treatment recommendations and study previous documentation from a referring facility.

Evaluation in occupational therapy provides a baseline on which to plan treatment and initiate a program. It is the process of obtaining and interpreting data necessary for treatment. Methods used in occupational therapy include, but are not limited to, standardized tests, performance checklists and activities or tasks designed to evaluate specific performance abilities. For a patient with arthritis, the evaluation may be broken into different sections including:

a. Hand and wrist assessment
b. Upper extremity range of motion and strength
c. Trunk involvement and posture
d. Foot assessment and limitations caused by lower extremity involvement
e. Activities of daily living
f. Vocational (including homemaking) and avocational or leisure time
g. Psychological considerations

Re-assessment is the process of obtaining and interpreting the data necessary for revising the goals and treatment planning with the patient who has rheumatic disease. The time periods between re-assessments differ according to the stage of the disease, the health care setting requirements and the progress or problems which the patient has experienced in occupational therapy. Portions of the initial evaluation or assessment may be administered as well as documentation taken from progress notes of individual sessions. The occupational therapist may decide that more frequent re-evaluations are needed because the patient is progressing faster than the program envisaged, or may find additional problems that the patient was reluctant to discuss during initial assessment that should be added to the treatment goals.

Occupational Therapy Goals and Modalities in Relation to Specific Stages of Rheumatic Disease

Acute Phase

During the acute phase of inflammatory joint disease, whether there is single or multiple joint involvement, the role of the occupational therapist is four-fold: (a) To reduce pain and inflammation, (b) To maintain range of motion and joint integrity, (c) To maintain strength and endurance and, (d) To assist the patient in maintaining a positive outlook and a good psychological balance.

Reducing Pain and Inflammation: Patience education begins during the inflammatory stage as the patient and those assisting are taught methods for lessening the pain, permitting complete rest and preventing deformities. Proper posture for lying or sitting must often be taught. The therapist should advise the patient to use a firm mattress with a simple bedboard, if necessary. Use of a hospital bed may be needed. The patient should learn to lie on a small pillow placed just under the neck so that the head is not forced forward. A butterfly pillow allows the individual to move more easily while keeping the head and spine in correct alignment. There should be no kneed pillows and the patient must be instructed in the great dangers of propping the lower extremities, leading to knee contractures. When using a hospital bed, the mattress must be kept flat under the knees.

The occupational therapist is usually called upon to splint or position specific joints for complete rest. These include wrist/hand resting splints, posterior leg or ankle splints, and proper support for the neck and back while lying or sitting in bed. A soft neck collar may be indicated while sitting. Footboards are helpful in elevating bedcovers so feet are not forced into plantar flexion. In home care, heavy cardboard may be used to construct a suitable footboard. A variety of materials allow construction of splints at the bedside.

Unnecessary joint stress is eliminated through adequate rest in bed or a chair for the lower extremities, and instruction in energy conservation and joint protection methods given for the upper and lower extremity involved joints. Appropriate transfer methods and ambulation may also be stressed for hospitalized and home-bound patients.

The occupational therapist may occasionally be asked to relieve pain secondary to joint inflammation and protective muscle spasm by application of ice compresses, heating pad or hot packs. In such instances, safety techniques in the use of heat must be stressed.

If there is temporomandibular involvement, the occupational therapist will also instruct the patient in exercises to maintain jaw mobility, and watch that the diet encourages proper chewing. Deep breathing and postural exercises may be indicated to help the person maintain thoracic and scapular joint mobility during the acute stage. Finally, it is essential that within a multi-discipline health care setting, the team members coordinate their activities to allow adequate rest by the patient.

Range of Motion and Joint Integrity: Maintaining range of motion (ROM) and joint integrity may be the role of the occupational or physical therapist. Gentle passive or active ROM to the point of pain, without stretch, is given twice a day. The therapist may teach the patient to do effective self-ROM of the neck, elbows, hands, knees and ankles. But, it is usually necessary to assist the patient in gentle passive range of the shoulders and hips, and passive ROM is necessary to allow the greatest relaxation of muscles.

Strength and Endurance: Performance of self-care and feeding activities as well as isometric exercises encourage the patient in maintenance of strength and endurance. Isometric exercises of one to three full contractions per muscle group per day are recommended if the patient can tolerate them without muscle spasms. Strengthening is not started while the patient has systemic illness, and the therapist will be directed by the physician's orders and philosophy as well as by the patient's condition.

Maintaining a Positive Outlook: Both the adaptation of basic utensils for self-feeding and grooming as well as patient education regarding future treatment plans will assist the patient in maintaining a positive outlook and psychologic balance. The importance of understanding the individual's fears and frustrations, and of giving reassurance, cannot be overstated. The talents of the occupational therapist as a counselor are as important as the physical exercises during the acute stage.

Subacute Phase

During the subacute phase, the occupational therapist continues to aid the patient in reducing both pain and inflammation, through splinting and proper positioning to rest involved joints. At this point in patient education, the individual is feeling better, wants to do more, and the therapist moves into discussion of joint protection methods, planning for adequate rest and use of assistive aides, such as the raised toilet seat and hand rails to reduce stress on the lower extremities, especially the knees.

When maintaining ROM and joint integrity, the therapist can now begin to apply gentle pressure through manual assistance or graduated activities to insure that the patient achieves a complete range of motion. Exercises while lying prone will help insure full hip ROM.

As the patient begins to do more, he or she will also require more re-education in proper positioning, whether sitting and reading, watching television, writing or doing handwork. A seating arrangement must be designed to keep the back and neck supported in straight alignment, with the knees in full extension (while in bed), and the ankles supported at right angles whether lying or sitting. The individual should be encouraged to extend the fingers while at rest. The therapist may recommend a lapboard that permits complete rest of the hand and forearm for use with bed, chair or wheelchair.

Graduated activities in occupational therapy will maintain muscle strength and improve endurance for persons with systemic disease. Patients also require education in work simplification and energy conservation techniques. The therapist will evaluate with each patient the daily schedule, emphasizing the need of adequate rest.

Chronic-Active Phase

At this point, there is still synovitis which makes supporting joint structures vulnerable to joint deformity. Patients are anxious to do more, and the occupational therapist must focus education on maintenance of joint integrity. Joint protection techniques, assistive or self-help aids and splinting, are all important in preventing deformity. Exercises to improve muscle strength and increase ROM may also be started. Again, careful supervision is necessary to make sure the patient does not substitute or overdo.

Implications for Occupational Therapy in Juvenile Rheumatoid Arthritis

Occupational therapy has a broad role when working with children with juvenile rheumatoid arthritis. The major therapeutic goal is to allow the growing child to function as normally as possible to assume a full role in society. Maximal activity within the confines of the disease is encouraged. Translating the goals to parents, gaining both their understanding and involvement is a critical aspect in patient education. Parents must understand that promoting good health, following directions for exercise programs to maintain ROM and muscle strength are paramount to the child's complete functioning.

In the presence of temperomondibutes joint arthritis, the occupational therapist should encourage the child to eat normal foods. The parents must understand that if they allow the child to adjust the diet to increasingly soft foods, even to sipping through a straw, both diminishing range of jaw movement and development of subsequent adhesive capsulitis may occur. Jaw movement and normal eating habits should be encouraged.

Implications for Occupational Therapy in Ankylosing Spondylitis

Patient education that stresses balanced rest and activity are as important for the ankylosing spondylitis patient as for the rheumatoid arthritis patients. The therapist will stress proper positioning at rest, with a firm mattress and small or contoured pillow no larger than necessary to support the normal lordotic curve of the cervical spine. In addition, a home program to maintain range and strength will be combined with breathing and posture exercises. The patient must learn to avoid activities which place stress on the back.

Since many of these patients are young, prevocational testing and counseling may be part of the occupational therapist's role. Adaptations within the work place, i.e., correct seating and relation of work surface to the body, should be done through an on-site visit.

Implications for Occupational Therapy in Post-Operative Rehabilitation

Hands severely deformed by arthritis are often quite functional despite their appearance. Reconstructive surgery, therefore, is indicated only if further function can be restored or increasing deformity prevented. The most common surgical procedures for the hands are tendon transfers and correction of contractures.

Other procedures include arthroplasty and the implantation of prosthetic replacements. In all instances, the occupational therapy program focuses on coordination and range of motion during the early post-operative period. When arthroplasty is performed at the elbow to increase motion and relieve pain, a careful program to maintain muscular control is indicted. Muscle re-education will aid in return of supination.

Reconstructive surgery of the lower extremities is far more advanced than that of the uppers. The post-operative rehabilitation program focuses on ambulation. The occupational therapist may see these patients for prescribing of aids while recuperating and for training in activities of daily living, especially tasks requiring bending and ambulation.

Implications for Occupational Therapy in Non-Inflammatory Joint Disease

Non-inflammatory joint disease is treated in occupational therapy the same as the chronic-inactive stage of inflammatory joint disease. In this degenerative or "burned out" phase of rheumatoid arthritis, the therapist teaches that prolonged static positioning leads to joint stiffness, and that exercise is important to avoid or overcome disuse atrophy. The program may assist the patient in developing better endurance, which was lost because of inactivity or systemic involvement. Proper positioning, both in terms of posture and of using tools, continues to stress joint protection to reduce muscle spasms and pain as well as to work within residual deformities and to prevent further deformities.

Those with chronic inactive rheumatoid arthritis and non-inflammatory joint disease are often candidates for transition to community activities. This outreach role is one assumed by occupational therapists who realize that rehabilitation within the home or hospital is not adequate for the patient to attain a full or balanced life-style. The files of an OT must, therefore, contain information on community resources and contacts with persons involved in groups, from Senior Center to volunteers and special transportation programs for the handicapped and aging.

Joint Protection and Energy Conservation

> "Tell me and I'll forget.
> Show me and I might understand.
> Involve me, and I'll remember."
> —A Chinese Proverb

Patient education in the intertwined areas of joint protection and energy conservation is a major role of the occupational therapist. To simply tell a patient and then expect that principles will be assimilated into tasks of daily life is not realistic. Programs through clinics and audio visual demonstrations help carry the message. Reinforcement by repletion by various disciplines helps. But, the only way to really educate a patient is to do each activity he or she is called upon to do in daily life, showing the principles each time.

Joint protection training, then, is *showing* the patient how to perform tasks with a minimal amount of stress to involved joints. The goals are to: (a) Respect and reduce pain, (b) Preserve joint integrity, and (c) Conserve physical resources or energy. The concepts of anatomy, kinesiology and the pathology of rheumatic disease must be so carefully translated to the patient that they mesh with daily activities in a manner that preserves both physical status and level of functional ability. The patient can learn to: (a) Reduce the force, (b) change the method, (c) use energy-saving equipment, aids or an orthosis, (d) eliminate the activity, and (e) take intermittent breaks.

Special techniques for protecting the hands, which are emphasized in occupational therapy include:

1) Encourage movement of each joint at maximum range of motion and strength consistent with the disease process. Maintain ROM of extension of the wrist and supination of the forearm.

2) Avoid ulnar deviating forces at the metacarpophalangeal joints, strains which abduct the phalanges of the thumb and cause lateral strains on interphalangeal joints. (Eliminate manual jar opening and small manual can openers.)

3) Avoid the internal stresses of strong grip. (Examples are using a screwdriver or extended writing.)

4) Avoid prolonged positions of deformity, such as flexion of the fingers and wrists, knees and hips, and avoid external pressures and internal pressures in their direction.

5) Use each joint in its most stable anatomical position or functional plane, i.e., work with the wrist in slight extension.

6) Avoid holding. Set objects down and slide them instead of lifting.

7) Use the strongest joint available for the activity, i.e., lift with the elbows and proximal parts of the forearm, not the wrist. Instead of overworking the fingers, use the palm, the ulnar side of the hand and the bend of the elbow to push, hold, pull.

8) Avoid muscle imbalance, i.e., perform activities, such as weaving, that call into play both extensors and flexors.

9) Hold objects in hand parallel to the knuckle, and not across the palm diagonally.

10) Never attempt an activity that cannot be stopped immediately, if it proves beyond your power to complete it.

Orthotics

Splinting of a limb affected by arthritis may be indicated at various stages of the disease for different reasons.

During the acute stage, complete immobilization of an inflamed joint reduces inflammation. With proper support of the joint, the muscles relax and pain through motion is eliminated. The occupational therapist may fabricate splints for any part of the body, including the lower extremities, although the most common is for the hand and wrist.

From the acute through the chronic-active stages, an orthosis may be prescribed to prevent further deformity by splinting the hand and wrist in a functional position with optimal joint alignment. Deformities which are minimized or protected through application of a wrist and hand orthosis include metacarpophalangeal ulnar drift, subluxation of the wrist and swan-neck deformities.

An orthosis to allow improvement of function may be designed by the therapist for use during the sub-acute to the chronic-inactive stages. The most common type of orthosis here is wrist stabilization, which minimize pain during the grasp and leads to increase of grasping power.

Finally, orthoses are indicated following surgery to: (1) maintain surgically achieved mobility and alignment, (2) assist post-operative strengthening and (3) prevent or minimize post-surgical adhesions.

Before determining the value of and type of splint to be applied, the occupational therapist does a complete hand assessment. Main foci include the current status of hand function, types of grasp used, how tasks are performed (ease, effort, pain, speed and dexterity), and uses to which the patient will be putting orthosis. The patient must simultaneously be instructed in the value of the splint, the reasons it is to be worn and for what activities.

Following fabrication of the orthosis, the therapist is responsible for checking fit over a period of time, making adjustments as needed, training the patient in its use including donning and removing, and following up at a specified time period to make sure orthosis is being used correctly. It is important for the therapist to see the orthosis in use, as immobilization of one or more joints can transfer stress to other joints and muscles. For example, splinting a weak wrist may require the shoulder to perform more work than previously done. If the shoulder is also involved, pain from stress can ensure and even be translated to the back with shifts in posture trying to compensate.

Aids to Independent Living—Assistive Devices and Environments Planning

Self-help aids and environmental planning help the patient with arthritis overcome barriers that could otherwise limit function. The occupational therapist works in both areas to allow the individual complete independence as well as adequate joint protection.

An assistive device may be indicated for one of several reasons:

1. To support and protect
2. To serve as a functional replacement or aid to a functionally inadequate body part
3. To serve as a means of conserving energy
4. To insure safety

A single device, such as a jar opener or lever handle on a door, may fill needs in more than one category. Both of these aids protect the hand and wrist joints from over exertion which could lead to further deformity, replace lost strength in the hands and conserve energy otherwise fruitlessly expended.

Self-help aids for patients complement rather than substitute for a well-planned rehabilitation program. They are kept to a minimum lest they encourage reduced exercise and activity by the patient. Each aid is prescribed with a specific goal in mind. Many times the goal may be a preventative as well as a functional one, in that an assistive device helps a patient do something independently at the same time it protects joints from over stress. This is especially true of home adaptations, such as tub bench or a raised toilet seat to reduce stress on hips and knees, or the use of a wheeled carrying unit to reduce stress on the hands and arms.

Prescription or application of assistive devices requires analysis by the therapist of the utensil as well as the job. For the patient with rheumatoid arthritis, cutting with scissors is an activity that can increase deformity, especially ulnar drift. Small scissors which require gross grasp work well for cutting threads and small mending chores. For longer term projects, electric scissors are occasionally the answer. A better solution is the spring-open scissor which works by palmar pressure, when placed on a stand, allowing the fingers to remain in extension.

With the availability of work-saving products, the therapist can often find answers in the commercial market. For items that must be constructed, publications are available that give both ideas and plans.

Patient education involves first telling the patient the purposes of the device, i.e., to increase function and/or protect joints, then teaching the patient how to use it. Often the need for a device will have to be restressed as that it is understood that, although a task may be done without the aid, the purpose is conservation of energy and joint protection.

Keeping a large supply of aids on hand is both expensive and impractical for the therapist engaged in home care or non-hospital based work. A sampling of the most useful aids are listed in Table 18-1.

Daily Living Skills

Dressing: As part of the evaluation process, occupational therapy deals with problems with dressing that the patient may be experiencing due to limited range of motion or poor hand function. A three-fold approach may be taken: (1) Application of techniques and modifications which reduce the effort required, (2) Prescribing of simple aids to overcome permanent or temporary limitations, and (3) Recommendations for selection of easy-to-handle clothing.

A new technique may be all that a patient needs. Lying on the bed, for example, is often an easier way to put on a girdle or trousers. The feet may sometimes be brought up within reach to slip on socks. Putting the more affected arm into a sleeve first leaves the more mobile extremity for the other tighter sleeve. For handling back zippers, a rigid zipper-pull made from a dowel with a crosspiece for a handle is easier to use than a cord-type-pull. A bra may be put on backwards, the elastic straps slipped over the shoulders after it is fastened and turned.

Simple modifications include Velcro tabs under buttons to eliminate buttoning, especially at collars, elastic thread on cuff buttons, Velcro or hooks at waist openings, loops or rings added to zipper pulls. A dressing stick (closet hook attached to a dowel) slips sweaters over immobile shoulders, helps pull up pants and gets items out of the closet. Large buttons with shanks or a button hook may be used when hand function is impaired. A long-handled shoe horn and a sock/stocking device extend reach. Shoe adaptations may be made by the therapist or a local shoe repair shop to allow fastening footgear for proper support when walking. The therapist may also be asked to make foot orthoses or shoe inserts to achieve correct balance in the shoes themselves.

The occupational therapist may recommend some general principle in making future purchases of clothing. Front closures are always preferred. Some sweaters come with large front zippers. Purchasing clothes one or two sizes larger than usual makes dressing easier. "V" necks are easier to slip on as are raglan sleeves. A slippery lining of silk scarf put over the hand allows one to don a coat with greater ease. Thin insulated linings reduce weight of winter outdoor clothing. Ponchos and capes are stylish answers. As part of patient education the therapist may suggest sources for easy-to-handle clothing.

Ambulation

Although ambulation training is mainly the province of the physical therapist, the occupational therapist may be involved in the adaptation of walking aids, i.e., adapting forearm crutches. The OT will also be working with the patient learning to manage functional tasks while ambulating. It is at this point that carrying items, performing vocational or household tasks must be tested for safety and adaptation.

Homemaking

Homemaking activities are an excellent way of continuing occupational therapy in the home. Whether in a hospital or a home-based retraining program, the occupational therapist stresses the following in-patient education:

1. Attention to Diet: Help with planning for good nutrition with any recommendations or restrictions ordered by the physician. Overweight, which adds stress to the lower extremities and increases fatigue, is to be avoided. Writing out meal plans with the patient is a first step to diet modification.
2. Avoiding Fatigue Through Simplified Methods of Work and Schedules

Which Allow for Adequate Rest: Younger patients with heavy family responsibilities may need assistance in delegating or reducing the number of jobs they do. Older individuals with arthritis may require just the opposite—lots of encouragement to do more.

3. Maintaining Posture Through Correct Seating: The person with arthritis will have to learn to change position frequently, alternating sitting with short periods of standing, grasping large-handled tools with intervals of extending the fingers and relaxing.
4. Joint Protection, Both in Selection of Correct Utensils and Handling of Activities: Education includes showing how to close drawers with fingers extended, pushing up from a chair with fingers extended, using a sponge rather than a dish cloth, using a dusting mitt and rolling pins, all with fingers extended.

Within the homemaking areas, the occupational therapist should see that hand-operated can openers are replaced by electric units or manual units with large built-up handles for greater leverage. Installing a simple wedge-type jar opener eliminates the stress caused by the most villainous job in the kitchen. A knife with a built-up perpendicular handle allows the user to translate the action of the arm to the knife blade, rather than putting stress on the wrist and fingers.

New methods of doing tasks should be tried, such as turning a rotary egg-beater backwards to reduce the tendency towards ulnar deviation. If a jar opener is not accepted, then the patient must learn to open jars with the right hand and close them with the left. Stress of lifting is reduced by using both hands. The therapist should prepare a list of suggestions for the patient to follow on his or her own, or provide appropriate literature.

5. Adjusting to Limitations: A home visit is most important to assist the patient in making practical as well as therapeutic changes. When on the scene, the therapist can help select and adapt a chair from those available in the home, choosing one that is higher and firmer and affords the best sitting posture. The storage needs of the patient, from kitchen to closets, can be assessed more easily with recommendations for rearrangement or provision of a reaching device. The most commonly used utensils may be built-up for safe grip and the angle of grip adjusted for efficient, safe use. Opening containers so that the hands are protected from stress should be tried. Taking items in and out of the oven should be tested and the patient cautioned about proper clothing while working near the stove.

Reaching is helpful to encourage shoulder flexion and elbow extension. Bending encourages both flexion and extension of the knees, hips and back. Neither "exercise" should be eliminated, but accommodations made to allow for both "good and bad days."

Bedmaking requires careful evaluation as it places great stress on the back, lower extremities, arms and hands. Learning to cut down motions may help. Recommendations of lightweight thermal, electric or dacron-filled blankets reduces the amount of stress. Bedmaking and especially bed changing may be delegated to another member of the family, or fitted sheets can be adapted with one corner opened and Velcro strips added to close it. This eliminates the need to lift the mattress. If the client insists on tucking in blankets "a peole" a wooden bread spade makes an excellent tucker-in-er.

Leisure-Time Activities

Life cannot be balanced if a person is denied participation in leisure-time and social pursuits. This creates further depression, dependence and lack of motivation. An occupational therapy program, therefore, takes into account the leisure desires of the patient. Sports, gardening, crafts all are possible with some adaptations.

Gardening may become a more important year-round activity with starting of seedlings, planning or raised beds, use of a wheeled-seat and lightweight tools. Crafts such as knitting, which tend to be harmful to the hands, can be replaced with more exciting possibilities such as weaving on a flat or table harness loom, which increases range of motion, knitting on a round frame, bargello or large-point needlework.

Card playing and reading are more restful if the person knows how to sit comfortably and uses a card or book holder. Two inexpensive book holders will support a newspaper. A styrofoam pellet-filled lap desk supports a book and holds paper for writing. A felt tip pen makes for easier writing, especially if a foam curler is slipped over the shaft.

Automobile Travel

Transportation to and from shopping, medical appointments, community activities and visiting is often limited for the patient with arthritis severe enough to make handling various aspects of the car stressful. Evaluation of needs in this area can make auto travel not only more pleasant but can keep a patient involved in the world around rather than chronically home-bound.

The therapist may find that a new technique to open the car door, such as using the side of the hand, or prescription of a car door opener, is the first step. Getting into a car, as passenger or driver, may be painful. A swivel cushion seat eliminates the need to lift the buttocks and thighs while turning and reduces stress on joints and muscles. Assist handles on the roof gutter aid in attaining a standing position. A firm backrest permits better posture while riding or driving. A built-up key holder unlocks doors and turns on the ignition with ease. Automobile controls may be adapted to meet the needs of various degrees of disability. If an occupational therapist is not familiar with these modifications, help and often evaluation may be obtained through a State Registry of Motor Vehicles office.

Trained inspectors recommend equipment and test drivers to assure safety on the road.

Patient Education and Counseling

The occupational therapist is one of the team members responsible for a patient education program so clearly defined and tailored to the individual's needs that it becomes an integral part of daily life.

Throughout the disease process, specific major topics will be discussed and refined with the patient. The major areas, discussed earlier, are prevention of deformities, proper posture and positioning and time-management, whether at home, in school or on the job.

The occupational therapist, in conjunction with the social service department, works towards a transition to the community. Far-sighted planning and the utilization of volunteer and community agencies can permit an individual to live an even fuller life perhaps than before hospitalization. The therapist working in the home has an even greater opportunity to tap into community resources to assist the patient in transition to increased participation in the world.

Within the school system, the occupational therapist assists in translating the needs of the student to the educational staff. Where problems in proper seating within the classroom, handling of materials, such as writing implements, books or typewriters, or architectural barriers, i.e., too-heavy restroom doors, inaccessible water fountains, and unsafe hand railings exists, the therapist may help with solutions. It is, moreover, often by the student that these "small" problems are raised during an occupational therapy session. Such problems then may be brought to the attention of the parents to carry to the school or directly by the therapist to the student's counselor, school nurse or teacher.

Funding

Finding finances for equipment, home modifications, training and services is a serious obstacle with which occupational therapists and other health professionals must contend. Knowing what agencies will pay, is crucial. A current list of Medicare-approved equipment may be obtained from a surgical supply firm. Involving the family and friends often turns up individuals skilled and eager to help construct and even purchase, aids or home alterations. Other resources from which the patient may be eligible for assistance include equipment lending services, as part of or in conjunction with Visiting Nurse Associations, local chapters of the Arthritis Foundation, senior citizen centers and other such organizations. Shopping and transportation volunteers are available through the Red Cross and Friendly Visitors groups as well as other community organizations. Local organizations, such as the Rotary and Kiwanis often support individual cases. Contractor's association may make home changes. Local high school talent may be harnessed to make self-help aids in shop classes, to help out a home-bound person as part of a club activity. The same is true of college and university groups. Local chapters of the Arthritis Foundation may have special endowment funds, such as the Jerry Walsh Fund in Connecticut, for help in financing patient services, clothing modifications and equipment.

The occupational therapist needs as much imagination and ingenuity here in finding and funding as in designing the therapeutic program itself. A constantly up-dated file helps speed the process. Brain-storming the problems and needs with other health professionals gives new leads.

Resources

The occupational therapist has a wide variety of resources for help and sharing of ideas. Most active is the Arthritis Health Profession Section of the Arthritis Foundation. It has regional as well as national meetings. Local chapters of the Foundation also sponsor meetings on topics of relevance to those involved in the treatment of rheumatic diseases. For those interested in research in rheumatic disease, they offer a limited number of Traineeships and Research Grants for non-physician health professionals in clinical disciplines relating to arthritis.

The American Occupational Therapy Association has special interest groups which include aspects of arthritis and the rheumatic diseases. AOTA also distributes literature on arthritis.

The Arthritis Clearing House provides materials, both printed and audio visual, including curricula for establishing programs in patient education. Among their materials is a bibliography on exercise, daily living and clothing.

Resources are limited only by one's imagination. Occupational therapists often discover when searching for the solution for patients with rheumatic and other diseases, that the answer may be right before our eyes in popular literature and publications.

SUGGESTED READINGS AND INFORMATION SOURCES

The Aged Patient: A sourcebook for the Allied Health Professional. Eds. N. Ernest and H. Glazer-Woldman, Year Book Medical Pub. Co. 1983.

Aids and Adaptations. The Occupational Therapy Department, The Canadian Arthritis and Rheumatism Society, British Columbia Div., Vancouver. Individual sheets free from the Arthritis Society, 920 Yonge Street, Suite 420, Tornot, Canada M4W 3J7.

Aids to Independent Living: Self Help for the Handicapped. Edward W. Lowman and Judith L. Klinger, McGraw-Hill, N.Y. 1969.

Arthritis. Practice Div., The American Occupational Therapy Association, Rockville, Maryland. Revised March 1983. Personnel resources, organizational resources, bibliography, audiovisuals. OT reporting and evaluation outlines.

A Handbook of Assistive Devices for the Handicapped Elderly. Joseph M. Breuer, Haworth Press, N.Y. 1983.

Care of the Arthritic Hand. Adrian E. Flatt, 4th edition. C.V. Mosby, 1983.

Help for Your Arthritic Hand. Semyon Krewer with Ann Edgar. Simon and Schuster, N.Y. 1982.

Home Care Programs in Arthritis: A Manual for Patients. Subcommittee of the Education Committee of the Allied Health Professions Section of the Arthritis Foundation, Atlanta, Georgia 1969. Illustrated exercise program, information on managing at home and self-help aids. Free from local arthritis chapters.

How to Create Interiors for the Disabled: A Guidebook for Family and Friends. Jane Randolph Cary, Pantheon Books, N.Y. 1978. Well illustrated with line drawings and sources for assistance and equipment.

"Joint Protection, a responsibility of the occupational therapist." Joy Cordery, Amer Journal of Ooccupational Therapy 19:285–294, 1965. (Whole issue is devoted to arthritis and occupational therapy.)

Living and Loving: Information About Sex. Available from local chapters of the Arthritis Foundation.

Manual for Allied Health Professionals. Professional Manual Subcommittee of the Education Committee. N. Coyne, Chairman. The Allied Health Professions Section of the Arthritis Foundation, Atlanta, Georgia 1973. Available from national office and local chapters of the Foundation.

The Mature Years: A Geriatric Occupational Therapy Text. Sandra Lewis. Slack, Thorofare, New Jersey 1983. Includes psychosocial changes, primary diseases of the elderly, and community OT programs.

Mealtime Manual for People with Disabilities and the Aging. Judith Klinger with the Institute of Rehabilitation Medicine, New York University Medical Center. Campbell Soup Company, Camden, New Jersey 1978. 2nd edition. From Mealtime Manual, Box 38, Ronks, Pennsylvania 17572.

Non-Operative Hand Management of Adult Onset Rheumatoid Arthritis. P. MacBain, N. Galbrain and F. Brady. The Arthritis Society, Vancouver, B.C. 1981.

The Patient at Home. M. Barnes and C. Crutchfield. Slack, Thorofare, New Jersey 1971.

A Model for Planning Patient Education: An Essential Component of Health Care. Report of the Committee on Educational Tasks in Chronic Illness. Public Health Section, American Public Health Association, U.S. Dept. of Health, Education and Welfare (3rd printing) 1975. Publication Number: HRA 76-4028. From The Superintendent of Documents, U.S. Govt. Printing Office, Washington, D.C. 20402.

Patient Education in Arthritis. "How To" Packet, prepared by the Arthritis Health Professions Section. The Arthritis Foundation, Atlanta, Georgia 1977.

Rehabilitation Gazette. Gazette International Networking Institute, 4502 Maryland Avenue, St. Louis, MO 63108. Articles on attaining independence in all areas of life by those with disabilities and professionals, plus reviews of new literature.

Rheumatic Disease: Occupational Therapy and Rehabilitation, 2nd edition. Jeanne L. Melvin, F.A. Davis. Philadelphia, PA 1982. An excellent complete resource for the occupational therapist and other professionals on background and procedures of treatment. Well-illustrated.

Scorable Self-Care Evaluation. E. Clark and M. Peters. Slack, Thorofare, N.J. 1984. Method to measure a variety of self-care skills in a brief amount of time.

Self Help Manual for Patients with Arthritis. The Task Force to Revise the Self-Help Manual. The Arthritis Health Professions Section of the Arthritis Foundation. Judith L. Klinger, editor. The Arthritis Foundation, Atlanta, Georgia 1980. From the national office or local chapters of the Foundation. Basic information on joint protection and managing at home, aids and techniques for various areas of daily living, with sources. Well-illustrated.

RESOURCE ADDRESSES

The American Occupational Therapy Association, Inc.
1383 Piccard Drive
Rockville, Maryland 20850

The Arthritis Health Professions Section
The Arthritis Foundation
1314 Spring Street NW
Atlanta, Georgia 30309

The Arthritis Information Clearinghouse
P.O. Box 9782
Arlington, Virginia 22209

The Arthritis Society (CARS)
British Columbia Division
895 West 10th Avenue
Vancouver, B.C. Canada V57 1L7

TABLE 18-1
TYPICAL OCCUPATIONAL THERAPY AIDS

Foam curlers to use as built-up handles
Swivel spoon
Large-handled mug or commuter cup
Flexible drinking straws
Several sizes of elastic cuffs with Velcro closures and palmar pockets
Tapes and rubber bands for handles of small utensils
Velcro, rings for zipper tabs, large hooks
Elastic shoelaces
Long-handled shoe horn
Gutter stocking and sock aid
Cup hook on a dowel for lacing shoes and doing zippers
Closet hook on a dowel for dressing
Assorted reachers
Raised toilet seat and toilet bars
Adjustable height commode
Adjustable height tub bench or seat
Portable shower unit
Wooden transfer board
Pull-up aid to attach to bed
Wedge-type jar opener
Sponges to adapt an electric can opener
Sponge cloth to stabilize a bowl, plate or other objects
Book holder
Card holder
Adapted breadboard
Swedish or similar knife with angled handle
Door handle lever
Suction brush
Swivel seat cushion for car transfer
Car roof gutter grip
Car door opener

CHAPTER 19

SOCIAL WORK

Enid Engelhard, MSW, CSW

INTRODUCTION

The basic tenet of the discipline of social work is to treat the person—in the situation. It is the social worker's task to engage the strengths that will help those so disabled adapt to the chronicity and uncertainties of their illnesses. In rheumatic disease care, social work incorporates and utilizes a multi-level system of interventions. It is an eclectic approach that draws on all the varied skills of the profession. Ever present is the challenge of meeting the special needs of people, each one an individual, each suffering in a different way.

The following is based on my clinical experience among such patients. It should be noted that, where necessary, I will use the feminine rather than the masculine pronouns, largely because so many of the rheumatic diseases are more likely to occur in women.

The First Imperative: Patient Assessment/Evaluation

Assessing and evaluating the social, familial, financial and societal environment of the patient is not merely the starting point, but probably the most important part of the overall treatment plan. What this assessment does is to immediately focus on the individual needs of the patient.

A demographic profile is taken to obtain all the relevant data: age, sex, income, education, marital status, occupation, presence and ages of children, etc. Psychographic factors are explored as well; these include assessments of ego strength, cognitive ability and degree of adaptability both to the environment and to the crisis of chronic illness. As shall be seen, these factors as they interrelate form the groundwork upon which the social worker builds in helping the client come to terms with rheumatic disease.

A review of Erik Erikson's theory of development offers a most useful framework for understanding the differing demands of adaptation to disability. Briefly stated, Erikson speculates that each life stage presents a variety of tasks to be mastered before proceeding to the next stage. The school child's task is to develop a sense of industry and competence; the adolescent's to form an identity through peer interaction while at the same time reaching for independence; the young adult's is to develop a sense of intimacy leading to a capacity for relationships with another. Clearly, these expected roles and tasks are necessarily interrupted by the limitations of a disabling or chronic illness.

In fact, when rheumatic disease strikes, a patient's whole life and, to a great extent, the lives of the people around the patient can be said to be interrupted. Appropriate intervention by the social worker to help the patient get on with her life will depend on the specific demographic and psychographic considerations obtained in preliminary and ongoing evaluations.

Referring back to Erickson, the adult patient has differing responsibilities from those of the adolescent patient and, thus, age is a very important variable to consider. But no matter what age, the limitations which the effects of the illness place on the patient's responsibilities must be viewed within the family system. Family members' roles, as well as their expectations, might well need to change as they too confront the crisis of disability.

Marriage poses both problems and positive resources. Always, however, roles within the marriage must be redefined. As responsibilities must of necessity be shifted onto the able-bodied partner, the patient must still feel needed and the patient's spouse must feel appreciated. While this can more easily happen in the case of a young couple, in the case of an elderly one, shared life with a spouse can be totally disrupted if the able bodied husband is physically or otherwise unable to care for the disabled wife. For this kind of patient as well as for the alone elderly, lack of a well partner may force placing the patient with an adult child or in a nursing home.

Sex of the patient, coupled with lifestage, has its own considerations for determining intervention. For the adult woman, there may be child rearing, homemaking responsibilities, or, in today's world, employment and career demands to bear in mind. For all women, adolescents and unmarried young women in particular, there can be the problems of self-image to deal with: worries about the illness itself, worries about weight gain or about disfigurement can be mighty threats to self-image. Not that these worries do not confront male clients, but an even more important consideration for males can be the loss of self-esteem that can result if or when his traditional roles as breadwinner and head of household are taken from him by rheumatic illness. Not only can both males and females lose these roles, they can lose the fruit of them, the income which heretofore supported themselves and family members and which also supported senses of self worth.

Evaluations of psychographic factors such as ego strength, cognitive ability and adaptability are in a sense the social worker's bottom line. Depression which is a common component of the chronic pain of rheumatic illness can alter thought processes and cause such problems as illogical thinking, particularly self deprecation and self blame. In turn, depression can lead to other maladaptive cognitive difficulties and learned helplessness. Adjustment will depend on premorbid personality patterns. And, as might be expected, the greater the ego strength, the better prognosis for adjustment.

Concerns Brought to the Social Worker

Worry, and attendant depression, whether evidenced to the social worker or not, is uppermost in the minds of patients newly or long diagnosed to have rheumatic disease. The social worker's role is to bring these worries to the surface so that they are less able to sap emotional strength. Typical concerns include the uncertainties and unpredictability of pain level that may be experienced in the short and long term. Moreover, with some rheumatic diseases there are indeed life-threatening levels of illness to be concerned about, as can be the case with systemic lupus erythematosus, scleroderma or, more rarely, rheumatoid arthritis.

For almost all of the one hundred rheumatic diseases, there is the reality that reduced activity may be an eventual necessity. Even short term absenteeism is a major fear whether it relates to occupation, school, family obligations and responsibilities or social activities. However, as noted above, the financial stress brought on by possible or real loss of employment can be the most difficult worry to deal with of all.

Helping to Facilitate Necessary Role Changes

Loss of independence and loss of mobility can lead to feelings of dissatisfaction, anger, resentment and frustration. Even so, as an example, if the patient is a young mother who can no longer care for her child, others must take on at least the physical aspects of this role. Here, the social worker in open discussion with client and family members can facilitate task division, letting the mother retain the child-rearing tasks she is still able to perform and reallocating those she cannot, thereby helping her to overcome feelings of worthlessness or worse, withdrawal from family life. In dealing with the necessity of role changes, it is a maxim that inhibition of communication between patient and social worker and, most especially, between patient and family members can slow the process of adaptation to the disability on the part of all concerned.

The Impact on Social Life

The physical restrictions of rheumatic disease on social life are a valid concern because of broken plans and, more importantly, because of the frequent inability of significant others to deal with chronic illness, as it affects their own social lives. Generally speaking, people are able to nurture, help, rescue and be useful in an acute illness situation; the acutely ill either pretty much recover completely or otherwise. On the other hand, people are far less able to cope with illness that is chronic and not immediately, if ever life-threatening. After all, they see their social lives being curtailed too, and for the very long term.

It is the social worker's job to see to it that the well family members do not give up their favorite activities and that the patient is encouraged to maintain her connections with the larger society to the extent that she can. In these efforts, the social worker's thrust is to continually reinforce a patient's feelings of worth in society. As an example, one patient of mine had to be told over and over again that her friends are her friends not because she is so accomplished in gourmet cooking as well as in about everything else, but because people love her for what she is inside, a warm person. She had to be convinced that they did not want to be shut out.

Sexual Function and Dysfunction

Rheumatic disease may or may not interfere with sexual function. Certainly, physical limitations or lack of responsiveness related to overriding worry may very well constrain sexual activity. In one case of mine, the able bodied partner avoided intimacy because of fears that it would cause his wife pain or discomfort. The wife thought she was being avoided because her husband thought her unattractive because of her disease. As is the case with many well couples, this unhappy couple was unable to communicate their sexual problems not only to their physicians but also to each other. It took separate meetings where these feelings could be aired to finally straighten all this out. In this connection, it is important for the social worker to "permit" the family to express feelings that they might consider socially unacceptable and to listen to them in a supportive and accepting way. For patients with sexual difficulties related to their illness, group therapy is sometimes indicated and recommended as it provides the opportunity for an exchange of ideas and problem solutions with others who have experienced similar difficulties.

Bolstering Self Image

The way one views one's body is an integral part of a person's identity. This is especially true of adolescents who so desperately need peer approval. With the side effects of steroid treatment as well as with the ravages of the disease itself, the bodily changes that result can be devastating to a patient's self image. Many of my patients, young and old, have expressed despondency, despair and depression to me over their weight gain or loss, hair loss, joint deformity or skin lesions. The emotional side effects, e.g., self-consciousness, lowered self-esteem, social withdrawal and isolation, are often far more devastating than the physical ones. The social worker can help the patient cope with these problems and find solutions, as with wigs, an adaptable wardrobe and covering make up. Empathetic, practical advice of this nature frequently helps to preserve dignity.

Dealing with Feelings of Loss

The psychosocial impact of rheumatic disease includes major issues of loss. Primary is the loss of good health for all time. As with the description of the mourning process described by Elisabeth Kubler-Ross in her book on death and dying, the patient and family members will need to grieve for the loss of the former self. The process Kubler-Ross describes includes periods or stages of denial, anger, guilt, bargaining and finally acceptance. The social worker can help the patient with rheumatic disease reach the final stage of acceptance by leading her and her family members to recognize that all such stages or emotions are normal and necessary to experience, as they are valuable coping mechanisms in the process of mourning the loss of good health.

Other impacting losses include not only the earlier described feelings of lowered self-esteem, but losses of power or control over one's life and loss of independence. These, combined with anxiety, a sense of isolation and a fear of the future can lead to an insecurity which the social worker must understand and help to overcome.

Dealing with Stress

Extraordinary emotional stress is experienced from the first awareness of symptoms to the eventual diagnosis of a chronic, painful, debilitating and sometimes disfiguring disease. Further, whether rheumatic disease has yet been diagnosed or not, stress seems to both exacerbate and trigger its symptoms and effects. To counter these deleterious results, stress management programs, individual counseling, family counseling, group therapy, biofeedback, guided imagery, relaxation techniques and prescribed breathing techniques are all useful treatment modalities.

An assessment of the individual's needs and problems will determine the type of intervention as well as its frequency and the necessary duration of intervention. In assessing the alternative choices, variables such as severity, extent or progression of disease activity as well as the patient's lifestyle, interpersonal relations, ability to work, support systems and ego strengths should all be taken into consideration.

The Use of Groups as Therapy

The group situation, used as therapy, psychotherapy or as a support system, has gained great popularity in the past few years due to the success it has enjoyed.

Low expense for the patient is a not inconsiderable benefit of group therapy. Groups can be conducted by professionals among both hospital and outpatient populations, either independently or as part of a comprehensive rehabilitation program.

Basically, groups offer emotional support. Other key attributes of groups, chosen for their appropriateness for our purposes are from Irvin Yalom's book, The Theory and Practice of Group Psychotherapy. Briefly addressed, groups offer *altruism:* helping others help to raise self esteem. *Cohesiveness or interaction:* we know that socially active patients fare better than those who are isolated. *Universality:* seeing the, "We're all in the same boat" reality in action. *Guidance:* via the suggestions or help in problem solving proffered by group members. *Catharsis:* the learning how and the ability to express or ventilate anxiety and negative feelings in a safe environment. *Identification:* as some of my clients have put this, "I found someone in the group I could pattern myself after," or "I'm trying to be like someone in the group who was better adjusted than I," or "Being in the group was, in a sense, like being in a family, only this time a more accepting and understanding family." *Instillation of hope:* or, put by a patient, "Knowing that the group had helped others with problems like mine encouraged me." *Existential factors:* such as the recognition inspired by the commonality of the disease in the group that life is, indeed, at times unfair or the building of inner strength that comes from seeing it in others.

Not all group therapy experience is positive, however. When a group member dies, becomes hospitalized or becomes obviously more disfigured, the reaction of others might be, "Am I next?" This kind of situation requires careful handling. These situations may stir up suppressed feelings and fears. The social worker must provide support and control, to open and maintain communication about the situation and provide opportunity for clarifying, coping and eventual acceptance.

The first death in our lupus support group was of an eighteen-year-old girl who had been hospitalized frequently from onset of disease. The group experienced grief over the loss of this member and concern for their own mortality. The following five group sessions were devoted to expression of their previously latent, unexpressed fears. Catharsis was encouraged. I found that the crisis situation strengthened the already cohesive nature of the group. The group concluded that whenever anyone they knew died, they always reacted to the evident fact that one day they also would die from one thing or another, but not necessarily from their illness. In this case, the group provided a means for encouraging expression of significant feelings and developed a desensitization to previously disturbing topics.

Two of my patients expressed concern about joining the group for fear of seeing patients "worse off" than themselves, but eventually did join the group and, after a significant number of sessions, reported no negative feelings. I have found that crises from moderate to severe has motivated the group to progress and strengthen.

From my experience, an open, ongoing group with readiness to welcome newcomers works best. Especially helpful is bringing in expert guest speakers from the medical and health professions who can elicit and answer questions that often weigh heavily on patient's minds. An additional and very important benefit of group therapy is that by providing a supportive network of fellow sufferers, it helps share and to thereby decrease the physical and emotional burden of the client's illness for spouse, family and friends.

The Use of Guided Imagery

Guided imagery is a psychological technique that can enable an individual to modify bodily functions. It is a process of imagining or conjuring up pictures or scenes in the mind's eye. This process has been successfully used to alleviate discomfort for both physiological and psychological problems. In a related tension-free environment, the person imagines a pre-determined, remembered pleasant scene as vividly as possible and imagines they are there, experiencing the pleasant environment with all their senses. Some imagery can be a creative imagined treatment, such as lubricating a stiff painful joint with an oil can. Some people describe it as daydreaming, others as a form of self hypnosis. The social worker finds it an extremely useful tool in enabling clients to live better with the side effects of chronic illness.

The Social Worker's Role Vis a Vis the Patient's Physician

The social worker acts as a liaison between the patient and the patient's primary physician. As a "broker," the social worker may actually refer patients to physicians or, conversely, may be called upon by physicians for assistance in complementing the patient's overall treatment management. As a member of this three party team, the social worker monitors progress of the illness and takes many of its burdens off the shoulders of both physicians and their patients.

This team approach incorporates complementary but different disciplines. Health care professionals learn about specific cases from each other, physicians from social workers and vice versa. What the social worker learns in intimate relationships with patients and communicates to physicians can ease the interaction of the patient and her family with the doctor and other medical health professionals involved in the case.

Physicians' initial communication of the diagnosis of chronic illness to patients is frequently incomplete communication or even misunderstood communication, especially given the anxiety which patients can bring to this situation. Also, even given long term relationships, people are often afraid to ask questions of their physicians. They may feel their questions are not intelligent ones or that the doctor's time is too limited to listen. Helpful to both patient and physician is the social worker's knowledge about the diagnosed disease and its control along with the social worker's ability to take time to fill in much of the missing communication.

In fact, the social worker's well-founded knowledge about the patient's specific disease is a most important adjunct to helpful treatment, for the more the patient knows about her disease and its treatment, the more she can allow the doctor to help her. This will help to enable the doctor-patient relationship to become the "partnership" it should be.

As the patient's "teacher," the social worker can instruct how to make medical appointments beneficial for both doctor and patient. Some ways this can be done are to teach patients to keep daily journals of symptoms to report, as well as to write questions that pertain to medications or other medical aspects of the treatment plan. As suggested above, the patient is often all too aware of medical office time limitations. Nevertheless, she still has a right to voice concerns and issues such as the inability to cope with activities that arise in daily living.

When deemed necessary, the social worker must make the patient recognize that a crisis situation or exacerbation of symptoms should not wait for the next scheduled appointment, but rather be reported to the physician at once. Unfortunately, some people believe that "M.D." stands for "medical deity" and do not perceive their physician as human, but, rather, as a god who should never be bothered. In a doctor-patient partnership that works, the patient shares the responsibility of her care with the physician. It is the responsibility of the patient's to obtain as much reliable medical information about her illness as possible and be able to communicate openly and honestly with her physician. She must carry out the treatment program, adhering to proper use of prescribed medications, follow physician's instructions as to rest and level of activity, report any unusual or new symptoms or bodily changes. In fully participating in her care, she is "co-manager" with her physician. Above all, the patient must trust her physician's judgement. If not, both the patient and the physician should have the willingness to undertake additional consultation for a second opinion. The physician's responsibility is to make proper diagnoses through careful evaluation and to formulate and supervise individualized treatment plans including medication, exercise, rest, physical therapy and other forms of medical management.

Overall, it is the social worker's role to offer listening time and in so doing, supportively encourage the patient to communicate all questions, some of which should be addressed to physicians, others of which the social worker can answer. This opportunity to confide can effectively lower the damaging effects of internal stress and may also foster compliance with physician's recommendations.

The Social Worker as Part of the Larger Team

An interdisciplinary team of health care professionals representing not only medicine, but also nursing, mental health, education, occupational therapy, physical therapy, nutrition and recreation can and does offer support to those with rheumatic disease. As "broker" or "facilitator," the social worker can identify, contact and help the patient utilize all these many available resources.

One important benefit of access to these resources is that they provide the patient with human contact with people who because of their expertise help with specific problems, but who also, in the process, become friends with whom the patient can socialize. As they are trained to do, all members of the health care professions working with the chronically ill must be ever alert to the social isolation affecting both the patient and her family, and must recognize that the patient's relationship with both her physician and with themselves helps to sustain hope. At the same time, in coming to terms with her illness and with these new relationships, the patient will also need time to mourn the loss of some old and comfortable ones and time to learn to deal with a changed set of expectations. Perforce, health care professionals working on the team meet a good deal of sorrow and anger and have to be better friends to the patient than the patient often is at first to them.

The Social Worker's Role in Dealing with Employment Issues

As touched on earlier, the eventuality that the chronically ill patient may be unable to work is a crucial issue for patient and family, one which the social worker must confront from many points of view. First of all, the social worker must deal with the frustrations and anger of a person who was financially independent, but who now finds herself dependent upon family, government assistance or alternate sources of income. It is a time to facilitate trust and openness in all communication and a time to guard against demoralization and loss of self esteem, not to mention the hardship of the new financial realities for the patient and her family that may force stringent budget moves. Secondly, the social worker as "facilitator" may be called upon from homes, etc. to identify the appropriate sources of financial assistance and supplementary services.

The social worker in the role of "broker" should be well able to connect the patient to all the entitlements which are available for persons disabled by illness. However, in doing so, there is a delicate balance for the social worker to maintain between care giving and encouraging independence. Also, clear goals to which the patient agrees must be set, for connecting a patient to available entitlements can be a very sensitive area of intervention. The cultural and societal mores of the patient's orientation and her value base will be determining factors.

To explain, although all people share common financial needs, their willingness to accept help that is offered can very well differ. For some, because self-support and self-respect are synonymous to them, there is profound discomfort and even humiliation experienced in applying for and receiving financial assistance. For such people, it is sometimes helpful to point out that entitlements are not charity or welfare but rather a source of assistance which they have earned and contributed to from previous years of employment. Explanations like this can enable the social worker to shift patients' attitudes and see assistance as a right to which they are entitled, but not obligated to use.

Another issue to be recognized is the loss of socialization which the patient's job previously provided. By encouraging the patient to maintain established, particularly worthwhile friendships and to develop new ones by getting her involved with local support groups or foundations that serve her particular illness, the social worker can help make up for this.

The Social Worker as Networker

Networking is the social worker's most valuable tool for acquiring resources in and beyond the community. For those working with people with rheumatic disease, affiliation with or membership in the Arthritis Foundation and the Allied Health Professional Association opens many doors. The conventions, seminars, workshops and literature sponsored by these organizations offer opportunities for continuing education and enhancing skills. Socialization with colleagues either in the work situation or in association meetings also broadens the social worker's network and results in additional resources.

Opportunities to develop support groups and self-help groups are provided through networking with local chapters of foundations to which people who suffer from some specific rheumatic diseases and social workers who work among such patients have contact. Examples of these are the National Lupus Foundation of America, the Scleroderma Foundation, the Multiple Sclerosis Foundation, and the Moisture Seekers (Sjogren's disease). Current and updated information about work that such organizations are doing are available through their newsletters, seminars, workshops and conventions. It is wise for the social worker to be on as many networking and professional mailing lists as possible. Most resource catalogs, especially self-help clearinghouses, list names, addresses, services and contact persons offered by just about every organization in existence. As an example, the Arthritis Information Clearinghouse, supported by NIADDK, (National Institute of Arthritis, Diabetes & Digestive and Kidney Diseases) offers a vast compilation of information, literature, publications, bibliographies and references that cover every aspect of rheumatic diseases.

IN CONCLUSION

When working with those with rheumatic disease, the eventual goals hoped for the patient must always be kept in mind. They are five-fold:

1. to foster compliance and adherence to the physician's treatment;
2. to maintain as much independence for the patient and family as possible;
3. to encourage self-management and help sustain the patient's competence in problem solving;
4. to help the patient adapt to lifestyle changes, particularly in maintaining or redirecting socialization;
5. to assist with financial management.

The intangible rewards of working among those who have rheumatic disease are many. Enabling people to adapt, live useful lives, and triumph over chronic illness and its disabilities provides self-fulfillment far more enriching than any financial rewards. Although the goals are clear-cut, the end result of achieving them—a patient who has maintained or has had self-respect restored to her—is accomplishment indeed.

SUGGESTED READINGS

Eisenberg, Myron G., Jansen, Mary A., and Sutkin, LaFaye C. *Chronic Illness and Disability Through the Life Span*. New York: Sprinzer Publishing Company, 1984.

Erikson, Erik H. *Childhood & Society*. New York: W.W. Norton, 1963.

Ferguson, K. and Figley, B. "Sexuality and Rheumatic Disease: A Prospective Study" in *Sexuality and Disability* 2 (2) Summer 1979, Human Services Press, 1979.

Golan, Naomi. *Treatment in Crisis Situation*. New York: The Free Press, 1978.

Kubler-Ross, Elisabeth. *On Death and Dying*. New York: MacMillin, 1969.

Mailick, M. "The Impact of Severe Illness on the Individual and Family: An Overview," *Social Work in Health Care*. 5 (2) Winter 1979.

Siegel, Bernies, M.D. *Love Medicine & Miracles*. New York, Harper & Row, 1986.

Simonton, O.C., Simonton, S. and Creighton, L.J. *Getting Well Again*. New York: Bantam Books, 1984.

Yalom, Irvin D. *The Theory and Practice of Group Psychotherapy*. New York: Basic Books, Inc., 1975.

APPENDIX

EMPLOYMENT RESOURCES

Employment: An Ongoing Issue for People with Disabilities, 1986
Senator John E. Flynn, Chairman
Senate Select Committee on the Disabled
Room 307, Legislative Office Building
Albany, New York 12247
(518) 455-2096
(518) 455-2097 (HY)
Reviews the Federal and State statutory guidelines. Legal framework to establish access to equal opportunity and employment.

Federation of the Handicapped
211 West 14th Street
New York, NY 10011
(212) 242-9050
(212) 206-4200
Rehabilitation specialist and services.
To elevate, train and secure employment for homebound disabled people in the skill areas of telecommunication—based transcription typing and automated office practice. Transportation, equipment and wage compensation provided. Ancillary services.

International Center for the Disabled
340 East 24th Street
New York, NY 10010
(212) 679-0100
Job placement, consultation, comprehensive vocational employment, rehabilitation.

Just One Break
373 Park Avenue South
New York, NY 10016
(212) 725-2500
Jobs for the disabled, employment opportunity.

Tap Center #7
2715 Webster Avenue
Bronx, NY 10458
(212) 733-1500
Testing, assessment, programming, vocational referral agencies.

ORGANIZATIONS

ACES
Area Center Entitlement Specialists: public assistance. Beekman Hospital, Beth Israel Medical Center, Hospital for Disease/Orthopedic Inst., New York Hospital, St. Luke's–Roosevelt Hospital Center, St. Vincent's Hospital & Medical Center of New York.

Arthritis Health Profession Association (AHPA)
1314 Spring Street, N.W.
Atlanta, Georgia 30309
(404) 872-7100
Rheumatology related issues of practice, education and research. A coalition of professionals that offers access to new developments, national, regional and local forums, meetings, study groups, etc.

Arthritis Information Clearinghouse NIADDK, U.S. Department of Health and Human Services, Public Health Services, NIH
P.O. Box 9782
Arlington, VA 22209
(703) 558-8250
Identifies, collects, processes and disseminates information about print and audio-visual educational materials concerned with arthritis and related musculoskeletal diseases: areas of patient, public and professional education. Abstracting and indexing for database information storage and retrieval system. Development of biblio—profiles, bibliographies, directories and reference sheets. No charge for services to health professionals.

Coalition on Sexuality and Disability, Inc.
853 Broadway, Suite 611
New York, NY 10003
(212) 242-3900
National organization of professionals committed to social integration of disabled people—opportunity to network.

Coming to Terms with Disabilities
Senator John E. Flynn, Chairman
Senate Select Committee on the Disabled
Room 307, Legislative Office Building
Albany, NY 12247
(518) 455-2096
(518) 455-2097
A compilation of Vocabulary Relating to Visible and Non-Visible Disabilities, special programs and services, State and Federal laws, and contact groups for information and support.

The Community Council of Greater New York
275 Seventh Avenue, 12th Floor
New York, NY 10001
(212) 741-8844
How to Secure Help: A guide to social and health services in New York City
Help Yourself: A guide for young people in New York City
Network: Information exchange, current information about social, health and human services, programs and entitlements
Guide for Emergency Services in New York City: Information about shelter, food and clothing

Health Resource Center
1 Dupont Circle, N.W., Suite 800
Washington, D.C. 20036-1193
(202) 939-9320 (Voice/TDD)
toll free (800) 544-3284
Higher education and adult training for people with handicaps. A fact sheet describes financial aid programs, process of applying for aid and the financial aid programs. State programs and private scholarships included.

National Center for Education in Maternal and Child Health
3520 Prospect Street, N.W.
Washington, D.C. 20057
(202) 625-8400
A major link between sources of information/services and the professional in areas of maternal and child health. The Center offers network, services, resources, publications and clearinghouse.

PUBLICATIONS

ARA Membership Directory
ARA Executive Office
17 Executive Park Drive, NE
Atlanta, Georgia 30329
(404) 633-3777
Contains names, membership classification, professional addresses, telephone numbers, and specialty/practice codes.

A Directory of Mutual-Support Resources
New York Institute of Technology
Self-Help Action Center, Inc.
Long Island Self-Help Clearinghouse
Old Westbury, NY 11568

Directory of Resources for the Disabled in New York City
Paula Girden, Legal Asst.
CALS Legal Support Unit
355 Broadway, 5th Floor
New York, NY 10013
(212) 431-7200 (VOICE ATTY)
Lists: Advocacy and consumer groups, auxiliary aids, emergency services, employment and vocational rehabilitation agencies, government agencies, New York City legal services, publications and transportation.

Directory of Self-Help Groups in New York City
New York City Self-Help Clearinghouse, Inc.
186 Joralemon Street
Brooklyn, NY
(718) 852-4290

Help Yourself to Health, Ulene, Art
Perigee Books, G.P. Putnam & Sons
200 Madison Avenue
New York, NY 10016
300 publications that contain information about health; 200 locations where you can obtain free services; guide to health organizations, self-help groups or support groups; organizations that offer free or low cost health care services. Index is cross referenced with 15,000 entrees.

Rare Diseases: A Resource Directory
(NTIS Accession #PB86-180262/AS)
U.S. Department of Commerce
National Technical Information Service
5285 Port Royal Road
Springfield, Virginia 22161
The directory is a guide to voluntary organizations and federal agencies with specific emphasis on their scope of services, and availability of printed and audio-visual materials for use by consumers and health care professionals.

Social Security Administration:
—A Brief Explanation of Medicare, publication #05-10035
—SSI For Aged, Disabled and Blind People, publication #05-10029
—Social Security Strengthened, publication #05-10055
For further information about Social Security or Supplementary Security Income, contact your local social security administration office.

The Source Book, R.R. Bowker Co., New York: London
Director, Service Agency Inventory System
Greater New York Fund/United Way
99 Park Avenue, 4th Floor
New York, NY 10016
OR
Director, Information and Referral Systems
Human Resources Administration
Department of General Social Services
250 Church Street
New York, NY 10013
A single comprehensive, authoritative and reliable source of information about the multitude of providers and services available in the New York City area. The largest single information source of its kind, containing up-to-date information of 1,721 agencies operating 11,861 service programs at 4,472 locations.

IV SOCIAL, PSYCHOLOGY AND CULTURAL ISSUES

"To ward off disease or recover health, men as a rule find it easier to depend on healers than to attempt the more difficult task of living wisely."

Mirage of Health by R. Dubos, Harper and Row, 1959, p. 24.

CHAPTER 20

COPING WITH PAIN AND DISABILITY

Martin V. Cohen

INTRODUCTION

A senior rheumatologist once told me about a conversation that he had when he was a young intern. He remembered asking a well-respected attending physician what was the most important thing to do when first seeing an arthritis patient. The older doctor thought for a moment and then replied, "Scoot out the back door before he sees you!" We certainly have made great progress in medical and adjunctive treatments so that health professionals today are better equipped to help the patient who is coping with chronic arthritic pain and disability than ever before. While we are not able to cure the patient, we do have much to offer. Nevertheless, anyone who has ever worked with patients who have arthritis, or had a family member or close friend who suffers from this chronic illness, is well aware of the very real struggles in daily living and loss in human potential that it can create.

Arthritis is certainly more than a disease of the joints, as it is often discussed and perceived. It is a chronic illness and as such has considerable psychological ramifications. For instance, most patients who are dealing with the effects of chronic pain, discomfort, disability, and fatigue—the major symptoms—will also be struggling to cope with a chronic depression which varies from mild to severe in its effects. In fact, for many patients it is often very difficult to experience, no less report, to what degree their overall sense of pain and discomfort results from specific inflammatory and structural problems per se, or from these very real secondary psychological factors.

Typically, a very negative feedback cycle develops which characterizes the chronic pain syndrome. For example, the patient's joints may be inflamed, resulting in sensations of pain, discomfort, and fatigue. This is depressing in itself. However, there is also a typical restriction of normal activities and behaviors in response to the physical symptoms. This often results in fewer social, intellectual and emotional contacts and pleasures for the individual, which, in turn, isolates and further depresses him. This depressed patient often does not have the energy or morale required to exercise properly, take medication as directed, or seek out and comply with other potentially helpful medical and adjunctive treatments. There is even some recent data in the emerging field of psychoimmunology and in the arthritis research literature itself that strongly suggests that chronic depressive states may even in some more direct biochemical way further the disease process.

The implication here has its positive features. By interrupting this destructive pain-depression cycle, we may be able to significantly limit the overall sense of suffering caused by the basic inflammatory disturbance or disability per se.

It would seem most important, then, for health professionals working with arthritis patients to be sensitive to these mind-body connections. However, given the high degree of technical expertise that is required to master the various specialized modalities of health care, most professionals are not trained to understand or work with psychosocial factors in their clinical work. Similarly, the realistic time pressures that exist in office and hospital practice often create a situation where attention to 'the person' behind the presenting physical symptoms is often minimally attended to. Significantly, though, studies have shown that in those situations were chronically ill medical patients do have the opportunity to receive, for example, even a brief series of psychological consultations, their number of physical complaints and office visits significantly diminish, surgical recoveries are quicker and have less complications, compliance with treatment recommendations increases, and overall sense of well-being is markedly improved. This happens with not only the more emotionally troubled patients but also those 'healthier' individuals who themselves often recognize the crucial importance of dealing with the psychological manifestations of their illness.

Nevertheless, since only a minority of arthritis patients will have the benefit of seeing a mental health worker who has the training and time to comfortably sit down and thoroughly discuss their adjustment to this illness, it is most important that other medical and health care professionals have an appreciation and understanding of this dimension of chronic arthritis.

It is certainly true that arthritis patients can often pose significant challenges to the health care professionals they see. This is particularly true of those patients who seek out the services of allied health professionals. They are the individuals who for the most part have not been able to achieve a complete remission or control of their symptoms via basic medical treatment. In addition to the considerable organic pathology that they often have, such patients can present significant personal needs and demands to the health care professional as well. After all, patients with chronic pain and disability have already experienced a major disappointment with the medical system; they have discovered that they cannot be cured. When they arrive at the offices of physicians, seeking second opinions, or to the physical therapist, occupational therapist or social worker, they are often suspicious, angry, frightened, depressed and anxious. They may still cling to the hope that you will be the 'great doctor' or miracle worker who will somehow, finally, be able to release them from their pain and make them feel 'whole' again. How the health professional responds to these intense emotions and expectations, which may be either directly or subtly expressed, will be crucial in influencing the effectiveness of their work and the satisfaction it engenders, for patient and professional alike. For example, will the worker be overwhelmed by the patient's despair and tension? Will they feel intimidated by the patient's unrealistic demands and retaliate by withdrawing their interest or best care? Will they feel a need to 'rescue' the patient who feels hopeless? Or will they be able to transform these and other negative presentations into a constructive therapeutic relationship that engages the patient in a realistic approach to coming to terms with their illness?

This chapter, then, will now focus on the 'inner world' of the arthritis patient—how he/she experiences the illness and how it affects his/her perceptions of daily life, sense of self, and even the treatment process itself.

THE INNER WORLD OF THE ARTHRITIS PATIENT

Over the past seventeen years I have worn two hats regarding my interest in arthritis and the problems of coping with chronic pain and disability. As a clinical psychologist, I have consulted with hundreds of individuals, couples, and families who are trying to constructively confront the realities of living with physical illness. I have also had to come to terms with my own painful, disabling arthritis condition, ankylosing spondylitis. Both my professional and personal experiences have heightened my appreciation of how very important psycho-social factors are in understanding just how any given person will experience and cope with his or her illness. One striking impression that I have had is that despite what appear to be similar levels of disease activity or physical handicaps, some individuals who have arthritis are able to maintain a generally positive outlook on life, finding meaning and pleasure in their daily experiences and relationships, whereas others are truly overwhelmed and immobilized by the very real stresses that this chronic illness presents.

In addition to the extent of the medical problems involved, then, a person's overall adjustment to his/her illness appears to be mediated by the following major psycho-social factors: (1) social support system—e.g., Is this an individual who lives alone, with few close friends available for practical and emotional support, or is this someone who is happily married and assisted by mature, helpful loved ones? (2) unique talents, interests and coping abilities—e.g., Does this person have few interests, or is this an individual who has a broad range of activities that give him/her pleasure which do not require considerable physical capacity for their enjoyment? (3) economic and vocational issues—Is this a single parent who has little job security or is this a professional person who has adequate health insurance, financial resources, and a rewarding job that can be adapted to meet his/her physical needs? (4) personality factors—Is this someone who even before getting arthritis had a history of unstable, immature or rigid behavior, or is this an individual who has successfully faced hard times before and has the inner strengths required to cope with the real stresses of chronic illness?

While the above psycho-social factors can help the professional to predict and understand how different patients will adjust to their illness, there are nevertheless certain very basic, common emotional and cognitive reactions that all arthritis patients who experience chronic pain and disability face.

I will discuss some of the major ones here.

Anxiety

Arthritis presents a very real threat to a person's capacity to function, to take care of themselves and their loved ones. Simple, daily activities like lifting oneself up out of bed, turning on a faucet, trying to dry one's back with a towel, tending to urinary and bowel needs, wiping oneself, putting on socks and shoes, and bending down to pick up or help a young child are just some of the basic tasks required in the first hour of the day that can create considerable functional difficulty for the chronic pain/disabled arthritis patient. It is certainly quite normal, then, for people to be frightened by the loss of capacity that their symptoms may generate or even begin to suggest. Any new ache or pain or increased feeling of fatigue or stiffness, however minor or transient it may seem to the professional, and in fact be, may set off considerable anxiety. Or, as one patient stated, "Whenever I feel a new twinge or tenderness in one of my 'good' joints, I start to worry and think, is this the beginning of more pain and disability for me?"

The frightened patient will need considerable reassurance and experience to come to see that their worst fears about becoming helpless and dependent are, in fact, primarily fears. While arthritis certainly presents a threat to one's sense of independence, the great majority of patients are able to adapt to their disability in ways that enable them to maintain considerable autonomy. While the health professional who has seen hundreds of patients knows this, the individual patient does not. When professionals are relatively silent, impersonal or 'cool' in their examinations and treatments, scared patients tend to fantasize the worst. The person who has arthritis is very comforted to know that one's physician, physical therapist, social worker, etc. is very aware of his/her desire and need to maintain the capacity to function as normally as possible. In fact, most every arthritis patient treasures any words of reassurance in this regard that the professional may offer, no matter how stoical, brave, or resigned about the illness they may appear. Similarly, when exercises, occupational and social work services, etc., are presented and carefully explained to the arthritis patient in terms of how they will specifically increase that person's functional capacity, they are much more likely to be met with enthusiasm and compliance.

Another source of anxiety for many people who have arthritis relates to their fear of being viewed as unacceptable to others. When an individual looks in the mirror and sees his/her body perhaps disfigured by the ravages of this potentially deforming illness or by scars of surgical treatments, he/she may feel unattractive, ugly or even repulsive compared to "what they once were." If the individual's self-esteem had, in fact, been greatly uplifted by their former grace and beauty, even minor changes in their body-image can be particularly distressing. The patient may fear that if anyone sees them unclothed, be it a spouse, lover or even a physician or physical therapist, they will be 'turned off' and/or "cringe at the thought of touching them." Rather than face this vulnerability the person with crippling arthritis may withdraw from intimate relationships and in some cases even from professional treatments. Similarly, the individual may be concerned as to whether people will be willing to make the continued adjustments and accommodations that are often required to enable them to participate in social activities. For example, a single woman with rheumatoid arthritis may wonder how much she can reasonably expect a new date to modify plans and intimacies in order to be with her. Or similarly, will an employer begin to phase out or even find an excuse to fire a male worker once he learns that his limp is a symptom of a chronic arthritis problem? Just how open can one be? These very real interpersonal anxieties, of course, will exaggerate and be exaggerated by any insecurities about one's self-worth or 'loveability' that the person may have had to begin with. The individual with arthritis, then, can often become hypersensitive to any sign of disapproval from others, be they based on real or imagined concerns. Unfortunately, this stress is often 'resolved' either via more social withdrawal or via an angry, combative, yet equally alienating posture. I will talk more about this later.

For many chronically ill patients, the health professionals whom they continue to see become among the most important relationships they have. The professional, then, often comes to have considerable personal impact upon the arthritis patient. For example, the physician or allied health professional will convey in his manner of relating to the patient very important interpersonal messages and feedback. It is often not what the health professional says, but how he says it that has the deepest effect. The vulnerable patient is often highly sensitive to these 'communications.' For example, is this person with arthritis worth carefully listening to, worth touching in a gentle, compassionate, unhurried way, worth reassuring and supporting, worth believing in? This interpersonal relationship, then, between professional and patient is often very important in influencing the latter's attitude toward themselves, their acceptability, and to what they can expect from others. It has the potential to bolster or hinder the person's confidence, morale and hence overall adjustment to the illness, quite apart from the effectiveness of the clinical treatments per se.

A third source of anxiety experienced by most, if not all, arthritis patients emanates from the treatment process itself. While the lay public often has the impression that arthritis is an illness of old people, in fact this is not the case. For many young adults and early middle-aged patients and the 1/4 million children afflicted with the illness, this may be the first time that they go to see a medical specialist or other health professional, visit a hospital, get extensive and repeated blood tests, X-rays, or are instructed to take medication on a daily basis. Many of these procedures and instructions may be totally unfamiliar and disturbing to them. Furthermore, there may be side effects to medications such as stomach upsets, dizziness, mood changes, insomnia, etc., or in some cases more serious reactions or perhaps no effective response at all. This may warrant further tests or consultations until a satisfactory treatment regimen is arrived at. At some point the patient with more serious illness may be advised to wear a splint, utilize other prosthetic devices, or perhaps even consider their first hospitalization for joint replacement surgery. Unfortunately, there may not be sufficient time taken to carefully explain all of the interventions. This can understandably all be quite stressful. With each new treatment that is tried and with each new specialist that is seen, the patient experiences an anticipatory anxiety. Many will think, "Will this help me, or instead will new problems be seen or develop?" Also, there is the fear of being disappointed again, if numerous unsuccessful treatment efforts have, in fact, occurred before. And finally, as the arthritis patient sits in the waiting area outside the health professional's office, he/she often has ample time to observe other patients, some of whom may be further "down the road" than he. The person may wonder what lies ahead for him with this truly unpredictable illness.

Depression

We have mentioned the reality of depression in the lives of virtually all chronic-pain patients. It is often a neglected issue in the treatment of arthritic disorders, and yet it is frequently the most disabling aspect of the illness. As mentioned, it also threatens to impede the patient's capacity to maintain the positive attitude and sense of hope that is necessary in order to follow through with health care recommendations.

What, then, is the basis for the prolonged depressive reactions that frequently characterize arthritic illness? Psychologists have noted that people often get depressed when they feel helpless to cope with the problems they face. The considerable physical, emotional, interpersonal, social, sexual, financial, and other adjustments that one is continually required to make in living with this chronic illness can, understandably, be quite overwhelming. Similarly, whenever the grace and pleasure of body movement is impaired, or whenever an activity that a person enjoyed must be given up, or whenever one's overall sense of well-being is compromised, a very real disappointment and feeling of deep sadness naturally occurs. A grieving process begins that furthers a healthy way of dealing with all loss and transition. This both reminds and prepares us to accept our basic vulnerability and eventual death. However, for the person with arthritis, whose illness is chronic and progressive, this grieving and adjustment process is often so protracted and recurrent that he may experience a chronic state of loss and mourning.

There is also a physiological aspect to the depressive symptoms of this illness. For example, for those patients whose arthritis is characterized by a systemic illness (e.g., rheumatoid arthritis, lupus, scleroderma, ankylosing spondylitis, etc.), their overall energy level is indeed 'depressed' by the underlying inflammatory process. Patients often describe the feeling as similar to having "a virus or flu that doesn't go away." It is often reassuring for patients and loved ones to be aware of these 'real' depressive effects of disease activity, so that they don't feel that it is 'all in their mind.'

I have already mentioned the tendency of the chronic pain/disabled patients to withdraw from life. They may stop calling friends and friends may stop calling them. Spouses tend to complain that their partners who have arthritis can become less communicative and show less interest in entertaining, planning vacations, or going places. Single people may isolate themselves from dating and new experiences. Instead, the chronic pain/disabled patient can become totally preoccupied and self-involved with their symptoms and illness. Instead of feeling like a person who happens to have arthritis, they begin to identify with their illness and 'become the arthritis.' This results in a corresponding drop in self-esteem.

In the diagnostic and treatment situation the focus is understandably on what is wrong with the patient, their physical symptoms. However, the patient with a chronic illness may be very sensitive to this perspective. They may resent or feel threatened by being viewed so clinically. Intuitively, they know that they will need to see themselves more fully if they are to survive. The health professional who does not lose sight of, and can convey, that he sees this person as more than a bundle of painful, worn-out joints will certainly help to support the patient's will to live. Of course, for those patients who seem quite stuck in a self-defeating depressive reaction, it is most appropriate to suggest that they speak in greater depth with someone specially trained to deal with this aspect of the illness.

Other patients, who are having similar difficulties coping with the illness, may express this same underlying depression via more hostile, aggressive behaviors. They feel angry at life for the 'rotten deal' they feel that they have gotten. They were always good, honest people; why should they have to deal with chronic pain? Some individuals may think that perhaps they are 'bad,' 'guilty,' or so 'emotionally disturbed' that the arthritis is a just punishment or manifestation of such character weaknesses. Others may search outside themselves for someone to blame—e.g., a parent, ex-spouse, doctor, God. They may even discover (as all chronic-pain patients at times will) that if they succeed in being able to make people around them feel as miserable and as powerless as they do, they can enjoy some temporary sense of self-affirmation and control with this uncertain, unpredictable condition. However, this pleasure is certainly short-lived and generally results in guilt, isolation, and more depression.

As mentioned earlier, people who seem to make the best adjustment to their arthritis are those who are able to avoid this depressive cycle. They are able to keep the arthritis in some perspective. One way that helps them to do this is by making themselves available to people and situations that continually validate and support the healthy, vital aspects of who they are and what they have to contribute. They have arthritis, but they do not feel that it totally defines them. When people feel that they are needed and valued, it is a great push to overcome whatever depressive undertow the illness may have. I will discuss this further in the following section on acceptance.

Acceptance

Individuals who have a chronic illness and disability like arthritis are often told by loved ones and professionals alike that they need to "learn to accept" their problem, and indeed they do. The daily struggle required to cope with pain, fatigue and physical limitations requires considerable mental clarity, emotional composure, and an underlying sense of purpose or faith. To the extent that an individual's energy and attention is focused instead on negative feelings, thoughts and behaviors, his/her choice of effectively dealing with a disability is reduced, regardless of the quality of one's medical and health care per se. What then is required or what must the patient do to facilitate a constructive acceptance of their illness?

It is important to remember that accepting a chronic disorder like arthritis is an ongoing process, not a final state that one achieves. As the person's life experience with the illness and personal maturity develop, new, often deeper levels of acceptance are required and made. Acceptance is a dynamic process which demands considerable flexibility, openness and risk-taking ability on the part of the patient in order to prosper. If the patient does not choose on some level to engage in this active learning process then the acceptance will not occur, no matter how long they live or suffer with their problem.

I would like to discuss, then, some of the essential aspects of this process of acceptance, as it has typically unfolded with patients in my clinical practice and in my own life as well. One of the initial steps in developing a constructive acceptance of an illness like arthritis involves coming to terms with the unpredictable and often frightening, chronic nature of the physical symptoms. As I have mentioned earlier, patients are often overwhelmed to think, for example, that "every day for the rest of my life I will feel some degree of pain and/or physical discomfort." It is understandably an alarming thing for someone who has previously been active and healthy to fathom. Patients initially react to this consideration in various ways. Many may deny that they even have an illness. While for some this denial may take the form of an avoidance of professional treatment or basic self-care, others go through the external steps of proper management, and yet internally cannot believe that they have a chronic illness. However, if the denial is chronic and all-pervasive it certainly can seriously impede the patient's ability to realistically deal with the illness. It is important to remember, though, that at times denial can also serve a valuable, necessary function. It enables the patient to regroup forces, garner support and slowly integrate the notion of imperfection into his/her self-concept. This is most vital in the process of self-acceptance. I must say that even today, seventeen years after experiencing my first muscle spasms, joint pains and disability, which have continued and slowly progressed with time, I still find it hard, on some level, to believe that I really have arthritis. I notice that as I feel more self-confident in coping with the illness, clearer in the knowledge that it will not destroy me, I am able and willing to let in more of the awareness of my true limitations and needs.

Some patients will react to this fear, which the chronic, progressive nature of the physical symptoms can suggest, by mobilizing all of their efforts to cure the illness. They cannot envision living with the problem, and so eliminating it becomes the only viable option. Since the current state of medical science cannot offer such a prognosis, these patients will often seek out, at considerable expense and effort, 'alternative' or unproved remedies that keep alive the possibility of finding such a cure. Apart from its potential benefits, such a search gives many patients the hope that they may need to go on, to, similarly, bide for time, until they are ready to feel and believe that the arthritis is something that they can truly learn to successfully live with.

This aspect of the process of acceptance, not being terrified by the illness and thereby having the strength to realistically face it, often takes time. It cannot be rushed by family members or by professionals. It also takes a willingness on the part of the patient to stay awake, involved with people and the activities of daily living. As the patient comes to see, for example, that the pain does come and go, that there are good days as well as bad ones, that the symptoms do not have to wreck their lives, that they are not socially ostracized or condemned by 'healthy' people, that their worst fears most often do not occur—then the person comes to fear the symptoms, their chronicity and the illness less.

The individual who is not overcome by psychological shock, numbness or desperation about their illness can better begin to seriously consider just how they can go about effectively learning to deal with it. This stage of the acceptance process, then, involves the patient's making specific, very basic accommodations and adjustments that improve the comfort and quality of his/her daily life. For example, the individual may buy a firmer mattress to facilitate better sleep, rearrange closet space to avoid having to make painful bends, find time during the day to take rest breaks or naps. While none of these individual actions will 'cure' the illness, they do 'add up' and also help to improve morale and self-confidence. This experimental process of trying to discover and create ways of enhancing daily comfort and function extend into interpersonal relationships as well. For example, behaviors such as asking a loved one for a hug or massage (instead of withdrawing with one's pain), requesting that a neighbor help with some difficult project (perhaps in exchange for something the patient can do in return), explaining to an employer just what restrictions and considerations one's arthritis entails (instead of falling victim to public fears or stereotypes about the illness) are all ways that reflect and further one's inner acceptance of the illness. More personally, the patient may discover that, if they are able, at times, to cry, sob, appropriately 'let out' pent-up emotions and learn techniques of relaxation, they can generate a greater sense of well-being and relief. At this stage, patients are often most receptive to the different kinds of help that allied health professionals can offer, rather than seeing the latter as reminders of the hopelessness (i.e., 'incurability') of their conditions.

I often share with my chronic pain/disabled patients something that Helen Keller once said: "...that when God closes one door, he opens another..." Unfortunately, many people with illnesses like arthritis spend considerable time banging angrily at the closed door, or else sitting resignedly in front of it. Indeed, the active acceptance of a chronic physical problem is clearly enhanced when the patient is able to discover and develop untapped potentials that are still within their range of capacity. For example, one patient, a 35-year-old semi-professional athlete who developed rheumatoid arthritis, was able to redirect his interests into a successful career in sports broadcasting. An older patient who developed a painful osteoarthritis of the spine was able to replace a lifelong love of outdoor hiking by cultivating a dormant interest in nature photography. For other patients who are able to successfully 'work with their illness' the gains are quite personal. For example, one young woman who was struggling with lupus was able to make friends again with her parents, after years of tension and separation. The arthritis forced her to feel her deeper needs for compassion and support; and so, she was now able to accept her parents for their shortcomings and able to appreciate what they did have to offer. This also proved to be a pivotal step in her ability to accept a man for his limitations and get married.

People who have the required flexibility and courage to meet the challenge of having arthritis often report that it has been a most important motivator for their self-development and maturity. Certainly whatever unresolved personality 'hang-ups' a person has do come into sharp focus when having to cope with a chronic illness. For example, very stubborn, rigid individuals, who have always had to have things their way, will be forced by the illness to become more patient, compromising and adaptive if they are to survive. Individuals who tended to be very self-contained, aloof or impenetrable, will be encouraged by the illness to see that they need to become more vulnerable and communicative if they are to lead a more meaningful life. Similarly, the individual with chronic pain or a disability gets very immediate feedback in their highly sensitive, vulnerable body as to which people, places and things are 'good for them' and which result in greater stress and discomfort. The arthritis, then, can become an important 'guide' or teacher that continually provides the knowledge and motivation as to what new risks need to be taken (or avoided) and which new capacities and skills need to be developed in the person's life. By encouraging and supporting patients' efforts in these new directions, friends, family and health professionals can help insure that the difficult task of 'learning to live' with a chronic illness, like arthritis, will be a challenging opportunity and not merely an empty slogan.

SUGGESTED READINGS

Barber, J and Adrian C. Psychological approaches to management of pain. N.Y., Bruner Mazel, 1982.

Bogin, M. The path to pain control. Houghton Miffin Co., Boston, 1982.

Cohen, MV. Arthritis and the family in the National Arthritis News (Arthritis Foundation). Summer 1984, pp. 4–5.

Cohen, F and R. Lazarus. Coping with the stress of illness in Health Psychology: A handbook edited by G. Stone, F. Cohen, N. Adler and Associates, San Francisco, Jossey Bass Publishers, 1979, pp. 217–254.

Cousins, N. Anatomy of an illness, N.Y. W.W. Norton, 1979.

Holden, E. The arthritis survival book, Phoenix A2, Ernest Holding Publishing, 1983.

Wright, B. Physical disability. A psychological approach. N.Y. Harper, 1960.

CHAPTER 21

COOPERATIVE CARE APPROACHES TO PATIENT CARE

Mary Betty Stevens, M.D.

INTRODUCTION

No longer can "arthritis" be properly viewed as simply an inevitable consequence of the aging process about which little or nothing can be done. During the past two or more decades, rheumatology has emerged as a distinct subspecialty in medicine; and with its identity, expanded interest in rheumatic disease has been the focus of clinician and investigator alike. A cadre of health professionals broadly cross-secting disciplinary lines has been developed. Not only has increased insight into mechanisms of disease resulted but new interventions for suppression, control and correction of the clinical consequences have been developed. In this setting, the "health team" concept of management of patients with rheumatic disease, especially in its chronic and systemic forms, has come to replace the "doctor-only," isolated, treatment tradition of the past.

For presentation elsewhere are specific roles of specific disciplines/professionals in the problem-solving for patients with rheumatic disorders. To be emphasized here is their necessary interaction which collectively effects optimal patient care. At the outset, it must be stressed that there is no single formula for interdisciplinary care which must be tailored to disease process, individual patient and overall clinical and socioeconomic setting. Nonetheless, the key determinants or common denominators for satisfying rheumatologic need(s) merit outline for their adaptation to individualized health care programs.

Rheumatic Disease Processes/Problems

The rheumatic disorders encompass a broad array of articular and periarticular conditions, disease of bone and even non-organic syndromes which are expressed in musculoskeletal or systemic terms (Table 21-1). These processes and their clinical problems may be acute, in some instances recurrent, and often chronic and indolent. Thus, management programs and their demands of the health professional team vary enormously with chronicity (or not) as well as specific tissue involvement.

Of the numerous types of arthritis, relatively few (e.g., osteoarthritis; septic, traumatic and microcrystalline arthritis) affect the joints alone. Most acute and intensely inflammatory are septic and microcrystalline-induced arthritis with the latter presenting recurrent problems in the absence of appropriate therapy. Most indolent and progressive is degenerative joint disease or osteoarthritis which presents increasing problems of pain and/or joint dysfunction with time. In those with arthritis associated with extra-articular lesions (e.g., psoriasis, Crohn's disease, neoplasms), treatment is directed as much, if not more, against the extra-articular process as the arthritis itself. Finally, there are the large group of arthropathies which really are systemic or potentially systemic disorders in which the arthritis may dominate the clinical course (e.g., rheumatoid arthritis and its variants) or the synovium represents but one end-organ involved in a multisystem inflammatory process (e.g., the connective tissue disorders, sarcoidosis). Perhaps the subset of patients with systemic rheumatic disease presents the major challenge to the health professional team relative to the issues of comprehensive management and continuity of care.

The periarticular inflammatory conditions (e.g., bursitis, tendonitis) are acute, even self limited and infrequently recurrent. Nonetheless, more subtle soft tissue processes and tendon shortening with resultant joint contractures may present needs for prolonged and continuing rehabilitative care. Similarly, the problems arising from metabolic bone disease with its recurrent pathologic fractures and ischemic bone necrosis with its surgical consequences are recurrent and longstanding. Finally, of no less importance and need, are those patients with functional illness (especially depressive reactions) which is expressed as musculoskeletal pain syndromes or even generalized, multisystem and constitutional illness mimicking connective tissue inflammatory disease.

Thus, the first step in appropriate management design is the sorting-out, diagnostic process which is the obvious responsibility of the physician (e.g., family practitioner, internist/pediatrician or rheumatologist). Nonetheless, "problem-solving" rather than "disease-labelling" is the key approach to management; and the problems presented by the spectrum of rheumatic disease and the general goals in their resolution are shown in Table 21-2 which emphasizes several major determinants to successful outcome. First and perhaps most important, there must be constant alertness to the fact that not all clinical problems arising in patients with established rheumatic disease are a consequence of that disease process. Secondly, once diagnosed, the inflammatory process must be suppressed or, if irreversible as in the case of osteoarthritis, the symptoms relieved. Thirdly, the earlier the diagnosis and institution of therapy, the better is the chance for preventing tissue damage and functional loss. Finally, irrespective of specific rheumatic disorder, general medical health and mental stability must be maintained and negative psychosocial factors reversed if optimal comprehensive care is to be assured.

From both diagnostic and management points of view, the patient with chronic musculoskeletal and systemic rheumatic disease presents continuing and varying needs over time. Clinical problems change and the therapeutic team must be responsive and change with them as illustrated by the following medical precis:

> Patient E.S., a housewife and secretary, was referred to the Johns Hopkins Arthritis Clinic in *April 1964*, at age 34, with a five month history of an additive, symmetrical polyarthritis and associated morning stiffness lasting two or more hours. Otherwise, her medical history was one of excellent health. She had active inflammation of multiple PIPs and MCPs, both wrists, both knees and the right ankle. Laboratory tests revealed mild anemia, an elevated sedimentation rate and a positive Latex test (1:5120) for anti-IgG or rheumatoid factor. Radiographs revealed only soft tissue swelling and mild periarticular osteoporosis of the digits. With the diagnosis of rheumatoid arthritis, she was begun on salicylates and gold and a well designed exercise program to maintain normalcy of muscle strength and articular range of motion. She responded well to therapy; and, by fall of 1964, her disease was in clinical remission. She was continued on salicylates and monthly gold maintenance.
>
> In *January 1971*, she had her first major flare of disease with intense polyarticular synovitis in digits, wrists, elbows and knees which occurred in the setting of a family tragedy during the holiday period. Hospitalization was required for intensification of therapy. Periarticular subcutaneous nodules were first noted at this time. The patient was severely depressed. A balanced program of rest and physical therapy, intensified weekly chrysotherapy, low-dose corticosteroids, a dietary plan for weight reduction and psychiatric intervention were instituted. At hospital discharge, she was significantly improved; and by *May 1971* salicylates were substituted for corticosteroids and gold therapy returned to a monthly maintenance schedule.
>
> The patient continued to do well and work full-time despite waxing and waning of her arthritis until *June 1974* with the next major flare of disease again requiring hospitalization. In addition to active synovitis, pericarditis and peripheral neuropathy were noted, the latter a continuing although non-progressive problem through the present time. In *September 1976*, flare in synovitis of the right wrist was associated with almost simultaneous occurrence of a carpal tunnel syndrome and rupture of the extensor tendons of the fourth and fifth digits which were treated surgically without event. In *January 1979*, after months of progressive pain and limitation in the right hip refractory to medical and physical therapies, a total hip replacement was performed successfully; and in *April 1982*, after a dental procedure without heeded prophylactic antibiotics, she was re-admitted to the Unit with an infected right hip requiring eventual removal of the prosthesis. In *February 1983*, a leg ulceration refractory to local management required

> grafting which was successful. In *September 1983*, she developed dryness of the eyes and mouth; and the Sjogren's variant of rheumatoid arthritis was diagnosed.
>
> At the present time, the patient continues relatively well, still employed on a part-time basis and socially active. After failure or intolerance of multiple non-steroidal anti-inflammatory drugs, gold and antimalarial therapy, she is currently on low-dose, alternate-day corticosteroids and D-penicillamine. She continues daily an active physical therapy program which is periodically reviewed and redesigned as needed. Her general health and weight control are well maintained. Throughout the years, coping strategies have included regular follow by our clinical specialist in nursing as well as the physician team and intermittent intervention by psychiatrist and, more recently, clinical psychologist and social worker.

This 20-year profile of one patient with rheumatoid arthritis obviates the necessary variation in physician and arthritis health professional (AHP) dominance in management from one time to another as well as the continuing role of the core physicians (i.e., family practitioner or internist and rheumatologist). When the array of clinical problems associated with rheumatoid arthritis and other inflammatory and systemic forms of arthritis are considered, it becomes impossible to derive a single formula by diagnosis for the limits of the professional team required for optimal patient care.

The Management Team

There are two key factors in the team approach to comprehensive care, namely, the *coordination* of activities of concerned health professionals and the effective and continuous *communication* between health team members and with the patient; and not to be overlooked is the necessary inclusion of the family support system in management planning. In fact, the interaction(s) among team members becomes more critical to comprehensive care than the specific professional roster which will necessarily vary from one clinical setting to another and over time. In Figure 21-1, the course of Patient E.S. is schematically presented in terms of the physician and arthritis health professional input to the management of her rheumatoid arthritis with its variable clinical activity and complications. The consistent involvement of the internist (or family practitioner) and rheumatologist as well as nursing professionals contrasts sharply with the intermittency of others providing consultations and care. Thus, it becomes the pivotal role of the rheumatologist to orchestrate the team function and interactions.

However, it must be recognized that the vast majority of patients with rheumatic disease receive their care from professionals without subspecialty training in rheumatology; and the critical variable in achieving multidisciplinary team management is the availability (or not) of such a health care system. *Un*availability of the team approach results from multiple factors, some professional and others societal, including an absolute lack of specialized professionals and facilities in the region or the inaccessibility of the established program to

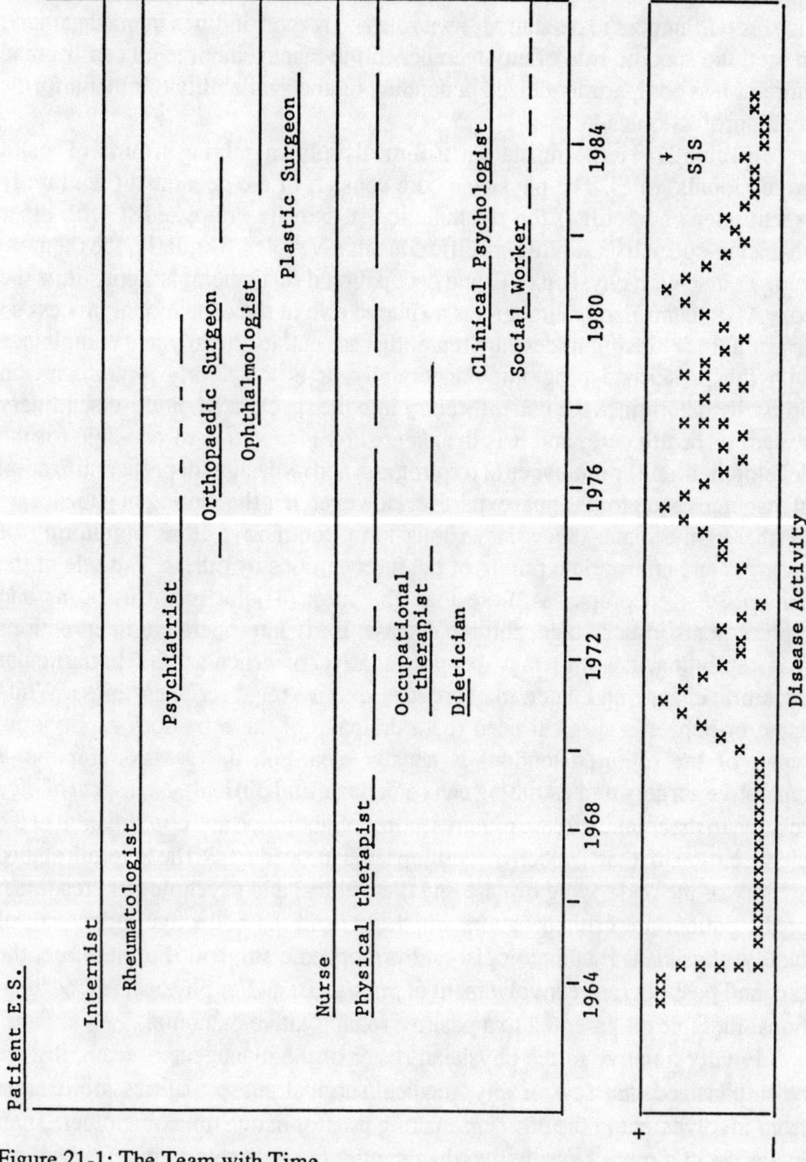

Figure 21-1: The Team with Time

patients by virtue of the common insensitivity of generalists to the referral need for specialized care, geographic separation or even cost/economic issues. For a large segment of the patient population, then, the necessary problem-solving (Table 21-2) and achievement of management goals, if realized, depend not only upon awareness of the generalist of the dimensions of comprehensive care but also his willingness to expand his own role and responsibilities in management. In fact, the specific role of any member of the management team can become more or less compartmentalized depending on the availability of other arthritis health professionals.

In Table 21-3 is the translation of clinical problem-solving in terms of health professionals' roles. The physician core consists of the generalist (i.e., family practitioner or internist) the rheumatologist and the orthopaedist with other physician-specialists serving specific consultative roles. Similarly, the rheumatology nurse with physical (PT) and occupational (OT) therapists constitute the core AHP team. Each member has an active role in the educational process so essential to achieving understanding of disease and its therapy and compliance with the prescribed program. Functionally, it is the *family physician* who primarily determines the patient's entry into the specialized, multi-disciplinary system of health care; and it is the *rheumatologist* who is responsible for the development and continuance of the program and its design for proper utilization of resources and professional expertise. However, it is the sharing of patient care by these physicians that assures long-term continuity, close monitoring of progress and appropriate timing of the interventions by others. The role of the *orthopaedist* encompasses more than the surgical joint reconstructions and replacements in late-stage, chronic disease. Early non-operative interventions (e.g., splinting, casting) may be preventative of articular and periarticular structural change and, later, may prove corrective (e.g., serial castings). While acute orthopaedic surgical need (e.g., drainage of the refractory septic joint, repair of the ruptured tendon) is usually clear-cut, the decision for major reparative surgery and its timing can be delicate and difficult. No aspect of care relative to rheumatic disease requires more collaboration and coordination of the physician-team than "elective" orthopaedic procedures. The overall status/activity of the underlying disease and the medical and psychological readiness of the patient are critical factors which demand the collective judgement of family physician, rheumatologist and orthopaedic surgeon. Furthermore, the pre- and post-operative involvement of *physiatrist* and/or physical and occupational therapies is essential to a positive rehabilitative outcome.

Finally, relative to the physician roster of the management team, it must be emphasized that few, if any, medical/surgical subspecialities are exempt from involvement in the decision-making process at one time or another. Their inclusion in a more consultative than continuing-care role is intermittent and problem-related as complications of the rheumatic disorder and/or its therapy arise.

With respect to the arthritis health professional (AHP) subset of the management team, by analogy, nursing along with physical and occupational therapy provide the core support. New extensions of old roles in patient care and education have emerged in recent years as increased focus on the total patient and comprehensive care has emerged. Perhaps nursing needs are most consistent and continuing irrespective of clinical setting. *Nurse-management* arms of the physician's office or hospital clinic have expanded the care system and offered greater availability to patients of professional resources to evaluate disease progress, monitor response to therapy, reinforce the physical medicine programs prescribed by others, and maintain general health surveillance. Furthermore, through subspecialty rheumatologic nursing, in-hospital intervention and home care programs have extended the potential of effective care at times of disease exacerbation and intercritical periods, respectively. The roles of *physical and occupational therapists* extend beyond direct physical management and can have major educational impact; and, again, all health team members maintain an educational role for patients and each other. A common denominator between these disciplines is their goal for prevention and, in some instances, correction of structural abnormalities and functional loss through well designed exercise programs. The involvement of the physical and occupational therapists early in the course of both chronic arthropathies and steroid-treated systemic disorders can provide an essential baseline for a continuing program directed to conserving energy and strength, protecting joints and periarticular structures, and maintaining the total functionality of the patient.

As with the full dimensions of the "physician team," the added potential members of the "AHP Team" are intermittently consulted in relation to essential planning and changing need. The *clinical psychologist* and *social worker* share in psychosocial assessment and interventions with patient and family. The matter of *vocational rehabilitation*, a pivotal issue for some patients, may require interplay between nurses, therapists, social worker and vocational counselors, depending on the specifics of the clinical and societal settings. The enormous value of the *clinical pharmacist* in sharing the educational process relative to the goals, mechanisms, and complications of pharmacotherapy for the hospitalized patient has been amply demonstrated on our specialized unit; and the contributory role of *laboratory technologists* and other support staff in providing necessary data for comprehensive and longitudinal evaluations must be emphasized.

As the scope of rheumatologic problems can encompass virtually all of medicine in the broadest sense (i.e., clinical and societal), the true, potential roster of the management team is endless. In the practical sense, the availability of professional disciplines ultimately dictates the composition of any health care team, but the concept of multidisciplinary health care can be fostered nonetheless through interchangeable roles/responsibilities if the goal of comprehensive care is maintained with top priority.

Team Function

Just as the management team will vary in its roster from one program to another, so will its manner of functioning vary with the clinical and geographic setting. The multidisciplinary team concept is comparatively easy to develop and implement for hospitalized patients but can be difficult to realize in relation to ambulatory care. It must be emphasized that, conceptually, the multidisciplinary approach must be a coordinated, unified program rather than independent actions of multiple professionals which are not inter-related or focused on a common goal. In the in-patient setting, the team conference is the ideal forum for interdisciplinary planning; and, when the weekly conference is coupled with unit rounds, monitoring of progress can be realized as well as program design. The usual geographic separation of professionals attending ambulatory patients requires an effective, systematic means of continuing communication to replace team conferences/rounds and assure the same outcome. In most settings (i.e., in-patient unit, clinic, multi-office...), the rheumatologist and/or the nursing specialist can best serve as coordinator with the pivotal role in the communication system. However, again, no single formula accommodates all practice situations but if multidisciplinary, comprehensive care is deservedly high in priority an effective inter-disciplinary system of on-going communication must (and can be) developed.

SUMMARY

Problem-solving in rheumatic disease, especially those disorders with a chronic course, requires the input of professionals across disciplinary lines. Sensitivity to the special nature of rheumatologic needs is required of all in addition to professional expertise; and a coordinated care program with well defined goals must be tailored for individual patients with regard to the total patient setting. Underlying patient care, professional growth, and optimal team function is the educational process in which all team members have shared responsibility to patients and to each other.

SUGGESTED READINGS

Bird, A., Le Gallez, P.H., II, J.: Combined Care of the Rheumatic Patient, Springer-Verlag, New York, 1985.

Epstein, D.: Breaking the barriers to communication on the health team. Nursing 4:65, 1974.

McCann, V., Philips, C.A., Quigley, R.: Preoperative and postoperative management—the role of allied health professionals. Orthopedic Clin. N. Amer. 6:881, 1975.

Rubin, I., Plovnick, M.S., Fry, R.E.: Improving the coordination of care, a program for health team development. Ballinger, Cambridge, Mass. 1975.

Sackett, D.L., and Haynes, R.B. (eds.): Compliance with therapeutic regimens. Johns Hopkins University Press, Baltimore, Maryland 1976.

Ehrlich, G.E. (ed.): Rehabilitation management of rheumatic conditions. Williams and Wilkins, Baltimore, Maryland 1980.

Meenan, R.F., Gertman, P.M., Mason, J.H.: Measuring health status in arthritis, the arthritis impact measurement scales. Arthritis Rheum. 23:146, 1980.

Liang, M.H., Jette, A.: Measuring functional ability in chronic arthritis—a critical review. Arthritis Rheum. 24:1, 1981.

Ziebell, B., Wickersham, E.A., Boyer, J.T.: Team arthritis consultation. Phys. Ther. 61:519, 1981.

Jette, A.M.: Improving patient cooperation with arthritis treatment regimens. Arthritis Rheum. 25:452, 1982.

Riggs, G.K. and Gall, G.P. (eds.): Rheumatic diseases: rehabilitation and management. Butterworth Publishers, Boston, 1984.

TABLE 21-1
RHEUMATIC DISEASE

I. Articular
   a. Joint involvement alone
   b. Arthritis with extra-articular lesions
   c. Systemic disorders
II. Periarticular
   a. Bursitis
   b. Tendonitis
   c. Fascitis
III. Bone disease
   a. Metabolic
   b. Ischemic necrosis
   c. Other
IV. Non-organic syndromes
   a. Musculoskeletal
   b. Generalized

TABLE 21-2
RHEUMATIC DISEASE PROBLEM-SOLVING

I. Diagnosis
   a. Specific rheumatic disease
   b. Presenting clinical problem
      1. Underlying rheumatic disorder
      2. Complications: disease, therapy
      3. Intercurrent illness
   c. Contributing psychosocial factors
II. Management
   a. Suppression of disease process and/or its symptoms
   b. Prevention/repair of structural damage or deformities
   c. Prevention/repair of functional impairment
   d. Maintenance of general medical/mental health
   e. Alleviation of psychosocial issues

TABLE 21-3
MANAGEMENT TEAM ROLES

Problem-solving Role	Generalist	Rheumatologist	Orthopedist	Other Specialists	Nurse	Therapists (OT/PT)	Psychologist	Social Worker	Other AHPs
Specific diagnosis	+	++	-	-	-	-	-	-	-
Pharmacotherapy	+	++	-	-	+	-	-	-	-
Deformity/dysfunction									
Prevention	-	++	+	-	+	++	-	-	-
Correction	-	+	++	-	-	+	-	-	-
Health Maintenance	++	+	-	+	++	-	+	-	+
Psychosocial Therapy	+	+	-	+	+	-	++	++	-
Educational Process	+	++	+	+	++	+	+	+	+

Role/responsibility primary (++), acceptable (+) or not expected (-)

CHAPTER 22

SEXUALITY AND FAMILY LIFE

Sheldon P. Blau, M.D.
Bette Blau, M.A., A.D.T.R.

Arthritis has long been recognized as a physical problem imposing pain and limitation upon the patient. Symptoms may be exacerbated by physical and emotional stress. The unpredictable course of the disease itself may also produce stress. It is therefore important to view arthritis in terms of the social and emotional impact upon the patient in relationship to his or her family.

The most important facility for the ultimate care of the arthritic is the patient's home and family. It should be the place where a continual program of rehabilitation and adaptation to the changes imposed by chronic disease is supported. The family must be viewed as part of the treatment team.

A series of adaptations is necessary to maintain a viable family life under the best conditions. A reasonable degree of flexibility, open communication and commitment to the family unit is necessary for any family group to maintain itself.

When faced with the crises of chronic illness, many family units disintegrate. Where stable relationships have existed prior to the onset of the illness, loved ones may be ready to face the anxiety associated with issues of dependency, pain, depression, anger, changes in life style, and fears for the future.

Acceptance of the diagnosis is itself a problem. Denial often postpones needed treatment and prevents the patient and their family from obtaining the factual information necessary to intelligently discuss aspects of the illness which will affect them all. Open and honest communication is necessary.

Family dynamics are altered. Illness may result in the patient's inability to fulfill their usual role. Other family members may have to take on additional responsibilities. The patient's need for rest is considerable and that factor alone imposes limitations on other family members.

Husbands, wives and children must be aware of their own anger and resentment; feelings that build as they experience limitations imposed by the requirements of taking over chores and meeting other needs of a loved one who is chronically ill.

Individuals who are afflicted with arthritis experience alterations in their bodies which can result in changes in body image. Adaptation to pain and alteration in functional capability is not easy. Success of adaptation depends upon the total personality structure of the patient and on family dynamics. Chronically ill people demonstrate an increase in self-observation and self-interest, resulting in a decreased interest in family and friends. Depression may result.

At the other end of the spectrum, are those patients who completely deny symptoms and the resulting limitations imposed by their illness, thereby damaging themselves further by paying no attention to the realistic goals of the treatment program.

Family counseling when used to facilitate supportive family interaction, is in certain cases, an indispensable part of the treatment program. The health care professional may refer the patient to a psychologist, social workers, psychiatrist or other certified therapist for individual and family counseling. A sexual therapist may be of value.

Sexuality, as a characteristic of being human, should be viewed as a major route of self-esteem and identity, an important element in human relationships, and a fundament in the family. Since sexual activity has implications for one's own body image and self-esteem, problems in sexual functioning becomes stressful in themselves, and may exacerbate other physical and emotional symptoms. As a consequence, sexual relations suffer further.

While much information regarding the medical diagnosis and prognosis of the rheumatic disease is available, little relating to the social sexual functioning has been written. Recently, as a result of the more open attitudes toward discussion of sexually explicit material, the sexual social problems of the handicapped has been recognized. Sexual interest and activity is of continued importance to the chronically ill, yet sexual expression may become more difficult. There is a decrease in the ability to initiate and maintain social contact. Where mobility is reduced, the ability to travel to places where social contacts can be made is lessened. Social isolation becomes a problem. The opportunity to establish and maintain a sexual relationship is diminished.

Physical deformities, especially in young patients who have not yet established a firm sexual image, may lead either to abnormally aggressive or reticent sexual behavior. When corticosteroids have been administered to the very young child, as in juvenile rheumatoid arthritis, growth retardation may interfere with realization of full sexual potential.

Actually, the physical deformity and ungainly movement which may be associated with arthritic disease is a deterrent to social interaction in members of any age group.

Limited sexual expression is often an effect of chronic illness. There is a decrease in libido. Sexual drive is commonly lessened in chronically ill people who experience acute pain and tenderness when moving. Pain or the fear of inducing it, effectively diminishes libido. It is not only the patient who may fear a sexual contact, but the sexual partner may lose desire if he or she is afraid of producing discomfort as a result of advancing intercourse.

Fatigue, depression, anxiety and general malaise are also effective deterrents to sexual desire. Besides the emotional and psychological components of rheumatic illness, the pain, limitation of joint mobility, disfigurement, fatigue and side effects of drug therapy, are factors also to be considered in the patient's response toward sexual intimacy. Medication, including cytotoxins, analgesics, diuretics, tranquilizers, sedatives, anti-hypertensives, steroids and anti-inflammatory drugs may suppress the disease process and its symptoms. While alleviating the pain and sleeplessness, and improving the physical ability to make love, it may decrease the desire to do so. (See Table 22-1.)

It is important for patients and their partners to know that drug side effects are possible, but that alternative forms of sexual relations are also possible. The site and nature of joint involvement effects the nature of sexual interaction.

Hip involvement, for example, may result in years of pain and/or avoidance of sexual intercourse. Hip replacement has produced dramatic results in alleviating problems. Arthritis of the hands and shoulders limits the ability to touch and embrace. It also prevents weight-bearing during sexual contact. Involvement of the lower limbs further curtails positioning. Spinal involvement may make genital contact difficult, and once achieved, may inhibit the movements involved in the usual mechanics of coitus. Foreplay and climax become difficult to achieve.

Where local lesions of the mouth, genitalia and/or anal areas are involved and ulcerations, inflammation, or dryness, as a result of lack of normal secretions occur, oral and/or genital sex may have to be curtailed until local lesions have subsided.

The sexual partner is affected, as well as the patient. While the patient may exhibit decreased libido, the partner may still maintain a normal sex drive. However, fear of producing distress in their chronically-ill mate by engaging in sexual relations often dampens inclination to initiate lovemaking.

Problems involved in anticipating mechanical difficulties, selecting predetermined body postures, curtaining foreplay and duration of sexual involvement as a result of fatigue is not conducive to the spontaneity or orgasm usually thought of as the resulting ideal. The mechanics of lovemaking become a focus which overshadows the importance of expressions of caring and tenderness.

A disabled partner whose libido is decreased may be fearful of freely expressing physical affection lest this be misread as a desire for further lovemaking which may lead to pain. Diminished physical attractiveness may foster a fear of rejections and desertion. Although the partner may feel sympathy, the frustration and unresponsiveness involved in sexual encounters leads to resentment and an assault on self-image as a lover. Irritation builds. The final consequences may include a total cessation of loving interactions and a withdrawal of all manifestations of caring.

How can the difficulties be ameliorated? The premorbid interpersonal situation is of vital importance for the future course of therapy. Some patients may be able to solve their sexual problems by themselves, but others require counseling. The importance of open, honest communication between patient, their partner and the health care professional is a necessary prerequisite for helping problems. Factual information concerning the disease prognosis, therapy and possible side-effects of medication must be discussed.

Patients should be encouraged to communicate freely and frankly so that activities which are comfortable and which produces pain can be identified and understood. The couple may then explore alternative positions and techniques which are mutually satisfying.

Suggestions can be made so that sexual partners can identify erotic areas of sensitivity and increased awareness of avenues of stimulation may be found. Manual and oral methods of gratification should be explored. Gentle massage, except when skin bruisability is a problem, as when steroids are administered, is often a sensual prelude to erotic encounters.

A hot bath or warm compress prior to sexual relations may help to reduce pain and encourage relaxation of muscles. Planning sexual activities around time of the day when the pain and fatigue is minimal is advisable.

Mutual exploration of alternative positions which put less stress on affected joints may add a new dimension to what may have become routine unimaginative encounters in the past. Lovemaking on a couch, chaise lounge, or water bed utilizing pillows for support, may prove more comfortable than an ordinary bed.

When pelvic thrusting is a problem, intercourse may be avoided. Kegel's exercises which strengthen vaginal musculature, may increase the strength with which the vagina can grip the penis and restore pleasure during intercourse. The pubococcygeus muscle is a sphincter muscle located in the pelvis. It is associated with female vaginal perception and participates in vaginal responsiveness by gripping the penis during intercourse.

Women can contract and relax this muscle at will. In order to identify this muscle, a woman may experiment with starting and stopping her flow of urine while seated on the toilet with her legs spread apart. Contraction and realization of the pubococcygeus muscle is the only way in which urine flow can be stopped in that position.

Once identified, women can learn to contract, hold and relax the muscles periodically during the day. It is suggested that the exercises be done twenty-five to fifty times per day and that the muscular contraction be sustained for about three seconds during each session. This exercise should be done at various times during the day rather than all at once, so that the muscle does not become "tired." Any muscle will become sore if previously unexercised and patients should be told that such discomfort is temporary. Kegel's exercises can be done any time or any place.

A second exercise which improves the ability of the vagina to utilize the pubococcygeus muscle for gripping the penis involves taking a deep breath while tightening the genital muscles. Then, the whole pelvic region relaxes as the air is exhaled. Bearing down, as if attempting to expel something from the vagina, followed by tightening of the vaginal muscle is a third exercise which can aid in conditioning the muscular apparatus of the pelvic area. These exercises strengthen and tighten the vaginal vault and provide for more friction during intercourse. Penetration for both partners in conjunction with rhythmic contractions may provide sexual pleasure, sometimes to the point of orgasm.

When vaginal dryness (sicca syndrome) is a problem, a water soluble lubricating jelly placed on the penis and/or in the vagina may help. Artificial saliva, for the dry mouth, associated with sicca syndrome, will also help to make sexual encounters more pleasurable. These substances are available over the counter, in the pharmacy.

If a partner is unwilling or unavailable to participate in sexual relations, masturbation should be discussed. The use of sexually explicit books, photos and magazines may aid in increasing interest.

Methods of contraception should be discussed, as the use of a diaphragm or condom may be difficult for arthritic hands. The non-affected partner may aid in applying these devices.

Chronically ill patients and their families require an understanding, accepting professional who is willing to give the additional time necessary to explore sexual attitudes and family interaction. One must be able to accept the healthy aspects of sexual activity so that non-harmful means of aiding performance can be encouraged. Of course, psychological limits and flexibilities as well as unique family relationship must be considered.

SUGGESTED READINGS

Blau, Sheldon and Blau, Betty. Sex and Systemic Lupus Erythematosus, in *Medical Aspects of Human Sexuality*. November 1976, pp. 93–94.

Blau, Sheldon. Changing the Lifestyle of the Lupus Patient. *Behavioral Medicine, Practical Information for Physicians,* Vol. 5, Number 10, October 1978, pp. 18–21.

Brecher, Edward M. *The Sex Researchers*. Little Brown and Company, Boston 1969, pp. 176–177.

Carrera, M.A. *The Facts, The Act and Your Feelings*. Crown Publishers, New York 1981.

Conine, Tali and Evans, Juli. Sexual, Reactivation of Chronically Ill and Disabled Adults, *Journal of Allied Health,* Vol. 11, Number 4, November 1982, pp. 261–270.

Hamilton, E.A. Sexual Problems in Arthritis Patients. *British Journal of Sexual Medicine,* Vol. 7, Number 6, 1978, pp. 19–23.

Robinault, I. *Sex, Society and the Disabled.* Harper and Row, New York 1978.

Schilder, P. *The Image and Appearance of the Human Body.* International University Press Inc., New York 1970.

TABLE 22-1
DRUG THERAPY AND SEXUAL FUNCTION

A. Drugs that have been associated with a high incidence of impotence:
   1. Antihypertensives
   2. Cardiac Antiarrhythmic Medications: Disopyramide (Norpace) may cause acute urinary retention in both males and females, as well as impotency in males.
   3. Analgesics: Meperidine (Demerol), Morphine, Dilaudiol, Codeine, Pentazocine (Talwin), Percodan, Dextropropoyxphene (Darvon).
   4. Immunosuppressives.

B. Drugs that have a variable effect on the libido:
   1. Tranquilizers
   2. Sedatives
   3. Muscle relaxants
   4. Steroids

C. Drugs that do not interfere with the libido:
   1. Aspirin
   2. Nonsteroidal anti-inflammatory drugs
   3. Gold
   4. Penicillamine

CHAPTER 23

UNPROVEN REMEDIES

Michael D. Lockshin, M.D.

INTRODUCTION

Recent studies indicate that over 90% of patients with rheumatoid arthritis *who are known to physicians in rheumatic disease clinics* will use some form of unproven remedy. It is likely that as many patients who eschew physicians, and who seek care outside orthodox medicine, also seek unproven remedies. The scope of the problem is enormous. This chapter will discuss the reasons patients seek unorthodox care, the types of remedies used, the risks and benefits of these remedies, and the role of the orthodox health care provider in confronting unusual forms of care.

Definition and Characteristics of Unorthodox Care

Unorthodox care may be outdated medicine, honest but naive treatment, truly inspired experimental medicine, or fraud. It is not automatically either misguided, dangerous, or criminal; it may be all three. Characteristics of unproven remedies that render them unacceptable to orthodox medicine are scientific dishonesty or sloppiness, inappropriate promotion to the public, excess cost, and absence of disclosure of adverse effects. Unusual fanfare, claims that "orthodox medicine is preventing the release of treatment X," suggestions that treatment X is 100% effective or has 0% adverse effects, are the usual hallmarks of quackery. There are unfortunate instances in which the release of reasonable new therapies has been delayed because the manner of presentation has been so unorthodox that serious scientists have refrained from studying the therapy or federal agencies from licensing it, but this sort of delay is extremely rare. Most often the style of the presenter is a good reflection of the substance of the presentation.

Reasons Patients Seek Unorthodox Care, and the Costs Thereof

An illness such as rheumatoid arthritis is highly susceptible to claims from unorthodox health care practitioners: the disease is painful and chronic; it is sufficiently common that friends and relatives are likely to know others with the disease about whom they can relate anecdotes; the disease can easily be confused with an even commoner malady, such as osteoarthritis or bursitis (which under normal circumstances is self-limited); the disease spontaneously waxes and wanes, and spontaneously remits; public perception of rheumatoid arthritis is that it inexorably progresses and cripples; untrained physicians tell the patient, "There is nothing I can do"; television advertisements belittle the severity of the illness ("the minor pain of arthritis"); and physicians' goals (prevention of disability) may be at striking variance with the patient's goals (wanting to feel better and have no pain). Thus there is ample chance for miscommunication.

The remittent nature of the disease provides a fertile ground for the unproved remedy weed. Anything done by or to a patient at the time spontaneous remission occurs will be credited with curative powers. This, plus placebo effects, account for most of the testimonial accounts supporting unproven remedies. To the scientifically untrained patient, the physician's casual discussion of probabilities, controlled studies, and remission frequency is irrelevant (if not unintelligible), if the patient is convinced that a given diet, procedure, application or other phenomenon caused relief of pain.

Unproven remedies have four types of costs. First and most noted, the dollar cost may be, for the individual patient, trivial to extraordinary; nationally, the cost is high. Second, there is the cost to health and life of a dangerous form of treatment. Both these costs must be weighed against the cost of orthodox medicine's alternatives. Third is the cost of wasted time and of abandoned potentially useful forms of therapy. Fourth is the emotional cost of wasted hope.

TYPES OF UNPROVEN REMEDIES COMMONLY ENCOUNTERED

Unproven Remedies of Trivial Cost and Danger

Copper bracelets represent the prime example of a harmless form of unproven remedy. In the author's office, approximately one-third of new patients are wearing or have recently worn copper bracelets. The bracelets have no known effect on the course of any form of arthritis, but their use has been so pervasive that formal studies have been done examining copper deficiency in rheumatoid arthritis (it exists), copper absorption through the skin from the bracelets (a small amount is absorbed), and supplemental dietary copper as therapy (not beneficial).

Many forms of *diets and ingested supplements, such as vitamins,* are also of trivial cost and danger. Periodically an individual patient appears whose arthritis appears to be triggered by a specific dietary item. In addition, many forms of allergies, food or otherwise, include joint pain among their symptoms. Current theories regarding the origin of rheumatoid arthritis allow for the central role of an agent foreign to the patient; foods could fit this role, and do, in at least one experimental model of a type of arthritis caused in monkeys by a product or contaminant of alfalfa sprouts. By interfering with eating or with gastrointestinal absorption, arthritis can directly induce malnutrition. Medications may interfere with nutrition both directly and, as in medication induced diarrhea, indirectly. Certain fish oils may provide chemical precursors to the bodies' mediators of inflammation and may, if taken as a food supplement, either decrease or increase the inflammation of arthritis. Thus open-minded physicians acknowledge the possibility that diets can modify the course of arthritis.

Formal studies of claims made for specific dietary supplements, such as vitamins, minerals, and a variety of food stuffs, have failed to show benefit in humans with spontaneously occurring disease. The converse, elimination diets, have similarly failed to be beneficial in formal trials. The formal trials, done as recently as 1983, included most if not all of the most popular "anti-arthritis" diets reported in the lay press.

There is not a great cost to the average patient of experimental diets *tried in moderation*. Occasionally a patient may become seriously malnourished by attempting a prolonged elimination diet (for example: living on rice alone for months on end). Vitamin poisoning with those vitamins capable of causing poisoning (A, D, occasionally C, and possibly B6 or E) occurs in patients addicted to "mega" vitamin treatment. Other dietary supplements are more bizarre. In specific tests, extracts from the green-lipped mussel failed to alter either osteoarthritis or rheumatoid arthritis. Superoxide dismutase (SOD, Orgotein), while interesting chemically, is digested by the stomach and pancreas; taken orally it is an expensive and tasteless way of supplementing the protein that would be more pleasurably be ingested as trout with almonds, pepper steak, or even chili.

Salves, topical applications, and acupuncture. Unpleasant sensations occurring on the skin may draw attention from (by reflex nerve pathways or by the endorphin [internal pain control chemicals] system) painful areas such as joints. The term describing these applications is "counter-irritant." It is likely that most topical balms, rubbing materials, applied dots, pins, electrical shocks, and the like work by the counter-irritant mechanisms. The relief they provide is temporary; pain is lessened, but the basic disease process continues. The majority of available remedies fitting this description are cheap, harmless, and unimportant. Patients have, however, unintentionally self-immolated by choosing to bathe in gasoline; turpentine or kerosene would have worked equally well were dramatic suicide, and not relief of pain, the intent.

Two remedies in the category of topical agents and applications merit special discussion. *Acupuncture* as currently practiced may not be cheap. There may be a specific set of personal characteristics, probably inherited, possibly related to the patient's own endorphin metabolism, that predict achievement of pain relief by acupuncture in some individuals and failure in others. In controlled trials, acupuncture has not altered, in any measurable way, the course of rheumatoid arthritis in any feature other than temporary pain relief.

Dimethylsulfoxide (DMSO) probably works as a counter-irritant. Unlike some of the other counter-irritants, DMSO is a remarkably powerful pharmaceutical. Highly concentrated, it burns the skin. In experimental animals it can obliterate an apparently normal immune response, and it can affect kidney and liver function. Its terrible smell does not appear to justify its uncontrolled use as an over-the-counter medication.

Unproven Remedies of Greater Danger: Vaccines, Venoms, Antibiotics, and Extirpative Surgical Procedures

An earlier generation of physicians thought focal infections, such as of the nose and throat, caused arthritis (the source of the *rheum* of rheumatoid arthritis). An earlier generation of patients underwent tonsillectomies, adenoidectomies, tooth extractions, and other procedures with no demonstrable effect on the arthritis. Occasionally such remedies are still offered; an occasional physician still treats with *antibiotics*. This latter course has some scientific support: it is likely that Reiter's disease and other forms of spondyloarthropathy (ankylosing spondylitis) may be triggered by infection. Lyme arthritis clearly is. However, formal trials of popular antibiotic remedies, specifically tetracycline in early rheumatoid arthritis, have shown no therapeutic effect.

The same theories have led other physicians to suggest mixed bacterial *vaccines*, flu vaccines, and other vaccines as therapy. The theory of their effect is flawed. No clinical trials of such therapies have demonstrated efficacy.

Bee, ant, and cobra *venoms* are said to have curative powers in arthritis. These substances have powerful biologic effects, are capable of altering both inflammatory and immunologic responses, and could potentially be useful. Serious scientific studies have investigated the possible effects of these treatments, but some elements of the lay press, encouraged by the proponents of these therapies, have exaggerated their worth. None of the venoms at this writing is acceptable therapy for any form of arthritis. Allergic reactions and toxicities of the agents make them potentially dangerous.

Unproven Remedies of High Danger: Fraudulent Cures Using Powerful Pharmaceuticals

Many widely-touted cures depend on common, powerful pharmaceuticals that are not identified to the user. An oriental herbal medicine, sold as a "natural cure," *chiufong-toukawan,* contains a collection of anti-inflammatory agents, some illegal in the United States because of their known toxicity. A "balanced hormone preparation," *Liefcort,* derives its miracle-like effects from its 15 milligrams of prednisone, a high dose for the rheumatoid patient. Contrary to the claims of its proponents, the addition of male and female hormones in this preparation do not reduce the side-effects of the corticosteroid. Remedies available from unorthodox practitioners on the Mexican-American border, on analysis by local and federal (United States) authorities as well as by the Arthritis Foundation, contain corticosteroids and a variable collection of anti-inflammatory drugs as well as tranquilizers, often in dangerous combination. The physicians dispensing these medications have denied in public statements the demonstrated contents of the medications, despite verified analysis of their contents, and patients have suffered expected side-effects.

Medications useful for other illnesses occasionally find favor among unorthodox physicians. *Clotrimazole,* an anti-helminthic agent, was used for rheumatoid arthritis patients, based on the incorrect observation of protozoa in rheumatoid joint tissue. A legally prescribable medicine (for people with worms), the drug found its way into the anti-arthritis pharmacopaeia of a highly visible physician who had previously treated patients with flu vaccines, yucca plant extracts, and intra-nasal cocaine. Other drugs have less dramatic histories but their use is no more firmly grounded in fact.

The Border Zone Between Orthodox Medicine and Quackery: Experimental Therapies, Folk Medicine, "Holistic" Medicine, and Tomorrow's Remedies

Personal attention, sympathy, concern for all components of a patient's personality and life-style, are important tenets of orthodox medicine, whether practiced or not. *"Holistic"* medicine acknowledges the importance of these tenets; it may err on the side of inappropriate denial of the role of pharmaceuticals or surgery. It is not intrinsically dangerous, and may be helpful; it often does not merit separation from orthodox medicine. Similarly, many *folk remedies* may provide common sense or standard physical therapy. Others, such as bathing in gasoline, of course, may be dangerous. *Chiropracty* at its best offers useful physical therapy. At its worst it may delay useful therapy and unnecessarily injure structures by ill-advised manipulation.

Experimental therapies in conventional medical institutions require approval by human rights committees and scientific committees; full, informed patient consent is required by law. Often publicity about these therapies understates the experimental nature of the procedure or drug; often as well the therapy finds its way into the market-place before its usefulness is proved. *Plasmapheresis,* as an example, is actively being investigated for a variety of forms of arthritis;

it quickly became available to the public, at immense cost. In some areas of the United States mobile vans offered to perform the procedure at the patient's home. In these cases the ethical issue is more confused. Frequently *informed* consent was not obtained or independently reviewed. Over-promotion of advantages and understatement of expected complications were characteristic of the promoters, but the identical treatment was available at university hospitals at the same time. The criticism is therefore more of style than of content: the implied promises, the lack of consent, the often outrageous and inappropriate cost, and the hucksterism. Other, less dramatic, examples include laser beam therapy and total nodal irradiation.

RESPONSE OF OFFICIAL AGENCIES

Municipal, regional, federal, and voluntary agencies have, in the author's opinion, generally responded appropriately to the challenges provided by unproven remedies and by their needs to serve multiple constituencies. When a public danger is identified, agencies have combined forces to apply existing laws. If a lay agency is functioning as an unlicensed clinic, if medications are being provided without physician prescription, or if diagnoses and recommendations are being made by an unlicensed provider, existing laws may be enforced, terminating promotion of the least safe remedies. If there is not a technical violation of law, local health authorities and the Food and Drug Administration will often inspect premises and analyze samples of medication; locally prepared reagents frequently do not meet purity, sterility, or labelling regulations. In some cases of high public interest, the Federal Government, at its own expense, has convened open hearings on the value of a given agent. A case in point is the Bureau of Biologics' response to the claim that a cobra-krait venom ameliorated rheumatoid arthritis and multiple sclerosis. Despite obvious deficiencies of manufacture and labelling, the physician and the provider of the venom were invited to a public workshop, which had experts from appropriate fields of biology, pharmacology, immunology and medicine. At the hearings it was apparent that the physician was weak in diagnostic skills, used anti-inflammatory agents routinely in conjunction with the venom, and kept no records. It was also apparent that the provider varied the content of the supplied venom mixtures and lied about the contents of the vials. Nonetheless the Bureau of Biologics successfully recruited sponsors and participants from the private sector to perform a scientifically valid trial. When the provider violated the agreement he had entered to perform this trial, the Food and Drug Administration brought suit to enforce a cease-and-desist order. The Arthritis Foundation and other private agencies cooperated with and supported each of these actions.

Private agencies, such as the Arthritis Foundation, are limited in their abilities to counteract unproven remedies, because of the volume of the problem and the high cost of litigation. Rather, private agencies serve as foci for identifying problems, and for doing the basic ground-work for state-of-the-art information. They provide information to the public and to law enforcement agencies and on occasion also provide a forum for a formal test of a potentially promising agent despite the naivete of the proponent or his or her lack of basic knowledge, finances, or laboratory support. In this author's opinion the process is biased toward identification of a potentially helpful treatment and biased against early rush-to-judgement or severe condemnation; it is more likely that a dangerous treatment will persist within the community than that an unsuspected cure will be repressed.

For treatments originating outside the United States, be they procaine *(Gerovital)* from Romania, green-lipped mussel from New Zealand, Liefcort from the Caribbean, or "natural" pharmaceutical cures obtained within miles of the international border, regulation is dependent on foreign authorities and immigration officials. Large-scale importation can be restricted, but individual treatments should be approached from a *caveat emptor* vantage point.

THE ROLE OF THE HEALTH-CARE PROFESSIONAL IN MEETING THE CHALLENGE OF UNPROVEN REMEDIES

What should be the role of the health-care professional in dealing with unproven remedies? The vast majority of patients try them: to deny this is unrealistic. Many, if not most, waste time, money, and hope, but are not intrinsically dangerous. Some are exceedingly dangerous. Scolding patients for participation in unproven remedies will likely induce reticence or cause the patient to withdraw from conventional care.

Open-minded discussion, *introduced by the health-care professional* (since patients will seldom introduce the topic themselves) is the recommended approach. The discussion should acknowledge the universal nature of exposure to unproven remedies from friends and family, should discuss the monetary, emotional, and health costs of individual remedies, and should display a willingness to evaluate and re-discuss any future questions. Negotiation with patients over essentially harmless remedies (diet? why not try it and see?) is not only courteous, but it invites the patient to participate directly in his or her health management. It also leaves open the possibility that, for the arthritis patient population in general, or for the individual patient in particular, an unproven remedy may become a proven one in time.

SUGGESTED READINGS

Brown JH, Spitz, PW, Fries JF: Unorthodox treatments in rheumatoid arthritis. Arthritis Rheum 23:657–8, 1980.

Fitzgerald FT: Science and scam: alternative thought patterns in alternative health care. New Engl J Med 309: 1066–1067, 1983.

Lockshin MD: The Unproven Remedies Committee. Arthritis Rheum 29:1188–1190, 1981.

Panush RS, Carter RL, Katz P, Kowsari B, Longley S, Finnie S: Diet therapy for rheumatoid arthritis. Arthritis Rheum 26:462–471, 1983.

Panush RS and Endo LP: Diet and Other Controversial Arthritis Remedies. Ch. 96 in Diagnosis and Management of Rheumatic Diseases, 2nd edition, 1988, JB Lippincott, Philadelphia.

Wasner CK, Cassady J, Kronenfeld J. The use of unproven remedies. Arthritis Rheum 23:759–60, 1980.

Ziff M: Current comment: Diet in the treatment of rheumatoid arthritis. Arthritis Rheum 26:457–61, 1983.

CHAPTER 24

PATIENT EDUCATION AND COMPLIANCE

James M. Corry, Ph.D.

INTRODUCTION

Paul Starr (1982) chronicled the transition of American medicine from a quasi-scientific, marginally influential profession to a profession having extraordinary influence on the social and economic well-being of the American society. Starr's story has also noted the transition of American consumer attitudes from that of disdain of the early citizens to that of awe and respect for medicine. Most recently the transition now seems to be to that of skepticism about medical care and the medical system, combined with a growing challenge to the authority of physicians as exemplified by the budding self care movement, the use of alternative therapies, and a questioning of the costs of medical care.

Given this background, it is perhaps inappropriate to use the word "compliance" when referring to patient behaviors necessary to cure or prevent disease, because the word "compliance" conveys an image of an all-knowing health worker ordering a patient to behave in a certain way.

Philosopher Albert Jonsen has commented on this situation as follows:

> "...the authoritarianism to which physicians are often tempted can be a serious error. Compliance it seems is best achieved in a partnership of understanding. The authoritarian physician, giving orders without preparing patients for their acceptance or supporting them in their observance, can undermine compliance. Of course, firmness, and, for some patients, benevolent paternalism may be quite effective, but, even then, an eventual partnership should be the goal."
>
> "I wish to criticize (the word) compliance because it suggests the ethical "blooper" (mistake) of blaming the victim. To refer to the problem as compliance is to pose it as a problem of behavior of patients, and, consequently, to seek its causes in the patient. In so doing, the sins of the careless, irrational, authoritarian physician are visited on the heads of his patients. Those who study and write about compliance know physician behavior is crucial but by naming their problem after patient behavior, they skew the picture." (Jonsen, 1979)

Sackett has also commented on compliance and writes that "mutual responsibility" must be part of any effort to increase compliance if the effort is to be considered ethical. Sackett lists four criteria for when it is ethical to increase compliance of patients via behavioral, organizational and educational techniques. These criteria include:

1. the diagnosis must be correct
2. the therapy must do more good than harm
3. there must be mutual responsibility of patient and physician for prescribing and taking the medication
4. and the patient must be an informed, willing partner in execution of any maneuver designed to alter compliance behavior. (Sackett, 1976)

Compliance then may be an inappropriate word to fully describe the act of patients changing behavior, but it is the word most used in the literature and so will be used in this chapter. However, when the word compliance is used it will be in the context Sackett listed, meaning *voluntary, informed behaviors on the part of patients that help them to improve their health.*

In this chapter a brief review of the extent and nature of compliance will be presented as well as factors that increase compliance. The review will include material specific to rheumatic diseases and material of a more general nature.

Because of the thin data base, the health worker interested in very specific strategies to improve compliance of rheumatic patients may be disappointed. However, a careful reading of this chapter should help the health worker to develop compliance-improving strategies based on the findings in other fields.

In the sections that follow, these topics will be explored:

- The Extent of Compliance,
- The Nature of Compliance,
- Compliance Improving Strategies.

THE EXTENT OF COMPLIANCE

Peck and King (1982) reviewed the literature concerning the extent of patient compliance and reported rather distressing findings. They found that compliance to important behaviors (i.e., medication-taking, appointment-keeping following screening and referral, and adherence to physician recommendations) was low. Boyd (1974) found only 22% of prescriptions given to 134 outpatients were taken properly and that 31% were being misused so as to be harmful. Blackwell (1972) reviewed 50 studies and concluded that complete non-compliance occurred with 25%–50% of all out patients. Davis reviewed the literature and concluded that 30%–35% of the patients do not follow their physicians recommendations. (1966)

Sackett and Snow (1979) reviewed 537 studies and concluded the following:

- Patients will keep approximately 75% of the appointments that they make, but only about 50% of those made for them.
- Compliance with short-term regimens declines rapidly.
- Only 50% of the patients on long-term regimens are compliant.

Regarding rheumatic disease, Jette reviewed the literature and reported the following: (1982)

- of 46 patients with rheumatoid arthritis of the hand, only one-third complied in wearing a hand splint (Moon, 1976)
- of another 66 patients with rheumatoid arthritis of the hand, 3% reported no use at all of the splint; 32% wore it less than half the time; 65% complied less than 50% of the time. (Oakes, 1970)
- 75% of patients in a third study did not comply by wearing a splint; 60% did not comply with suggested exercise regimens (Ferguson, 1979) and 22% did not comply with a drug regimen (aspirin). (Ferguson, 1979)

Physician Awareness of Patient Compliance

It is important to recognize that physician awareness of compliance as a problem can affect the extent of compliance by patients. An interesting study related to physician awareness of compliance as a problem was reported by Inui et al (1976). They reported a twofold increase in the number of patients taking 75% or more of medicine and achieving blood pressure control, after their physician attended a conference on problems of patient compliance and presumably became more aware of compliance problems.

THE NATURE OF COMPLIANCE

The term compliance can be inclusive of a vast array of behaviors ranging from appointment keeping, to diet adherence, to medication taking. Compliance may be to short term or long term regimens, each of which may result in different levels of compliance or different problems in assuring compliance. Similarly, a long list of other variables can affect compliance, such as the nature of the illness, certain economic barriers, family support, and physician-patient interaction.

For the purposes of this chapter, a review of studies of five factors which shed some light on the nature of patient compliance will be presented. They are: disease factors, referral process, clinical setting, treatment, and "human" factors.

Disease Factors

Haynes, in a review of the literature has found the following disease related factors to be of importance in determining compliance (1979). (1) *Diagnosis* and compliance, especially diagnosis of psychiatric conditions (schizophrenia, paranoid features and personality disorders). These patients are less compliant than other psychiatric patients, and they in general are less compliant than patients with non-psychiatric disorders. Deyo et al (1981) reported that rheumatoid arthritis patients were significantly more compliant than patients with other rheumatic diseases. (2) *Increasing symptoms,* contrary to logic and common belief, do not increase compliance. In fact, four studies showed that increasing symptoms had a negative effect on compliance. (3) *Disability* does appear to influence compliance in a positive manner. The greater the degree of disability, the greater the level of compliance.

The Referral Process

The single most important finding regarding referral is that time plays a role in compliance to referral appointments. "The longer the elapsed time between referral and appointment the lower the likelihood that the appointment will be kept." (Haynes, 1979)

Finnerty (1973) found that by decreasing referral waiting time of patients with hypertension from two weeks to one or two days compliance rates rose from 50% to 95%.

There are a number of other referral factors affecting compliance: Leprosy patients found in screening programs has a higher rate of default than those self-referred from other sources of care. (Hertroijs, 1974) In hypertension screening, letter referrals were more successful than phone calls or than direct referrals by workers at the time of screening. (Wilber & Barrow, 1972) Patients referred to a psychiatric outpatient department were more likely to attend if referred to a specific physician rather than just the clinic. (Hoenig & Ragg, 1966)

The Clinical Setting

Several studies confirm common sense notions about appointment keeping by patients: i.e., if patients have to wait long, or are assigned to an unfamiliar physician (or to no particular physician), their attendance will be low. Alpert (1964) for example, found that 29% of low attending patients reported waits of four or more hours. Only 10% of patients with good attendance records reported this problem.

Rockart and Hoffman (1969) examined the relationship between patient assignment and appointment keeping in a hospital out-patient clinic. When patients were block assigned, the average wait was 85 minutes, and there was a no show rate of 27%. Also, under this system both patients and physicians tended to be late. However, when patients were assigned at the same time but given to specific physicians, the waiting time was reduced to 57 minutes and lateness was also improved by this simple, administrative procedure. Lastly, when patients were given individual appointment times the average wait was 33 minutes and the no-show rate was 13%. Both patients and physicians tended to be early under this plan.

Treatment Plans

Features of the treatment plan affecting compliance include: type of medications given, the way they are given, complexity of the drug regimen, side effects of drugs, duration of treatment, cost, and packaging of the drug. Closson and Kikugawa (1975) studied the relationship between drug type and drug compliance, and found striking differences. They found a compliance rate ranging from 17% for antacids to 89% for cardiac drugs. Hemminki and Heikkila (1975) found an 85% rate for drugs for symptomatic relief. Deyo et al (1981) found an overall compliance rate of 36% for patients taking arthritis drugs, but that aspirin, when prescribed, was taken less frequently than prednisone.

It has been demonstrated that adherence to treatment decreases with time. (Haynes, 1979, p. 59) Similarly, the more treatments the lower the compliance rate. Some contradictory data however, has been noted by Haynes.

Side effects do not seem to adversely affect compliance. Two controlled studies (Latiolais & Berry, 1965) found no difference in the frequency of side effects between compliers and non-compliers.

Cost of the drug is a negative factor in compliance. Hemminki and Heikkila (1975), Alpert (1964) and Brand, Smith and Brand (1977) found that cost of medications is an important barrier to compliance for many patients. This effect is exacerbated when one adds in time for treatment, transportation costs, and time lost from work.

Another feature of the treatment plan affecting compliance is the way in which drugs are dispensed. Safety locks have been shown to have an adverse effect on compliance. (Lane, 1971) Locking caps are especially problematic for the elderly population. Another study relating to dispensing shows that community pharmacists dispensed less medication than was prescribed on 15% of prescriptions for a ten-day course of treatment for children with otitis media. (Litt, 1981)

Human Factors

The human factors found in patients and physicians undoubtedly play a role in compliance, but the exact nature of this is not well understood. For example, Becker et al. have described a Health Belief Model which attempts to show the relationship between a patient's value expectancies state (or the state of motivation) and that patient's health-related actions. Becker's model can be summarized as follows: a patient's perceptions of certain things will predict his health-related behavior. These perceptions include: (1) perception of personal susceptibility to a disease; (2) perception of degree of severity of the consequences of the disease; (3) perception of the benefits of certain health actions; (4) perceptions of barriers to the health action, such as cost, time, discomfort, etc. Becker's model also posits that a "cue to action" is important to get the patient to recognize his feelings and perceptions about health. Such a cue might be a heart-to-heart talk with his physician, or a message from the media, family or friends. (Becker, 1972)

Becker's health belief model has been tested and shown to be predictive of health behaviors. By manipulating various parts of the model, health-related behaviors have been improved in test populations. For example, assume a newly diagnosed patient with hypertension had a perception that his condition was not serious, and that since he had few or no symptoms, that he was not susceptible to the disease. By querying the patient about these beliefs, and then giving correct information to the patient, the physician may increase the likelihood of that patient taking appropriate action. Similarly, if the patient perceives there are too many barriers in his way, the physician may be able to confront this belief directly and make suggestions for over-coming the barriers. Incidentally, this confrontation can be a pleasant, constructive occurrence if the physician-patient relationship has been properly developed through good communication.

Another human factor in compliance reported by Litt et al (1982) is that of self-esteem and autonomy. They studied 38 adolescents by giving standardized instruments assessing self-image and autonomy, then contrasted results with serum salicylate measurements. Patient and disease related characteristics were also recorded and interactions with personality variables examined. They found that compliers have significantly higher measures of self-esteem and are allowed more autonomy than non-compliers. They also found that the longer the duration of disease and the more symptoms present at onset correlated with a poorer self-concept and hence lower compliance levels.

COMPLIANCE IMPROVMENT STRATEGIES

Overview

Figure 24-1 from Haynes' *Compliance in Health Care* (1979, p. 79) diagrams the organizational, educational and behavioral strategies that can be employed to improve compliance. Organizationally, it seems that providing consistent care (i.e., familiar physician), sending reminders, reducing waiting

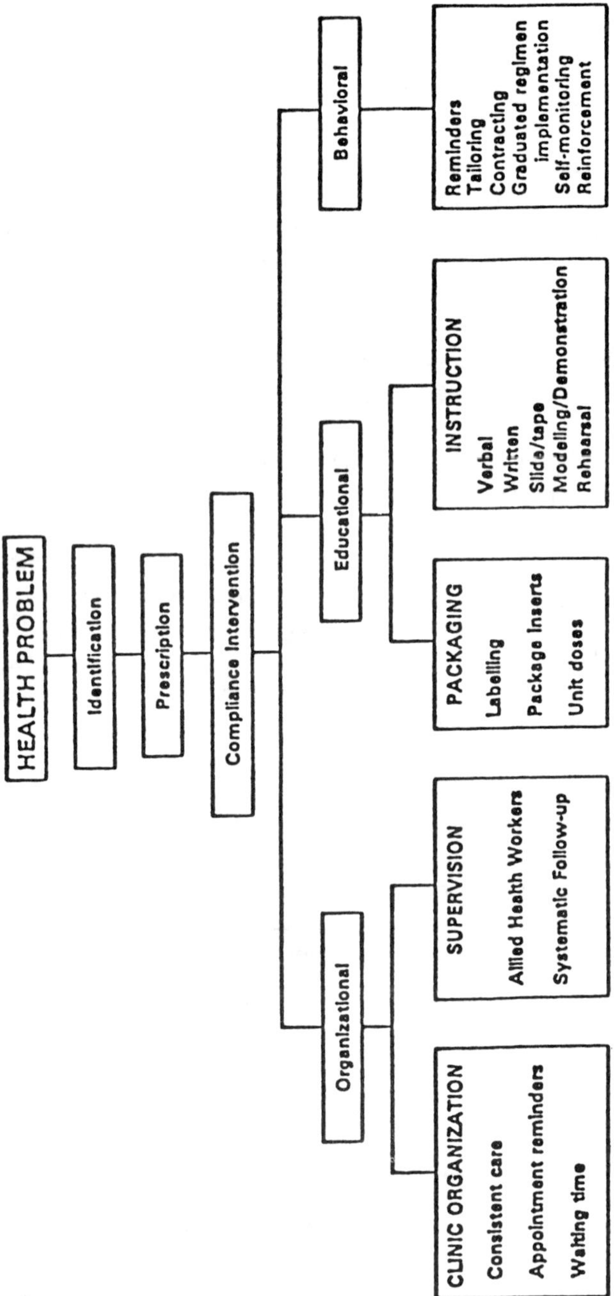

Figure 24-1: A process model of compliance intervention

time, using allied health workers to help supervise the compliance intervention, and keeping track of compliance via systematic followup, helps improve compliance. Coupled with educational interventions and behavioral interventions such as proper instruction, written directions, dispensing of drugs tailored to the daily regimen, and others, increases the likelihood of successful compliance.

Table 24-1 (also from Haynes' *Compliance in Health Care* p. 142) is an excellent summary of techniques related to four problem areas in compliance that are suggested from the research literature. To increase the chances of a patient keeping an appointment made after a referral four techniques help: Letter sent to the patient, referral clerk keeping track of contacts and attendance, patient instruction at the time of screening, and a short referral time. Appointment compliance is improved by mailed reminders, followed by telephone reminders and importantly efficient clinic scheduling. Explicit instructions help as well as pill packaging and pill calendars. Beyond tactics designed to encourage compliance, the critical factor is patient awareness.

Ron Anderson, writing in the *Archives of Internal Medicine* (1982) says:

> "Pragmatically, physicians must realize their limitations about assuming compliance in unsupervised settings. Therefore it is important to recognize and understand the role and responsibility of each in health care: the physician diagnoses and initiates the treatment regimen, and helps the patient to become a therapeutic partner by motivating, informing and educating the patient. This strengthens the patient to be a true partner."

This concept of patient as partner is very appealing, and is an earmark of ethical patient education. It is appealing because it recognizes the dignity and worth of individuals, and helps facilitate their growth as human beings. Also, it is not unreasonable to believe that doctors who appreciate the derivation of the word doctor (docure—to teach) realize that part of their role is to teach the patient how to be more responsible for his total well-being. But words and facts alone do not assure this happening. The act of teaching is the art of communicating sound knowledge.

Communication

Communication is defined as the sending of a message across a channel with the conscious intent of evoking a response in a listener. Good communication occurs when a person understands what is being conveyed.

"Noise" (i.e., interference or distractions that prevent the messages from being properly received) is the key problem in communication. Although noise may occur at any point in the act of communication, the principle place where noise occurs is in the receiver who may react to a message before it is complete, who may agree or disagree with the message during its transmission, who perhaps reacts emotionally to the message or the way in which it is being delivered. Interestingly, many receivers will react negatively to a speaker because the speaker's body sends a different message than his words. An example would be when a health worker's words convey empathy but his or her eyes dart away from the patient. Other sources of noise occur when senders encode messages improperly (e.g., using overly technical language, or neglecting a language or cultural difference) when speakers are inept at delivering or transmitting messages, or when the channel is jammed (e.g., a noisy air conditioning unit in a lecture room).

Some practices shown to improve communication include:

- Active, empathetic listening
- Trustworthy responses when warranted
- Congruency between spoken messages and body language
- Negotiated meanings of unclear messages
- Redundant messages
- Constructive confrontations

Active listening means the receiver works hard to eliminate internal noise. He does this by stifling brain chatter, attending fully to the speaker, and avoiding needless interruption. It may involve para-phrasing the speaker from time to time to let him know you are listening. This type of listening will in turn let the speaker know you care about him. It lets him know you have empathy for him, and this creates an atmosphere more conducive to problem identification and problem sharing because the patient feels he can trust the caregiver.

Trust is an important factor in solving the problem of compliance. For example, if an open atmosphere of concern has been created by good communication, this permits the health care worker to *constructively confront* a patient. Constructive confrontation, as the name implies, means bringing up a troublesome subject in a positive way to resolve it so things get better. Confrontation, when used to ridicule or to control a patient, can negatively affect compliance.

Congruency between spoken word and body language is vital to credibility, and to fostering trust. Negotiating meanings of messages is an easy process whereby the health worker can say: "...this is what I hear you saying...; am I correct?"

In summarizing this section on communications a quote by James McKenney seems appropriate: "Too often patient education is viewed as a lecture given to an attentive patient who understands the message and therefore adheres to the regimen. Nothing could be farther from the truth! Good counselors are interested not only in sending messages effectively but also in receiving them. They freely send and receive thoughts and feelings, both verbally and non-verbally. In this way they establish relationships with patients that engender trust and confidence and, therefore, foster patient compliance. Effective counselors specifically avoid negative confrontation, tension, attempts to control one another, or other factors known to impair the relationship. Their communication is clear, explicit, and reinforcing. The basic attitude of the effective counselor is one of concern and compassion with freely provided feedback to patients after the appropriate information has been solicited." (McKenney, 1979)

In a study on communication by Svarstad (1976), various characteristics of the patient-provider relationship were assessed and related to patient compliance among 221 patient encounters with eight physicians in an urban health center.

Characteristics that were analyzed included:

1. the amount of explicit instruction given regarding medication use;
2. the justification for the drug's use;
3. the friendliness or receptivity expressed by the provider toward the patient;
4. the exertion of medical authority;
5. the emphasis given to the patient's role in taking medications;
6. monitoring (or questioning) by the providers of previous medication taking behavior;
7. the responsiveness of providers to patient's complaints or admission of non-compliance.

Svarstad concluded that high levels of instruction, monitoring, justification, emphasis and motivation resulted in higher levels of compliance, and that the interactive effects of high instruction, high friendliness, and high motivational appeals resulted in the highest levels of compliance.

McKenney (1979) concludes that the manner of communication may be as important as the content of the communication at least insofar as compliance is concerned.

The next section on compliance complements McKenney's conclusion, i.e., that the form of patient education may be as important as the content of patient education. Some of the important documentation for this statement has been provided by Becker as mentioned previously. Most recently, Lawrence Green has presented an excellent model for assessing educational needs and developing strategies to assure compliance. This model takes into consideration the needs humans have for warmth and liking, the place of values and attitudes in their behavior, and the crucial medical information they need to have in order to behave in a healthy manner. This model is called the Precede Model, and will be described next.

Patient Education and the Precede Model

Scope of Health Education

Patient Education or health education should not be defined as merely informational exchange. Since the ethics of health education require participation and informed consent, this gives clues to the proper boundaries of health education vis-a-vis the overlapping technologies of communication, motivation, behavior modification and patient counseling. Each of these technologies has been confused as health education, and while health education incorporates techniques from each, health education is different because the student or patient is actively and voluntarily involved in an individually tailored learning experience that uses combinations of strategies to help the learner responsibly change his behavior. Note also that while many health personnel are called upon to share health facts with patients, this is not considered to be sufficient unto itself to change behaviors. The properly prepared health educator will conduct an educational diagnosis, then in consort with the patient choose learning experiences that have the highest probability of helping the patient to change his or her behavior.

Health Education then is defined as any *combination* of learning opportunities *designed* to facilitate voluntary adaptations of behavior conducive to health. (Green, 1979)

Green et al (1980) have devised the *Precede* model to assure that any health or patient education program meet the essential criterion of designed, purposeful learning. This criterion, requires that the methods employed have been developed or selected and combined on the basis of clearly delineated objectives derived from a careful diagnosis of the behavior in question. Educational intervention is more complicated than simply handing out a pamphlet and asking the patient to read it. A properly designed intervention must carefully examine the several factors contributing to a behavior.

It must also assess how the patient best learns (e.g., lecture?, reading?, film?, independent research?, conversation?, programmed learning?, written exercises?, etc.) and use the most appropriate pedagogical techniques *for that patient* which will increase his knowledge about his condition.

It must help the patient recognize his values and perceptions about his condition by using appropriate counseling techniques such as values clarification and constructive confrontation. It must include an inventory of resources—material and human. It must include skill work if that is necessary. The family and friends of the patient may also need to be involved in this intervention.

In short, whatever educational, counseling, communicative and motivational experiences that seem needed based on the educational diagnosis should be used to increase the chances of the patient voluntarily making a positive change in his behavior.

In summary, a serious health education intervention to increase compliance (change behavior) must include educational diagnosis and a customized educational plan if there is to be a chance of success. Many studies on educational interventions and compliance as reported by Haynes (1979) have showed poor results. Typically these interventions were naive in that they used only one strategy (usually lecture) to try to change compliance behavior. Green (1979), on the other hand, has reported good results in helping people change behavior when combinations of strategies are used after a proper assessment.

Before ending discussion on compliance, it is appropriate to ask who should do health education. The whole health care team can be involved based on their particular strong points as teachers, counselors, interviewers, trainers and resource experts. Roles should not automatically be assigned because of professional title. A nurse, for example, may be excellent at communication and building trust, and may be the logical person to perform an education diagnosis and perhaps constructive confrontation. On the other hand this same nurse may not be effective as a lecturer.

Ideally there should be one person who is trained in educational diagnosis, teaching, counseling, use of media, use of motivational techniques and evaluation and has knowledge of health and disease. This person can help develop the educational plans and coordinate the professional health care workers who deliver various parts of the intervention to patients. During the last 10 years the professional preparation of health educators in the United States has improved significantly and it is this new health professional who should be considered an ideal candidate to coordinate educational interventions in health care settings.

PATIENT EDUCATION RESOURCES

Several excellent resources are available for health workers interested in patient education. Below is a sample list of general materials and materials for health professionals working with rheumatic patients.

PERIODICALS

Patient Education Newsletter. Published by the University of Alabama-Birmingham, 930 South Twentieth Street, Birmingham, Alabama 35294. The PEN has articles by patient educators describing their programs and techniques for improving patient compliance.

Patient Counseling and Health Education. This Journal primarily includes research on patient education and counseling techniques. Published quarterly by Excerpta Medica, P.O. Box 3085, Princeton, N.J. 08540.

BOOKS AND MONOGRAPHS

R.B. Haynes (Ed) *Compliance in Health Care*. Baltimore: Johns Hopkins University Press, 1979. This is an outstanding book which examines the issue of compliance from an organizational, administrative and educational perspective.

N. Galli, A. Skiff, D. Urban and J. Corry. *Patient Education: A Better Way to Achieve Compliance in the Ambulatory Care Setting*. NY: Mount Sinai School of Medicine, 1982. Proceedings from a conference of the same name. Offers profiles of programs and an overview by Jeannette Simons on Patient Education.

L.W. Green, M.W. Kreuter, S.G. Deeds and K.S. Partridge, *Health Education Planning: A Diagnostic Approach.* Palo Alto, Calif: Mayfield Publishing Co., 1980. Describes in great detail the PRECEDE Model. Includes excellent chapters on the use of appropriate educational techniques.

Medicine in the Public Interest. *Learning to Live With Osteoarthritis*. MIPI 1983. Distributed by Pfizer Pharmaceuticals in the public interest. An excellent book for the layman on the disease, life problems associated with osteoarthritis and how to deal with these problems.

W. D. Squyres. *Patient Education.* Palo Alto, Calif: Mayfield Publishing Co. This book offers an overview of patient education—planning, administration, pedagogy and evaluation.

REFERENCES

Alpert, J.J.: Broken Appointments. *Pediatrics,* 34:127–132, 1964.

Anderson, R.J., Kirk, L.M.: Methods of Improving Patient Compliance in Chronic Disease States. *Arch Intern Med,* 142:1673–1675, 1982.

Becker, M.H., Drachman, R.H., Krischt, J.P.: Motivations as Predictors of Health Behavior. *Health Serv Rep,* 87:852–861, 1972.

Blackwell, B.R.: The Drug Defaulter. *Clin Pharmacol Ther,* 13:841–848, 1972.

Boyd, J.R., Covington, T.R., Stanaszek, W.F., et al: Drug Defaulting: II. Analysis of Noncompliance Patterns. *Am J Hosp Pharm,* 31:485–491, 1974.

Brand, F., Smith, R., Brand, P.: Effect of Economic Barriers to Medical Care on Patient's Noncompliance. *Public Health Reports,* 92:72–78, 1977.

Closson, R., Kikugawa, C.: Noncompliance Varies With Drug Class. Hospitals, 49:89–93, 1975.

Davis, M.S.: Variations in Patient's Compliance with Doctor's Orders: Analysis of Congruence Between Survey Responses and Results of Empirical Investigations. *J Med Educ,* 41:1037–1048, 1966.

Deyo, R.A., et al: Noncompliance with Arthritis Drugs: Magnitude Correlates and Clinical Implications, *J Rheumatol* 1981, Nov.–Dec. 8(6) 931–6.

Dunbar, J.J., Marshall, G.D., Hovell, M.F.: Behavioral Strategies for Improving Compliance in Haynes, 1979, op cit, p. 175.

Ferguson, K., Bole, G.G.: Family Support, Health Beliefs, and Therapeutic Compliance in Patients with Rheumatoid Arthritis, *Patient Counsel Health Educ,* 1:101–105, 1979.

Finnerty, F.A., Jr., Mattie, E.C., Finnerty, F.A., III: Hypertension in the Inner City: 1. Analysis of Clinic Drop Outs. *Circulation,* 47:73–75, 1973.

Green, L.W.: Educational Strategies to Improve Compliance with Therapeutic and Preventive Regimens: The Recent Evidence, pp. 157–173 in Haynes, 1979.

Green, L.W., Kreuter, M.W., Deeds, S.G. and Partridge, K.S.: *Health Education Planning: A Diagnostic Approach*. Palo Alto, Calif: Mayfield Publ. Co., 1980.

Haynes, R.B.: Strategies to Improve Compliance with Referrals, Appointments and Prescribed Medical Regimens, in Haynes, 1979, p. 142.

Haynes, R.B.: Determinants of Compliance: The Disease and the Mechanics of Treatment in Haynes (ed.) *Compliance in Health Care*. Baltimore: Johns Hopkins University Press, 1979, p. 51.

Hemminki, E., Heikkila, J.: Elderly People's Compliance with Prescriptions, and Quality of Medication. *Scand J Soc Med*, 3:87–92, 1975.

Hertroijs, A.: A Study of Some Factors Affecting the Attendance of Patients in a Leprosy Control Scheme. *Int J Lepr*, 42:419–427, 1974.

Hoenig, F., Ragg, N.: The Non-attending Psychiatric Outpatient: An Administrative Problem. *Med Care*, 4:96–100, 1966.

Inui, T.S., Yaortee, G.L., Williamson, J.W.: Improved Outcomes in Hypertension After Physician Tutorials. *Ann Intern Med*, 84:646–651, 1976.

Jette, A.M.: Improving Patient Cooperation with Arthritis Treatment Regimens. *Arthritis Rheum*, 1982, Apr. 25(4):447–53.

Jonsen, A.: Ethical Issues in Compliance, in Haynes *Compliance in Health Care*. Baltimore: Johns Hopkins University Press, 1979, 119–120.

Lane, M.F., Barbarite, R.V., Bergner, L., Harris, D.: Child-resistant Medicine Containers: Experience in the Home. *Am J Public Health*, 61:1861–1869, 1971.

Latiolais, C.J., Berry, C.C.: Misuse of Prescription Medications by Outpatients. *Drug Intell Clin Pharm*, 3:270–277, 1969, and Wilcox, D.R., Gillian, R., Hare, E.H.: Do Psychiatric Outpatients Take Their Drugs? *Br Med J*, 2:790–792, 1965.

Litt, I.F., Cuskey, W.R. and Rosenberg, A.: A Role of Self Esteem and Autonomy in Determining Medical Compliance Among Adolescents with Juvenile Rheumatoid Arthritis. *Pediatrics*, 1982 Jan: 69(1):15–7.

Mattor, M.E., Markello, J., Yaffe, S.J.: Inadequacies in the Pharmacologic Management of Ambulatory Children. *J Pediatr*, 87:134–141, 1975, also Pharmaceutic Factors Affecting Pediatric Compliance, *Pediatrics*, 55:101–108, 1975.

McKenney, J.J.: The Clinical Pharmacy and Compliance, in Haynes, 1979, op cit, 260–277.

Moon, M.H., Moon BAH, Black WAM: Compliancy in Splint-wearing Behavior of Patients with Rheumatoid Arthritis, *NZ Med J*, 360–365.

Oakes, T.W., Ward, J.R., Gray, R.N., Klauber, M.R., Mood, P.M.: Family Expectations and a Patient Compliance to a Hand Resting Splint Regimen, *J Chronic Dis*, 22:757–764.

Peck, C.L., King, N.J.: Increasing Patient Compliance With Prescription, *JAMA*, 248: 2874, 1982.

Rockart, J.F., Hoffman, P.B.: Physician and Patient Behavior Under Different Scheduling Systems in a Hospital Out-patient Department. *Med Care*, 7:463–470, 1969.

Sackett, D.L., Haynes, R.B. (eds.): *Compliance With Therapeutic Regimens*. Baltimore: Johns Hopkins University Press, 1976, 1–6.

Sackett, D.L., Snow, J.C.: The Magnitude of Compliance and Non-Compliance, in Haynes *Compliance in Health Care*, 11–22.

Starr, P.: *The Social Transformation of American Medicine,* NY: Basic Books, 1982.

Svarstad, B.L.: Physician-Patient Communication and Patient Conformity with Medical Advice, pp. 220–238, in Mechanic D. (ed.): *The Growth of Bureaucratic Medicine.* New York, Wiley, 1976.

Wilber, J.A., Barrow, J.G.: Hypertension—A Community Problem. *Am J Med,* 52:653–663, 1972.

TABLE 24-1
SUCCESSFUL COMPLIANCE-IMPROVING STRATEGIES

Compliance problem	*Strategy*
Referrals	Letter to patient Referral clerk Patient instruction (Short referral time)
Appointments	Mailed reminders Telephone reminders (Efficient clinic scheduling)
Acute medical regimens	Explicit verbal & written instruction Parenteral treatment Special pill packaging Pill calendars Extended-role nursing
Chronic medical regimens	Monitored drug levels Parenteral medications Increased supervision Behavior modification Physician instruction

CHAPTER 25

CULTURAL CONTEXT OF TREATMENT*

Meryl Sufian, Ph.D.

Lack of adequate health care is a problem for members of certain ethnic groups in the United States. These groups, which largely consist of Third World ethnic groups,[1] comprise a growing population in major urban areas that has significant health needs. Coupled with this is the growing problem of chronic disease which is the leading cause of disability and death among all groups today. Because chronic illness creates a special dependency of clients on professionals that may be inconsistent with the familiar conventions of their lives, members of Third World groups with chronic illness may find themselves in medical situations in which the clash of cultures is particularly significant in determining their health-related behavior. Our contention is that a conflict emerges between the culture of the health care system and the healing cultures of Third World ethnic groups. We are interested in the impact this conflict has on health-related behavior, especially on the patterns of utilization that emerge for Third World groups in relation to the healing resources that are available in urban areas. One way in which persons from Third World groups resolve the cultural conflict between systems is to engage in a pattern that involves the utilization of healing resources from both the mainstream health care system and a culturally sanctioned indigenous healing system. If this is the case, it is then incumbent upon the health care system and its practitioners, as far as policy is concerned, to become culturally sensitive on both a structural and interpersonal level in its approach toward healing and toward clients or potential clients of the health care system.

The following encounter is based on an observation by the author in the course of carrying out field work in the rheumatology ambulatory clinic at a major teaching hospital in New York City. The setting was one of the many examining rooms in which the physicians see clients. The client was a middle-aged

---

*I am grateful to Michael Brown, Charlotte Muller and Erol Ricketts for their individual contributions to this work.

Supported by the Multipurpose Arthritis Center, Downstate Medical Center, State University of New York from NIADDK-NIH, #AM20525-26 and partially by an Arthritis Foundation Research Fellowship.

black woman who was from the West Indies. She repeatedly told the physician that she did not feel well in the morning and, therefore, was unable to get out and go to work. The physician replied each time, "What do you mean?" This was repeated several times and both parties became increasingly louder and angrier with each exchange. Finally, trying to put an end to what had become a confrontation, the client raised her voice and exclaimed: "I don't feel good." The physician responded, while looking at her chart, "If you came when you had appointments and for the tests, I could help you." Later in the interaction, the client told the physician that she had been applying lemon to the rash on her arms. He asked if it was helping her. She immediately said that it did help. When he asked her to be more specific about how it helped, she admitted that it "really did not help" her, whereupon, he laughed. Throughout the entire interaction the client repeated that she wanted to work, but felt physically unable to. She said that she had been trying to obtain Medicaid since she could only afford certain tests that were needed if she received financial assistance. At the end of the interaction, on her way out of the room, the client exclaimed: "What kind of democracy is this?"

After she left, the physician commented: "She is a disaster. I try to help her. She's been trying to get Medicaid for over a year. I schedule her to come every three weeks and she shows up every six weeks. I'm glad she's leaving." He also said that her illness was not physical and that he did not know whether or not she was really sick. He concluded that there was something peculiar about a system in which people were on disability but worked despite that to make more money. "But that," he added, "seems to be the way it is here."

The question this encounter raises is whether the interaction of the parties represents an inability on the part of the client to participate in a rational process of diagnosis, or something more complex, perhaps a clash of different rationalities. From the standpoint of the physician the client was both self-serving and foolish. She could not answer specific questions about how she felt, could not listen to what was being asked, had failed to participate in a normal course of tests and diagnosis, had used remedies rooted in superstition, and was aggressive and self-serving. Even the researcher is tempted to adopt this perspective, since the research process is part of the same community of science as medicine. Yet, we are sufficiently familiar by now with what anthropologists have shown over and over again: the responses of people to situations may be unintelligible to observers from a different cultural background or may seem backward or unsophisticated, but there may be a rational basis for action rooted in that background that can become visible as such when it is made explicit. Indeed, sociology and anthropology have always had to deal with the problem of understanding others and the self-righteousness that so often accompanies contact with those whose experience and ways of organizing experience are in one way or another foreign. The example itself cannot provide an answer to whether or not the physician's evaluation is correct or adequate, but the fact that the encounter rapidly got out of hand and the fact that neither party seemed able to communicate with the other, or at least to establish a semblance of consensus, suggests that a deeper conflict than that of rationality with superstition and recalcitrance may have occurred. With this in mind, it seems at least strategically sound to suggest that the parties may have met in this encounter not as individuals—one seeking advice, the other an expert able to advise—but as members of communities whose cultures made it difficult for them to continue their interaction no matter how compelling or necessary it may have been for one or both of the parties. This model allows us to consider the possibility that the physician's problem was an inability to "hear" the client, and that the client's was a sense of violation due not to a preoccupation with democracy but due to a sense that there was no one to talk to, no one who could understand. One way of further investigating this, at least preliminarily, would have been to have observed the client in her community and to see how she speaks with others about her ailments and how she organizes the healing resources of that community in her own interest. That would at least have raised a presumption that there was a greater rationality on her part than the physician was able to grant. In any case, the model—of culture conflict—suggests that patterns of utilization can be understood as a sociological rather than as an exclusively social psychological problem. People who visit physicians do not cease to be members of a community any more than physicians and other health professionals they visit cease, in the medical encounter, to be part of the culture of professional scientific medicine, to which they, too, have been socialized and in which they participate.

SOCIAL AND CULTURAL FACTORS IN HEALTH CARE

> Broadly speaking, culture is a group's design for living, a shared set of socially transmitted assumptions about the nature of the physical and social world, the goals of life, and the appropriate means of achieving them.[2] At the heart of such designs for living are shared assumptions about the maintenance of well-being and appropriate means of achieving that state, however diversely it may be defined. Such assumptions relate not only to the nature of the material and social world but also to the nature of the biological world, i.e., to ways in which the human body is viewed and seen as functioning. Body image and anatomical knowledge are fundamental in this regard, as are ideas about disease causation, symptom, diagnosis, treatment and other facets of health.[3]

These shared assumptions refer to beliefs or belief systems.

> A belief is a hypothetical construct that involves the assertion of a relationship between some attitude object (a person, a situation, or a behavior, such as smoking) and some attribute of that object (e.g., causes of cancer).[4]

All cultures incorporate beliefs related to healing and illness. Therefore, if we view this fact cross-culturally, we find a variety of health beliefs and corresponding behaviors. Moreover, we shall argue that the health care system in the United States has its own healing culture that is dominant, namely scientific medicine. On the other hand, Third World groups living within the United States have distinct healing cultures which may incorporate to greater or lesser extents aspects of the mainstream health care system. More significantly, it is the contention here that there is a clash between the culture of the health care system and the healing cultures of Third World ethnic groups. The culture of the health care system, as represented by the biomedical perspective or scientific medicine incorporates assumptions and imperatives for its health care professionals. On the other hand, Third World groups (and all cultural groupings for that matter) have their own assumptions and imperatives for its members which are in conflict to varying degrees with the assumptions and imperatives of the culture of scientific medicine. As a result, each group may be resistant to the other's culture and cultural prescriptions regarding health and illness.

> When the practice of medicine involves the application of elements of the institution of medicine in one culture to the people of another, or from one subculture to members of another subculture within the same cultural group, *what is done or attempted by those in the healing roles may not be fully understood or correctly evaluated by those in the patient roles. Conversely, the responses of those on the patient side of the interaction may not conform to the expectations of those on the healing side.* To the extent that this occurs, the relationship may be unsatisfactory to everyone concerned.... When persons of widely dissimilar cultural or subcultural orientations are brought together in a therapeutic relationship, the probability of a mutually satisfactory outcome may be increased if those in the healing roles know something of their own culture and that of the patient and are aware of the extent to which behavior on both sides of the relationship is influenced by cultural factors. An even higher probability of satisfaction may result if the professional people are willing and able to modify elements from their medicine so as to make them fit the expectations of the laymen with whom they are working.[5]

In discussing the significance of understanding cultural differences for health and healing, Saunders has the following to say concerning what appears to be lack of adherence or ignorance on the part of the client who differs culturally with the practitioner:

> If such behavior can be seen and interpreted as an expression of cultural conditioning rather than as simply the whimsical result of individual

> deviance, it becomes possible to anticipate it and to devise effective ways of changing it or of adapting to it.[6]

Knowing the cultural orientation of the client and the possible bearing it may have on the client's behavior is important to the practitioner's strategy. The practitioner needs to know the extent to which cultural orientation influences behavior of clients.

> So equipped, he is able to see uniformities in and reasons for kinds of behavior that otherwise might be ascribed to individual perversity, indifference, apathy, or ignorance and to so direct his {sic} own behavior as to obtain the desired patient response.[7]

THE RHEUMATIC DISEASES

The etiology of arthritis and related rheumatic diseases is unknown and there are no known cures. Thus, treatment is aimed at the relief of symptoms that seriously interfere with the individual's well-being. Rheumatic diseases, unlike other chronic diseases such as hypertension or diabetes, typically manifest symptoms that are obvious to the afflicted person. There is variation among individuals as to the degree of disability, pain, and interference with daily activities. The desire to gain relief from symptoms supplies a strong motive to choose some course of action. The social and emotional consequences of chronic illnesses are major issues for the effective care of most people who have a rheumatic disease. They need explanations for what to expect and advice regarding reasonable strategies for coping effectively with their disease and for handling incidental problems that may arise. There is also a strong need for reassurance about the progress of the disease, in part because the medication prescribed, especially for a disease like osteoarthritis, often only ameliorates the symptoms. Consequently, a critical element in effective treatment is having clients understand their disease in terms that make sense to them and those around them and adjusting expectations to reality.

Aside from the physiological aspects of chronic illnesses, there are additional considerations that include sociocultural factors. Growing evidence indicates that social, cultural, and psychological factors have an important role in whether people become ill and in the duration of their disabilities and the intensity of their symptoms. Once a person is afflicted with a chronic illness, effective treatment of the disease often requires a modification of lifestyle and social relationships. Often a necessary component of this adjustment is that the person who is ill, along with family and friends, take a great deal of the responsibility for the care and the management of the illness. The extent of the change in lifestyle that the person may have to make will depend on the seriousness of the particular case. Ideally, the required lifestyle alterations would be discussed by health professionals with their clients. A successful outcome depends to a great extent on the quality of the practitioner-client relationship and the ability to communicate with each other.

Chronic illness requires an ongoing relationship between the client and the health care system. Having a chronic illness also creates a dependency and preoccupation with the body. The afflicted person's body is always implicitly involved in healing. Therefore, contact with physicians and other health professionals are unlike those for acute episodes of illness which have a defined duration. The ongoing treatment brings together individuals who may be from different cultural backgrounds. Given this set of circumstances, it is incumbent upon health professionals to familiarize themselves with the "whole person" including the social and cultural influences on the individual's life. The fact that a great number of people receive treatment outside of the health care system, either at home or by culturally traditional healers, should be recognized and incorporated in some fashion into treatment plans.

Since living successfully with a rheumatic disease involves establishing a meaningful exchange of information and ideas between practitioners and clients, a marked cultural distance, even independent of language barriers, makes the establishment of rapport and communication difficult, particularly around such sociocultural concerns as sexuality and diet. In addition, beyond the normative role of culture, it is likely that the symptomatology of the rheumatic diseases and the lack of a cure may encourage people to rely on culturally sanctioned or other alternatives to the health care system that are thought to be efficacious.

THE CULTURE OF THE HEALTH CARE SYSTEM

Let us now briefly examine the culture underlying the present health care system in our society. In addition to health care reflecting the norms, values, beliefs, and expectations of the larger society, the institutionalization of health care has generated its own culture of healing.

The approach of scientific medicine, or the biomedical perspective, focuses on objective and rational explanations and treatments for *disease*. It is only recently that an interest in health promotion or "wellness" has developed. Many physicians tend to see their patients, as objects for analysis rather than aspects of persons, and see themselves as specialists to distinct parts of the body and as experts about the body's condition. They, consequently, may be unable to grant rationality and relevance to clients' judgments and healing inclinations or to appreciate the significance of the social, cultural, and psychological factors that operate as inevitable and necessary features of the healing process.

There are several practical consequences of the institutionalization of the professional's culture and the establishment of the legitimacy of its control over healing. First, it becomes difficult to recognize that a valid and responsive healing program must be more than just a treatment plan. The health professional's culture could, therefore, exclude the healing inclinations and sanctioned healing practices established within the client's own culture: an exclusion the client might not accept. Further, it becomes difficult for the medical encounter to provide an opportunity for client and professional to reconcile their health-related cultural differences and, therefore, for the client to arrive at a rational—livable in his or her own terms—basis for adhering to the treatment plan. Indeed, the culture conflict dictated by an exclusively rationalistic approach to medicine may leave the client without an adequate basis for interpreting diagnosis and advice. Even more significant is the fact that this approach may force the client to decide between a medical regimen imposed from outside and one inextricably tied to the deepest moral values and practices of the client's culture. Finally, as can be seen from the encounter described at the beginning of this chapter, a failure of the health professional to find a basis for a cultural reconciliation may reinforce already existing biases making it difficult to adequately appraise the client's needs.

THE CULTURES OF THIRD WORLD CLIENTS

The fact that clients bring with them not only a presenting problem but knowledge, experiences, beliefs, and traditions is usually not taken into consideration in the practice of scientific medicine.

> In every way, the health institution is viewed as acting upon, impinging upon, or being introduced into communities or specific population groups to inject something into their lives that they do not already have. While this may be a laudable undertaking in the interest of sharing the specific health-related strengths of the orthodox system, the problem lies in the unicultural focus underlying such efforts. Reality is perceived in terms of introducing *something* where *nothing* of significance existed before. The acknowledgement that individuals and communities have *something* already, such as their own health cultural traditions, is not required by the concepts in current use by orthodox providers of health care.[8]

It is unquestionably true that clients or potential clients play active roles in their health and medical care. They make decisions based on their beliefs, self-perceptions, and the weighing of costs and benefits. If they seek medical advice, they choose whether and to what extent they will follow recommendations, and they decide the conditions upon which recommendations will be followed. In making these choices, clients cannot avoid conforming to the beliefs, expectations, values, and norms of their cultural settings. These decisions may involve seeking the advice of people outside of the health care system who are significant to evaluating their health and healing such as relatives, friends, and culturally indigenous and sanctioned healers, and engage in traditional healing practices.

The cultural imperatives that people adhere to may be largely derived from the culture of the ethnic group of which the individual is a member or in which one at least has his or her origins. The power and class relations associated with ethnicity are part of the development and experience of every individual in our society. Therefore, it is reasonable to assume that they are unavoidable features of practitioner-client interactions. This complex of factors is particularly important in the medical experience of Third World ethnic groups.

It has been well established by sociologists and anthropologists that Third World ethnic groups tend to maintain relatively independent cultural forms. Evidence indicates that a wide range of resources, including health care, are underutilized by this population. The causes of this underutilization are complex, partly because of the intricate relationships among subordinate status, political power, poverty, and education, and partly because of the effects of discrimination on attitudes and behavior. Studies in sociology and anthropology have suggested several important ways in which the cultural aspects of ethnicity influence health beliefs, perceptions, attitudes, and behavior. Third World ethnic group cultures, in particular, often approach health and illness in ways that differ from that of scientific medicine.

Traditional health beliefs and the culturally sanctioned utilization of traditional healers are well established in Third World cultures. The operation of these alternatives can be illustrated by a summary derived from previous research and field work by the author. In Latino communities many people adhere to a *caliente-frio* (hot-cold) theory of illness. According to this belief an illness will manifest itself when the body experiences an imbalance between hot and cold. In this scheme foods, medications, and herbs are classified as *caliente o frio* (hot or cold). When an imbalance occurs, the person must be given the appropriate items in order to restore his or her health. Arthritis is considered to be the result of an external cold that lodges in certain areas of the body. Therefore, appropriate treatments are medications, foods, and herbs that are classified as *caliente* in order to restore the body's balance. Someone who holds these beliefs may turn to a *botanica* (herb shop) as a source of care. A *botanica* is consulted for both herbal and spiritualist remedies. The person with arthritis may want to obtain herbs and teas or tonics that are *caliente*. In additions to, or instead of, an herbal remedy, the person might seek the help of a spiritualist, who is a medium, who may find a supernatural or psychic cause for the problem and recommend a strategy for eliminating it. A *botanica* may be used as a source of care either before or after consulting a physician or may be used simultaneously with a physician's care. It is not unusual for spiritualists, for example, to recommend to their clients that they see a physician along with their own recommendations for treatment.

Following are some of the ways in which culture and health are interrelated. First, concepts of illness including etiology vary according to cultural background. Social psychological, environmental, and supernatural influences may be emphasized in the etiology of illness. In addition, there are occurrences that are classified as illness in some cultures which are not found in others, for example, *mal de ojo* (evil eye) which is recognized in the Puerto Rican and Mexican cultures and cultures surrounding the Mediterranean.

Second, some cultural groupings recognize models of bodily functioning and good health that are different from and inconsistent with the biomedical model, for example, the *caliente-frio* model discussed above. Beliefs derived from these models lead logically to the use of traditional healing practices as well as of traditional healers, though not necessarily to the exclusion of scientific medicine. Third, cultural groups vary in their perception of and response to illness. For example, Zborowski has shown that the perception of pain and the response to it vary among different ethnic groups. Fourth, cultural background affects communication patterns between client and health professional as a result of both cultural distance and culturally influenced styles of interacting with other people.

Although we have been discussing the importance of cultural factors for health care, we must also recognize that differences exist within cultural groups as well. Health professionals should be able to use the cultural information they have about clients to provide general guidelines for evaluating the extent and the ways in which the medical encounter needs to be modified to fit culturally based expectations.

IMPLICATIONS FOR MEDICAL PRACTICE

There are several policy implications for medical practice on the interpersonal level between health professionals and clients and on the structural level of the health care system that follow from the ideas presented above. In general, health professionals should adopt a treatment style that is culturally sensitive. Practitioners need to be made aware that there are cultural differences related to health and healing among cultural groupings that must be respected if the client is to relate rationally to a treatment plan. A part of this awareness involves the recognition that scientific medicine itself has a cultural basis. Client innovations beyond the imperatives of scientific medicine or the expectations of health professionals may not be due to ignorance or lack of sophistication but to the need of the client to satisfy norms of well-being that are consistent with his or her cultural background. Once professionals in the health care system gain this awareness, they will be in a better position to care for not only Third World groups, but people in general since this general attitude would be helpful for other cultural groups as well as for women and older people who also experience discrimination.

If a practitioner should encounter a client whom he or she has reason to believe adheres to culturally grounded health beliefs or is engaging in traditional healing practices, the practitioner needs to be able to handle this situation effectively. That is, the practitioner needs to display a sensitivity to possible alternatives without being judgmental and without discouraging the client to the point where his or her health may suffer as a result. Strategies can be created whereby clients can utilize more than one system of healing as long as achieving positive results, i.e., improved health, is made the overall goal. Many practitioners may take the position that to entertain alternative forms of healing is irrational. However, psychology and psychiatry have recognized these issues on both the levels of research and practice as having great import. An obvious example of the achievement of greater sensitivity is that some mental health clinics that serve a largely Latino clientele have introduced the presence of spiritualists into their practice.[10] This strategy is one way of overcoming the cultural clash between scientific medicine and traditional healing systems.

The following suggestions are made toward achieving the goal of greater cultural sensitivity. First, genuine communication presupposes respect for the client as a person and rapport between practitioner and client based on such respect. In some cases, members of the client's family should not only be referred to, but should be included in the medical encounter and in treatment plans out of respect for cultural traditions. Second, an open non-judgmental attitude towards the client's beliefs, expectations, and values is part of the spirit of compromise that is essential for the client's full participation in treatment plans. Third, health professionals must do the interpersonal work necessary to reduce social, economic and cultural distance between themselves and their clients. Fourth, in cases where a community has well-established ethnic or cultural groups, the health care institutions and professionals in these communities need to become familiar with the cultures of those groups ahead of time, particularly with their beliefs and practices concerning health and healing. Fifth, as part of the medical encounter, the health professional should evaluate to what extent the client's medical condition needs to be interpreted in the light of culturally-determined concepts of disease and illness. If there is any reason to believe that the client's cultural background does figure importantly in his or her health beliefs and behavior, the health professional should elicit the client's conception of the problem. One of the inquiries that ought to be made is: "What do *you* think caused your problem?" The client should be encouraged to become an active participant in the encounter. Sixth, once the client's ideas are known, the health professional has to deal with discrepancies between the client's conceptual scheme and the biomedical perspective. In order to deal effectively with discrepancies, the treatment plan should be formulated in such a way as to include compromises to which all parties clearly agree. In addition, when treating clients who have indicated, verbally or otherwise, a preference for alternative modes of treatment, these should be incorporated into treatment plans. Seventh, when the situation calls for it, there should be consultation and cooperation between health care professionals and traditional healers, an approach which has been successful in the field of mental health.

Communication can be improved by several other practical strategies that deal with some of the more subtle aspects of the medical encounter. Since verbal communication is often limited in the medical encounter, clients look for other cues to gain information about themselves and their problems. The professional's nonverbal behavior is extremely important in conveying information and may, if not handled well, be a source of ambiguity. In order to create an atmosphere of warmth, caring, and understanding, and a sense of mutual respect, the health professional should establish good eye contact and use appropriate facial expressions, tone of voice, posture, and gestures. In addition, he or she may, if appropriate, shake hands or use a polite touch on the hand (not on the head) to reduce social distance and convey sympathy and understanding.

Furthermore, complications in communication arise when the client is not only from another culture, but speaks very little English or none at all. Initially, the health professional should not make any assumptions about language competence, but should ask the client what language he or she would prefer to use. If the person prefers his or her native language, a trained interpreter with a medical background should be available for interpreting—not a relative or a child or a convenient stranger. This is an important consideration because otherwise there are dangers of mistaken interpretation, violations of privacy and/or confidentiality, violations of cultural traditions, and the accidental introduction of extraneous and possibly detrimental information into the encounter. An even greater effort must be made to sustain rapport with non-English speaking clients using the guidelines listed above since there is a tendency to direct conversation to the interpreter when present and to neglect the client.

In summary, we have briefly explored the issue of social, cultural, and ethnic differences and how they relate to medical care. We are interested in knowing what happens when health professionals confront clients whose cultural orientations may be in conflict with the orientation of the health care system. We would argue that the differences in orientation which are manifested in a number of behaviors (e.g., lack of adherence to treatment plans, underutilization, etc.) are rooted in cultural explanations for beliefs and behaviors and not in lack of education or sophistication or in deviant beliefs and practices. Furthermore, it is our contention that social supports exist for the traditional cultures of Third World groups that do not necessarily exist for other groups in urban areas. Therefore, there are sanctioned alternatives for Third World group members to choose from for which they receive social approval.

REFERENCES AND NOTES

[1]Those ethnic groups whose members originate in Third World countries, i.e., countries in Africa, Asia, South America, and Latin America.

[2]Benjamin Paul, "Anthropological Perspectives on Medicine and Public Health," *Annals of the New York Academy of Political and Social Science* 346 (1963), quoted in Hazel Hitson Weidman and Janice A. Egeland, "A Behavioral Science Perspective in the Comparative Approach to the Delivery of Health Care," *Social Science and Medicine* 7 (1973):848.

[3]Weidman and Egeland, p. 848.

[4]D.J. Stang and L.S. Wrightsman, *Dictionary of Social Behavior and Social Research Methods* (Monterey, CA: Brooks-Cole, 1981) quoted in M. Robin DiMatteo and D. Dante DiNicola, *Achieving Patient Compliance* (New York: Pergamon Press, 1982), p. 123.

[5]Lyle Saunders, *Cultural Differences and Medical Care: The Case of the Spanish Speaking People of the Southwest* (New York: Russell Sage Foundation, 1954), p. 8; emphasis in the original.

[6]Saunders, p. 99.

[7]Ibid.

[8]Hazel H. Weidman, Miami Health Ecology Project Report: A Statement on Ethnicity and Health, vol. 1, University of Miami School of Medicine, 1978. (Mimeographed.) Quoted in Alan Harwood, ed., *Ethnicity and Medical Care* (Cambridge: Harvard University Press, 1981), p. 22; emphasis in the original.

[9]*Mal de ojo* is an explanation for the sudden onset of illness in a child which comes about when an adult, usually an acquaintance of the family, has shown the child an inordinate amount of attention.

[10]This has been achieved at Lincoln Hospital in the Bronx, New York.

SUGGESTED READINGS

Berkanovic, Emil and Reeder, Leo G. Ethnic, economic and social psychological factors in the source of medical care. *Social Problems,* 1973, 21:246–259.

Coulton, Claudia J. Factors related to preventive health behavior: implications for social work intervention. *Social Work in Health Care,* 1978, 3(3):297–310.

Delgado, M. Herbal medicine in the Puerto Rican community. *Health and Social Work,* 1979, 4(2):24–40.

DiMatteo, M. Robin and DiNicola, D. Dante. *Achieving Patient Compliance.* New York: Pergamon Press, 1982.

Galbis, R. Mental health service in a Hispanic Community. *Health and Social Work,* 1979, 4(2):24–40.

Glasser, Irene. Guidelines for using an interpreter in social work. *Child Welfare,* 1983, 62(5):468–470.

Harwood, Alan (ed.). *Ethnicity and Medical Care.* Cambridge: Harvard University Press, 1981.

Hautman, M.A. Folk health and illness beliefs. *Nurse Practitioner,* 1979, 4:23–24.

Henderson, George and Primaux, M. (eds.). *Transcultural Health Care.* Menlo Park, Calif.: Addison-Wesley, 1981.

Murillo-Rhode, I. Cultural sensitivity in the care of the Hispanic patient. *Washington State Journal of Nursing*—special supplement, 1979:25–32.

Press, Irwin. Urban folk medicine: a functional overview. *American Anthropologist,* 1978, 80:71–84.

Rautenberg, Ellen L. Ethnicity and health care. Institute on Pluralism and Group Identity. American Jewish Committee, New York, 1983.

Saunders, Lyle. *Cultural Differences and Medical Care: The Case of the Spanish-Speaking People of the Southwest.* New York: Russell Sage Foundation, 1954.

Suchman, Edward A. Sociomedical variations among ethnic groups. *American Journal of Sociology,* 1964, 70:319–331.

Sufian, Meryl. The influence of culture on health-related behavior. Unpublished Ph.D. dissertation, City University of New York Graduate School, 1985.

U.S. Department of Health and Human Services. Culture-bound and sensory barriers to communication with patients: strategies and resources for health education. Memorandum, Centers for Disease Control, Atlanta, Ga., 1982.

Zborowski, Mark. Cultural components in responses to pain. *Journal of Social Issues,* 1952, 8:16–30.

Zola, Irving K. Culture and symptoms—an analysis of patients' presenting complaints. *American Sociological Review,* 1966, 31:615–630.

CHAPTER 26

FOUNDATIONS AND THE GOVERNMENT

Dorothy Goldstein, M.S.

People create foundations and institutions to fight disease out of a variety of motivations. Sometimes, founders are health professionals who decide to band together to pool information and resources. Sometimes, the beginnings of a new foundation are the result of a personal loss or a traumatizing encounter with a specific disease. Sometimes, institutions develop in an apparently haphazard way in response to an urgent concern of the public. The various foundations and institutions that work, both independently and in concerted effort, to help eradicate and cope with the rheumatic diseases reflect all these different origins. What ties them together is the knowledge that it is alliance and cooperation which will ultimately help to surmount and outwit the magnitude of the arthritis problem.

THE ARTHRITIS FOUNDATION

The first professional group in the United States to organize because of a common interest in arthritis was the American Committee for the Study and Control of Arthritis. Formed in 1927, it worked with other national committees of the Ligue Internationale contre le Rheumatisme which had been founded in Europe. At its open meetings held prior to the annual scientific sessions of the American Medical Association, stimulating presentations attracted more and more interest. In 1934, the American Committee expanded its membership and changed its name to the American Rheumatism Association (ARA).

World War II interrupted ARA activities, but the end of the war and the return of physicians who had been trained in Army Arthritis Centers brought renewed enthusiasm to the organization. Realizing the need for financial support to carry on research projects and clinical service, a committee of the ARA was formed to study this problem.

They recommended that a voluntary health agency be organized with a primary mission to raise money for research projects. These research projects were to focus on finding the cause of arthritis, improving current treatment, and, ultimately, to search for a cure. In 1948, acting upon this recommendation, the ARA helped to form the Arthritis and Rheumatism Foundation.[1]

In 1958, the National Foundation–March of Dimes extended its interest to include arthritis. Under the leadership of Dr. William S. Clark, Director of Clinical Programs, the National Foundation created a network of medical centers involved in arthritis research. On September 1, 1964 they publicly announced their decision to relinquish their programs in rheumatology and transfer them to the Arthritis and Rheumatism Foundation. Shortly after this occurrence the name of the Arthritis and Rheumatism Foundation was shortened to the Arthritis Foundation, which by then had become the sole voluntary health organization dedicated to finding the causes, the cures and better treatments for the rheumatic diseases.

Dr. Clark, who left the National Foundation–March of Dimes to become the president of the Arthritis Foundation, helped to develop an agreement between the Arthritis Foundation and the American Rheumatism Association to work together more closely. In 1965, the ARA united with the Arthritis Foundation to serve as its medical and scientific section. Aware of the important role that professionals other than physicians play in the treatment of patients with arthritis, Dr. Clark was most anxious to form an additional professional section which would include nurses, occupational therapists, physical therapists, psychologists, social workers and other professionals with an interest in the rheumatic diseases. The Arthritis Foundation had already indicated its interest in the allied health professions by helping fund the American Occupational Therapy Association (AOTA) and the American Physical Therapy Association (APTA) to provide an advisory committee to the Foundation.

These two organizations were also demonstrating their concern for arthritis. A special issue on the rheumatic diseases was published by the Journal of the American Physical Therapy Association in 1963, and two issues concentrating on rheumatology appeared in the 1965 American Journal of Occupational Therapy. The AOTA had also developed a special interest group which met at their annual meeting to present up-to-date information relating to rheumatology.

Arthritis Foundation meetings took place to plan the formation of an additional professional section, and in 1967 saw the inauguration of the Allied Health Professions (AHP). As with so many other organizations it went through a name change to the present Arthritis Health Professionals Association (AHPTA).

As the sole voluntary health agency dedicated to the problems of arthritis, the Arthritis Foundation has worked to:

> Develop a nationwide research program to discover the causes and improve the treatment of people with arthritis.
>
> Establish fellowships to increase the number of qualified individuals who will engage in research and treatment.

Support medical centers devoted to research, teaching and treatment.

Promote professional education to enhance the ability of the medical profession to treat patients more effectively.

Increase public awareness of the magnitude of arthritis and its seriousness as a health problem.[2]

Today, the Arthritis Foundation consists of 71 chapters and divisions throughout the United States with a national headquarters in Atlanta, Georgia. Included in the organization, along with the American Rheumatism Association and the Arthritis Health Professions Association, is a membership group called the American Juvenile Arthritis Organization (AJAO) for people concerned with childhood arthritis.

One of the priorities of the national office has been to support individual scientists with postdoctoral fellowships and arthritis investigator awards. These have proven to be of great importance as evidenced by the fact that many of today's leading investigators and clinicians were once Arthritis Foundation fellows. In more recent years, the Foundation has also offered traineeship and research grants for non-physician health professionals working in an area related to arthritis. The traineeships are awarded to persons who are pursuing an advanced academic degree and are interested in research careers relevant to arthritis. Research grants are awarded to non-M.D. professionals with a research background for specific projects related to the management of arthritis and/or comprehensive patient care. In 1983, there were 128 awards given to M.D.'s, Ph.D.'s, persons with other equivalent postdoctoral degrees and to non-physician health professionals.

The Arthritis Foundation does not own any research facilities itself. However, it does provide funds to clinical research centers in medical institutions where there are arthritis programs in the three areas of research, teaching and patient care. In 1983, fifty-one centers across the United States and two arthritis pediatric centers were funded.

In 1985, the Arthritis Foundation and the American Rheumatism Association agreed to separate, primarily for organizational and tax reasons. Since that date the ARA has carried on its scientific and professional programs separately but with strong support from the Foundation. Each year the ARA sponsors an annual national scientific conference at which physicians, scientists and health professionals meet to share information and present studies about advances in arthritis research and treatment. Four regional meetings are also held throughout the United States, presenting up-to-date research results and in-depth discussions of topics considered to be of general interest to the rheumatology community.

In 1988 the ARA voted to change its name to the American College of Rheumatology (ACR) to better reflect its professional scientific, clinical and educational activities.

There are also arthritis organizations in other areas of the world, such as the

Pan-American League Against Rheumatism (PANLAR), the European League Against Rheumatism (EULAR) and the Southeast Asia and Pacific League Against Rheumatism (SEAPAL). The International League Against Rheumatism (ILAR) is a federation of these three regional leagues. Both the ILAR and the regional leagues conduct scientific congresses every four years.

As a vital part of its professional education program, the Arthritis Foundation publishes the monthly journal *Arthritis and Rheumatism* (A & R). Periodically, a special supplement or issue of the A & R will focus on a specific topic. Beginning in 1935, members of the ARA began review of the American and English literature covering research and clinical practices in the rheumatic diseases. They do so to this day. The *25th Rheumatism Review 1979–80* was published as a special issue of the A & R in 1983. Previous issues of the *Rheumatism Reviews* are available from the Foundation.

The *Bulletin on the Rheumatic Diseases* is distributed in the United States. It presently appears six times a year and each issue contains current thinking on a noteworthy topic in rheumatology. First published in 1950, it is also available in bound collections.

The ninth edition of the popular *Primer on the Rheumatic Diseases* was published in 1988. It briefly summarizes basic information about the rheumatic diseases with emphasis on clinical manifestations, pathogenesis, diagnosis and treatment. Discussions of recent microbiological research, clinical pharmacology and surgical management are also included.

Begun in 1965 and produced in cooperation with the National Library of Medicine, the *Annual Index of Rheumatology* includes a yearly index of the rheumatic scientific literature from journals that are cited in the *Cumulative Index Medicus.*

Audiovisual materials and cassettes are important resources provided by the Arthritis Foundation for the rheumatology community. They include the *Revised Clinical Slide Collection on the Rheumatic Diseases* which contains over 325 35-mm slides of clinical photographs, radiographs and micrographs of pathologic specimens of over 70 rheumatic diseases. The 195 page syllabus, included with the slide collection, contains a photograph and description of each slide. First issued in 1980, there is also an *Arthritis Teaching Slide Collection for Teachers of Allied Health Professionals.* It includes 198 slides covering clinical manifestations as well as the assessment and management of various joint diseases.

The 71 semi-autonomous chapters, branches and divisions of the Arthritis Foundation, were mainly organized by dedicated physicians and lay persons without whom the chapters could not function in any meaningful way. When the first chapters came into existence in 1948, there was little research being conducted, a minimum amount of money being spent for arthritis treatment, and a meager amount of time spent training students in medical schools how to treat arthritis patients. Today, the approximate size of the problem is known—36 million people—and the nature of the problem is better understood. The public is beginning to see that the chronic diseases of arthritis are one of our country's major health problems.

Originally in 1948, 13 local chapters opened in different sections of the United States. As the need for arthritis related services increased, more chapters were organized by concerned people in other areas. Today, there are chapters in almost every state, and those chapters that service a very large population usually have affiliated branches. Together, the various chapters provide a significant complement of services. However, due to limited funding and resources, some chapters are restricted in the range of services they can offer.

All chapters provide literature and current information on a wide array of topics for both health professionals and the public. They make referrals to rheumatologists, arthritis clinics, and other professionals who care for people with arthritis.

Newsletters are published to announce service programs and fund-raising events. Answers to important medical questions, and an article that addresses a specific topic may be written to help keep readers up-to-date about subjects of general interest.

A number of chapters can provide counseling for a variety of problems. Staff and volunteers are available to answer questions, to discuss vocational rehabilitation and psychosocial aspects of living with a chronic disease, and the problems of daily living, including where and how to get appropriate aids and devices, etc. Visits to homebound people and visits to those in the hospital may be available at certain chapters. When surgical correction has been recommended, there are chapters which can offer names of persons who have previously undergone a similar procedure. Discussing their personal treatments and outcomes with empathy and understanding can help a concerned patient gain the strength to make a difficult decision.

Exercise programs are available in many chapter areas. These help people increase their strength and flexibility, prevent loss of function, engender a sense of well-being and comfort with themselves, as well as provide the opportunity to meet others who share some of the same problems.

Another important program sponsored by many chapters is the "loan closet." This valuable service permits people to borrow needed equipment such as wheelchairs, walkers and canes.

The last decade has seen the growth of arthritis support groups which provide a secure place where persons with arthritis, their family members and friends can meet to learn more about arthritis and to share common concerns. Rheumatologists, psychologists, orthopaedists and other arthritis health professionals are often invited to participate in these programs. Some of these groups are for adults; others bring together teenagers who have arthritis; and, still others are for parents whose children have arthritis. Gathering together to share experiences and exchange ideas helps everyone to cope just a little bit better with the many problems that this disease engenders.

Speakers for public forums and organized community groups are coordinated by the chapters and feature trained volunteers and professionals who care for persons with arthritis. There is frequent participation in health fairs and other community events where there may be exhibits of literature, arthritis aids and devices and knowledgeable speakers.

There are some chapters which can provide small grants of financial aid. This aid is to be used by persons who are in need of something related to their disease which they cannot afford and for which they have no insurance. This can include transportation for medical care, housekeeping services, special equipment, etc.

An exciting new program called the *Arthritis Self-Help Course* has come into existence in many areas of the country. People who have arthritis or a special interest in arthritis have been trained to lead a course which includes six sessions, each one approximately two hours in length. During these sessions people learn more about their disease and how it can be managed. The popularity of this course seems to indicate that people want to help themselves in an intelligent way, and they are willing to commit the time necessary to become more informed.

One of the most important activities of chapters is the awarding of fellowships and research grants to physicians, scientists and allied health professionals. These grants are to further training in clinical rheumatology and to aid in the investigation of arthritis research projects. Some chapters support arthritis clinics and centers at medical institutions in their areas.

The programs of the Arthritis Foundation receive publicity due to the cooperation of the local media. Radio, television, newspapers and magazines carry stories, interviews, programming and public service announcements to help the Foundation inform the public about their available services and research efforts.

In order to pay for services and to support the research, patient treatment and training programs' chapters raise money from members of their communities. The Arthritis Foundation is depended solely on the goodwill and benevolence of its supporters in order to continue to maintain and expand its activities.

THE LUPUS FOUNDATION OF AMERICA, INC.

One of the more serious forms of rheumatic disease is systemic lupus erythematosus, frequently referred to as SLE or lupus. Lupus is a systemic disease because it can damage the body's vital organs, and it affects women about nine times more often than men. There are strong indications that SLE is also a disease in which the body attacks its own tissues and joints. A considerable amount of lupus research is involved in trying to understand the roles that antigens and antibodies play in the disease process.

The Lupus Foundation was created specifically to raise money to support research into SLE. The founders were members of families who were personally involved with the devastating effects of this disease. A little more than 10 years ago, three families were told that their daughters were extremely ill with what had been diagnosed as systemic lupus erythematosus. When one of these children died, her family decided to raise money for research into the cause of this mysterious and little understood illness. The other two families then spearheaded an effort to increase public and medical awareness of this disease. Acting out of a compulsion to do something about a sickness that had traumatized their households, these families attracted a small group of spirited people and the help of a sympathetic rheumatologist. Letters were written to everyone they knew soliciting time and money to support research and to educate people about SLE.

Before very long other groups formed, books and articles were written, and the Lupus Foundation had become a reality. Realizing the value of a national organization, a meeting was held in Boston in 1975 that resulted in the formation of the Lupus Foundation of America, Inc. Rapid growth followed, and there are presently 66 chapters, 37 groups with plans for future constituency with the national organization (located in St. Louis, Missouri), and 64 sub-chapters or support groups.

Lupus research today is being carried out at major universities and medical institutions as well as at the National Institutes of Health.

SCLERODERMA FOUNDATION

This disease was given the name "Skleroderma" by an Italian physician in 1836, and "Sclerodermie" by a French physician in 1847. It is presently called scleroderma, and it comes from the Greek words meaning "hard skin." It affects women more frequently than men, usually, but not always, appearing between the ages of 20 to 50. It is not yet known what causes this connective tissue disease. Some of the possible manifestations are swelling and puffiness of the hands and feet, thickening and tightening of the skin, joint inflammation, and involvement of organs such as the esophagus, intestinal tract, heart, lungs and kidneys. Raynaud's phenomenon is an early symptom, and is found in approximately 90% of the people at some time during the course of the disease. This phenomenon was named after Maurice Raynaud who first described it in 1962. It is an extreme reaction in the fingers, and sometimes the toes, ears or nose following exposure to the cold or emotional stimuli.

Scleroderma is also known as systemic sclerosis, progressive systemic sclerosis (PSS), and systemic scleroderma. But, whatever it is called, it can be a frustrating disease to both physicians and patients. Estimates range from 100,000 to 300,000 people who have scleroderma. To those who have been diagnosed it can cause anxiety and despair, and the urgent need for an emotional support system.

For this reason voluntary, non-profit organizations that focus on scleroderma have been established. They are dedicated to informing and educating the public about scleroderma, to supporting research to discover a cure, and to helping patients better understand and cope with their illness.

The first group to organize was the Scleroderma International Foundation, founded and organized in New Castle, Pennsylvania in 1971. There is also a national organization, the United Scleroderma Foundation, which was founded in Watsonville, California in 1975, and presently has 25 chapters in the United States. Other groups include:

Scleroderma Association of California, Inc.

Progressive Systemic Sclerosis Research Foundation, California

Scleroderma Foundation of Greater Chicago

Scleroderma Association—affiliated with the Massachusetts Arthritis Foundation

The Scleroderma Society, Inc. (in New York City)

Scleroderma Research Foundation of Pennsylvania and New Jersey

Scleroderma Foundation of Greater Washington, D.C.

All of these organizations provide literature and referral to medical care. Some of them offer individual and group counseling as well as support groups. They all work diligently to raise money in order to increase public awareness and provide funds for the research that is necessary if ever a cure for scleroderma is to be found.

MUSCULAR DYSTROPHY ASSOCIATION

Founded in 1950 the Muscular Dystrophy Association (MDA) has nearly 180 chapters in the United States and Puerto Rico. Medical services which include diagnosis and follow-up care are provided at 237 MDA clinics for people with 40 different neuromuscular diseases, including polymyositis, dermatomyositis and myositis ossificans. Currently, there is help for authorized medical services which are not covered by insurance plans or other community services, when approved by the chapter's executive committee.

Chapter services are also provided to help patients secure medically prescribed orthopaedic aids, respiratory equipment, certain appropriate drugs and transportation for specific needs. The chapters distribute literature and audiovisual materials and conduct educational programs for both professionals and the public. MDA-sponsored camp programs exist for children between the ages of six and twenty-one.

Advocacy is pursued in the schools to ensure that children with neuromuscular disease are participants in educational programs, and in legislation to increase accessibility for the handicapped.

The Association sponsors a worldwide research program whose aim is to further knowledge, and find cures and better treatments for the neuromuscular diseases. In 1983 the Association supported approximately 600 basic research and clinically oriented projects. Twenty-nine of these projects were focused on polymyositis, and 20 were concerned with dermatomyositis, at a cost of almost $1,300,000. One of the projects involves a study of patients with polymyositis at 25 clinics, and will form the basis of the first large-scale therapeutic drug trial study ever undertaken for polymyositis.

In addition, MDA supports a Task Force on Drug Development which searches for drugs that will be able to arrest or reverse the progression of muscular dystrophy and related neuromuscular diseases. It also maintains a Task Force on Genetics to help determine the causes of these diseases.

THE NATIONAL INSTITUTES OF HEALTH

There is one other institution that has mounted a major effort to fight arthritis, and that is the federal government. The origins of this involvement can be traced back to July of 1798 when the United States Congress passed a law to create a Marine Hospital Service. The Service was intended to provide sick merchant seamen with adequate medical care.

The United States Congress was by no means the first governmental body to concern itself with public health. There is abundant historical evidence that the earliest civilizations—including the Egyptians, Babylonians, Hebrews, Greeks and Romans—all created elaborate drainage, garbage and waste disposal systems. In addition, they tried to protect their food and water supplies from contamination. However, with the destruction of the Roman Empire the belief that the soul was more important than the body became dominant. Life in a European medieval town reflected this change in values. Sanitation was no longer a prime concern, and human dwellings became a breeding ground for disease. Dreadful epidemics and pandemics raged, but the populations did not respond by passing sanitation laws. Instead, many people believed the rampant spread of diseases was a punishment for sin handed down by divine will.

When the young Congress created the Marine Hospital Service in 1798, they were behaving with uncommon prescience. It was not until almost the latter part of the 19th century that it became fashionable, once again, to place emphasis on the preservation of health. The Marine Hospital Service was partially funded by a deduction of 20 cents per month from each seaman's salary, thereby initiating the unusual idea of a pre-paid medical care program. The President was authorized to appoint physicians in each port town to furnish the necessary care. However, demands for care became so time consuming that physicians found they needed to devote all of their time to the treatment of sailors. In response to the pressing need for hospital services, the first Marine Hospital was built at Norfolk, Virginia in 1800. Another was later built on Staten Island in New York, where the first medical research activities of the Public Health Service began in 1887 in a small Laboratory of Hygiene.

The small laboratory eventually developed into the National Hygienic Laboratory and finally into the original National Institute of Health which was located outside of Washington, D.C. in the town of Bethesda, Maryland. As years passed and the national concern for improved health mounted, congress passed funding for the establishment of a number of different institutes: a cancer institute, a mental health institute, a heart institute, an allergy and infectious disease institute and a dental research institute. The single National Institute of Health had evolved into the complex collectively called the National Institutes of Health (NIH).

Throughout this early development of our federal public health system, arthritis had not been considered one of the pressing problems facing the nation. By 1948 though, enough was known about the extent of its impact on the population of the United States for the American Rheumatism Association and the Arthritis and Rheumatism Foundation to have been created by medical professionals. The following year, at the International Congress of Rheumatology, the first to be held after World War II, Dr. Philip Hench reported his exciting experiences with cortisone which showed a potential for alleviating the effect of rheumatoid arthritis. It was an optimistic time. Concerted efforts were launched by scientists, physicians, and other concerned people to enlighten members of congress. In August of 1950, the Congress established and funded a new institute: the National Institute of Arthritis and Metabolic Diseases (NIAMD).

Up to this time, there had not been any institute whose primary mission was to conduct research into the causes of arthritis and to improve treatment of arthritis patients based on the results of clinical research projects. The mandate given to the new institute was to:

> "...conduct researches relating to the cause, prevention, methods of diagnosis and treatment of arthritis and rheumatism and other metabolic diseases,

to assist and foster such researches and other activities by public and private agencies, and promote the coordination of all such researches, and to promote training in matters relating to such diseases..."[5]

Since 1950, considerably more funding has allowed the Institute to expand its range of programs and activities. The NIH Clinical Center opened in 1953 as a research hospital providing for research studies with patients. In 1955, the Extramural Training Program was created to fund projects, programs, conferences and clinical trials that would be conducted at outside institutes such as universities and hospital-based clinical research centers. The name of the Institute was changed in 1972 to the National Institute of Arthritis, Metabolism and Digestive Diseases (NIAMDD) when attention focused on digestive diseases.

In 1974, acknowledging the vast latitude of the arthritis problem, Congress passed the National Arthritis Act (P.L. 93-640). This act provided for a National Commission on Arthritis and Related Musculoskeletal Diseases whose members were to put together a master plan for action against arthritis. The commission met for thirteen months, held public hearings, and in April of 1976 submitted to the congress a four-volume report entitled, *Arthritis: Out of the Maze*. In the report, the commission outlined an "Arthritis Plan" recommending the creation of Multipurpose Arthritis Centers to be located throughout the United States. These centers were to provide activities in three areas: research, professional and patient education, and community demonstration programs related to patient care. The "Arthritis Plan" also called for a doubling of the NIH research effort, a series of epidemiological studies, the development of a national arthritis advisory information clearinghouse and a national arthritis advisory board.[6] Shortly after the National Commission submitted its recommendations, congress passed P.L. 94-562, the Arthritis, Diabetes and Digestive Diseases Amendments of 1976. It also created the National Arthritis Advisory Board (NAAB) which was to make recommendations and to oversee the progress being made in research and treatment programs in arthritis.

The NIAMMD was given the primary responsibility for implementing the "Arthritis Plan," and in 1977 established the first 15 multipurpose Arthritis Centers. Nine more centers were subsequently established. It also organized the Arthritis Information Clearinghouse (AIC) in October of 1978 to collect, screen, store and disseminate information about materials and programs related to the rheumatic diseases. During the same year, it established an Epidemiology Program Office and provided support to a prototype research data system—the American Rheumatism Association Medical Information System (AMAMIS).

Professional training and development are also carried out through the NIAMMD grants program which endeavors to provide a sufficient number of trained investigators to maintain and augment the progress that has already taken place in arthritis research.

In recent years additional reorganizations and policy changes have led to further name changes of the "Arthritis Institute," first to the National Institute of Arthritis, Diabetes and Digestive and Kidney Disease (NIADDKD), and in 1986 to the National Institute of Arthritis, Musculoskeletal and Skin Diseases (NIAMSD).

NATIONAL INSTITUTE OF HANDICAPPED RESEARCH

To increase knowledge about the nature of musculoskeletal disorders, another organization, the National Institute of Handicapped Research (NIHR), was established in 1978. Its priorities are to support research which will result in improving the lives of people who have physical and mental handicaps. Twenty-seven Rehabilitation Research and Training Centers are funded to engage in rehabilitation research, to train professionals to work with disabled individuals and to provide service for patients. There are also eighteen Rehabilitation Engineering Centers which are involved in both developing and applying the most advanced technology to problems faced by handicapped individuals.

For more than 30 years there has been an evolving international program of cooperative research and demonstration projects that has now fallen under the auspices of the NIHR. This program involves the pooling of information and expert professionals, training programs for internal rehabilitation program specialists and technical assistance.[7]

DEPARTMENT OF HEALTH AND HUMAN SERVICES, DIVISION OF MATERNAL AND CHILD HEALTH

The Department of Health and Human Services, Division of Maternal and Child Health (MCH) provided an impressive increase in funding in 1983 when they awarded grants to six pediatric rheumatology programs in Colorado, Georgia, Hawaii, Illinois, Ohio and Texas. Prior awards had been conferred on centers in California, Pennsylvania and Texas.

It is expected that these grants will be used to provide team health care treatment, educational projects in cooperation with state departments of education and special programs geared especially for children with arthritis. These programs will, hopefully, lead to increased knowledge about juvenile arthritis, including the health team and the school system, and provide appropriate coordinated and comprehensive care for arthritic children.

A long range goal of the Division is to encourage and support the development of other pediatric rheumatology programs in the United States.

Because of their focus on the problems related to arthritis in children, the American Juvenile Arthritis Association (AJAO) has been actively engaged in seeking this government support and in multiplying its advocacy on behalf of the approximately 250,000 children with arthritis. Formed in 1981 for parents, relatives and friends of children with arthritis and for health professionals, the AJAO publishes a newsletter, provides information, and will, surely, redouble its endeavors on behalf of the children and families who will benefit from the grants given by the Division of Maternal and Child Health and other funding provided by the Arthritis Foundation.

CONCLUSION

In the short span of one-hundred-eighty-nine years since the creation of the Marine Hospital Service there has been enormous progress in federal support for medical research and training. Indeed, nearly every advance in rheumatology in the last half-century was supported to a major extent by federal funding through the NIH. Hopefully, more generous funding will result in improving the quality of the lives of all people disabled by a rheumatic disease.

All of these foundations and institutions were founded on the belief that it is possible to improve treatments and to find preventions and cures for the rheumatic diseases. Research scientists active in the arthritis field feel that the time process involved in the achievement of these goals can be shortened by an increase in the research effort. This effort is, of course, dependent on the amount of money committed by the federal and state governments and by concerned supporters. Within the limitations imposed by funding and resources, the foundations and institutions have continually tried to meet the broad range of needs of individuals and families who have been affected by the rheumatic diseases.

REFERENCES

[1]Freyberg, R.: *The Westchester Medical Bulletin,* Vol. 39, number 9, 1971.

[2]*Profile—The Arthritis Foundation,* The Arthritis Foundation, pg. 1, 1969.

[3]Hanlon, J.: *Principles of Public Health Administration,* St. Louis, The C.V. Mosby Co., pg. 15, 1969.

[4]Ibid, pg. 29.

[5]*The First Annual Report of the Director,* National Institute of Arthritis, Diabetes, and Digestive and Kidney Diseases, NIH Publication No. 82-2375, Department of Health and Human Services, Public Health Service, National Institutes of Health, pg. 4, 1982.

[6]National Commission on Arthritis and Musculoskeletal Diseases, *Arthritis: Out of the Maze,* Executive Summary, U.S. Dept. of Health, Education and Welfare, Rockville, Md., 1976.

[7]*A Comprehensive Program for Handicapped Research,* U.S. Dept. of Education, Washington, D.C., 1982.

SOURCES OF INFORMATION

American College of Rheumatology
(American Rheumatism Association)
17 Executive Park Drive, N.E.
Atlanta, Georgia 30329

American Juvenile Arthritis Organization Arthritis Foundation
1314 Spring Street, N.W.
Atlanta, Georgia 30309

American Lupus Society, The
23751 Madison Street
Torrance, California 90505

Ankylosing Spondylitis Association
511 N. La Clenega, Suite 216
Los Angeles, California 90048

Arthritis Foundation
1314 Spring Street, N.W.
Atlanta, Georgia 30309

Arthritis Health Professions Association
1314 Spring Street, N.W.
Atlanta, Georgia 30309

Arthritis Information Clearinghouse
P.O. Box 9782
Arlington, Virginia 22209

Council on Rheumatologic Care
17 Executive Park Drive, N.E.
Atlanta, Georgia 30329

Lupus Foundation of America, Inc.
11921 A Olive Street
Torrance, California 63141

Muscular Dystrophy Association
810 Seventh Avenue
New York, New York 10019

National Institute of Allergy and Infectious Diseases
9000 Rockville Pike
Bethesda, Maryland 20205

National Institute of Arthritis, Musculoskeletal and Skin Diseases
9000 Rockville Pike
Bethesda, Maryland 20205

National Lupus Erythematosus Foundation, Inc.
5430 Van Nuys Boulevard
Van Nuys, California 91401

Scleroderma Foundation of Greater Washington, D.C., Inc., The
2805 Ridge Road Drive
Alexandria, Virginia 22303

Scleroderma International Foundation, The
704 Gardner Center Road
New Castle, Pennsylvania 16102

Scleroderma Society, The
1725 York Avenue
New York, New York 10028

Sjögren Syndrome Foundation Inc., The
382 Main Street
Port Washington, New York 11050

S.L.E. Foundation, The
95 Madison Avenue
New York, New York 10016

United Scleroderma Foundation, Inc.
P.O. Box 350
Watsonville, California 95077

PUBLICATIONS

The following are available without charge from the Arthritis Foundation to interested health professionals.

Bulletin on the Rheumatic Diseases, published bimonthly

Primer on the Rheumatic Diseases
Ninth edition, 1988

CHAPTER 27

EDUCATION OF THE ARTHRITIS HEALTH PROFESSIONAL

Irwin Oreskes, Ph.D.

The goal of appropriate and quality arthritis patient care requires that health professionals be educated both in the basics of their professions and the latest medical, scientific and social developments of pertinence to the whole field of rheumatology. The purpose of this chapter is to briefly describe the diversity of educational pathways in the field, and how these pathways do or do not intersect with each other.

At the heart of this educational process are the nation's medical schools which train physicians-to-be and after four years graduate some six thousand new M.D.'s. In general, medical schools do not offer "majors" and all students take the same prescribed course. While medical schools have engaged in much curricular re-examination over the past few years, nearly all are strongly oriented to the natural sciences in the first two years. The second two years are devoted primarily to courses and clinical experiences in the major areas of medicine. In the clinical years, time devoted to rheumatology is quite variable. Indeed, one-third of schools do not teach musculo-skeletal examination, and 15% do not employ even one full-time academic rheumatologist. Elective opportunities vary and less than 15% of medical students participate in rheumatology electives.

For students who ultimately elect family or general practice, or most specialties other than rheumatology, this is all the rheumatologic education they may receive. Given that general practice physicians are often the first health professional seen by rheumatoid patients, this limited preparation is a matter of some concern.

To remedy this situation critics have suggested that all medical students spend at least three months in an out-patient setting where they will see patients with the more common rheumatic complaints. Regarding didactic training, they propose that more time be spent on rheumatology, nutrition and rehabilitation, if necessary, at the expense of other courses. At a more fundamental level, they argue that medical curricula should reduce emphasis on "disease" and place more emphasis on integrated "wellness" education. Whatever other educational reforms may be desirable, it is clear that there is a need for strengthening rheumatology education in medical schools.

Central to health care in rheumatology is the rheumatologist. For medical school graduates who wish to achieve this specialty, the route may typically include a one-year internship followed by a two-year residency in general internal medicine.

Specific training in rheumatology is normally obtained in a further two-year postgraduate fellowship. There are about forty such programs in the U.S., and they are typically offered by rheumatology divisions (usually subdivisions of department of internal medicine.) Details of these programs are quite variable, but generally they fall into three tracks: (1) clinical, (2) research and (3) combined clinical-research. The programs include, in varying combinations, clinic experience, hospital consultations, laboratory training, seminars and lecture subjects, which include immunology, biochemistry, pathology and epidemiology. Clinical work includes, in addition to rheumatology, orthopedics and rehabilitation. Much of the education is patient-centered, in that available hospital cases determine what topics are taken up. Thus, one element of a good program is the availability of large numbers of patients with different rheumatic diagnoses.

Rheumatology fellowships have typically stressed research training. In a new and rapidly changing field, this emphasis has helped clinically-oriented practitioners to understand the tentative and rapidly changing nature of rheumatologic knowledge. For a smaller number of research-oriented graduates, research experience has proved to be an effective gateway to advanced research training and to careers as full-time academic clinical investigators. Such investigators have played a crucial role in rheumatologic progress; they have also made major contributions in related fields such as immunology. Advanced research training in rheumatology is available via the National Institutes of Health Trainee Fellowships or Senior Rheumatology Scholar Awards.

To encourage qualified rheumatologists to develop or improve their research capabilities, a number of clinical research training programs have been devised under the auspices of the Pan American League Against Rheumatism. The goal is to encourage rheumatologists to become clinical investigators by improving their knowledge of research design, data management, decision analysis and biostatistics. Students participate in on-going research programs.

The N.I.H. has several programs to encourage advanced research training of physician-scientists. These are the Medical Scientist Training Program, and the Physician Scientist Award Program. Graduates of rheumatology fellowships participate in these programs.

Physicians who successfully complete rheumatology training will have passed both their internal medicine boards as well as the written certification examination given by the American Board of Rheumatology. They are then

"Board Certified." The examination was first given in 1972 and earlier fellowships graduates have been grandfathered. It is estimated that there are about 3,000 board-certified rheumatologists in the U.S. today.

Residency training for other medical specialties also follows the one-year internship. Typically such residencies are: three years for rehabilitation medicine and physiatry, and four or more years for orthopedics. The additional training required in orthopedics reflects the largely surgical nature of this practice. Upon completion of a residency and passage of a comprehensive examination, the candidate is then "Board Certified."

Residency programs are widespread in teaching hospitals and they vary so much that even a summary is difficult to make. In general, residencies are clinically (patient) oriented. Hospital rounds with senior physicians are an important element of this training as are case conference. Residents assume major responsibility for in-house hospital care of patients in their specialty. Some programs may include research training and experience. "Cross-over" experience in related fields may be encouraged, but seem to depend mainly on the interests of the resident. It is fair to say that one of the great strengths of American medicine is the very high quality of most residency programs and of their graduates. It is also fair to say that patients whose problems are less "interesting" may not always fare as well in the current system of specialist-driven health care. The integration of general and advanced care medicine still needs improvement.

In the past, mandatory education ended after certification, but now most specialists are required to participate in various forms of continuing education, i.e., journal reading, meeting attendance, taking of courses and, in some situations, re-examination to maintain their Board Certified status.

While residency and fellowship programs do an excellent job in the education of rheumatologists, there is increasing concern about the level of rheumatologic knowledge and sophistication among general practice and family practice physicians. After all, it is they who first see the vast majority of rheumatic patients. This question is of equal concern with specialty physicians not directly concerned with rheumatology. This problem is exemplified by a study carried out at a large metropolitan hospital. A rheumatology resident examined some one hundred general medical non-rheumatic patients and studied their medical records. More than 20% of these patients had evidence of objective rheumatic disease, yet no mention of this was to be found in their medical records!

Organized rheumatology is well aware of this problem and is responding in a variety of ways to improve rheumatologic awareness among health care providers. Among recent programmatic development are:

> The Arthritis Foundation sponsors a series of research award programs for medical students, for physicians and for non-doctoral health professionals.

They are intended to stimulate arthritis research and new directions in patient care and management.

The American Rheumatism Association develops or reviews programs directed to non-member physicians. Slide collections, videotapes, cable TV, seminars and courses are all utilized to deepen rheumatologic sophistication in the medical community.

The University of Michigan Arthritis Center, under the leadership of Drs. Stross and Bole, have designed and evaluated continuing rheumatology education programs for primary care physicians in small towns. A novel point was that the teachers were community physicians and not academic faculty. The investigators noted objective evidence of improvement in rheumatic care and concluded that this approach is of particular value in communities too small to attract a full-time rheumatologist.

At Case Western Reserve's Department of Family Medicine, investigators are developing a training program to improve rheumatic disease knowledge among family practice residents.

The Arthritis Center at St. Margaret's Memorial Hospital in Pittsburgh has instituted rheumatology training programs for various residents and medical students. The faculty consisted of allied health professionals and they emphasized such issues as patient referral, rehabilitative evaluation, therapeutics and expected outcomes. Eighty-eight percent of participating students rated the program as "good" or "excellent."

A group at the Southwest Arthritis Center of the University of Arizona College of Medicine, Tucson (Arizona), led by Dr. E.P. Gall and Ms. Gail E. Riggs, have developed a most unusual training program in rheumatology for medical students and practicing physicians. They employed, as instructors, patients with stabilized rheumatoid arthritis. These patient-instructors were first trained in anatomy, medical terminology, physical examination and health profession roles. Later, they combined the roles of patient subject and teacher. The argument behind this approach is that only a trained patient can tell if correct structures are correctly examined and can then advise the examiner. This fascinating on-going experiment raises the patient to "colleague" and, at the least, vivifies the diagnostic process.

This incomplete and somewhat random list of experiments designed to improve rheumatology education illustrates a variety of different approaches. Rheumatologists, family practice physicians, general practitioners, allied health professionals and patients all have been involved, in one role or another, in the educational process. We may conclude that many different approaches can serve to advance rheumatic disease understanding. Moreover, all arthritis health professionals have a role to play. This includes victims of rheumatic disease.

The educational work of other Multipurpose Arthritis Centers should be noted. A program established in fiscal 1977 has funded a number of centers across the country. Both the number of funded centers and the dollar appropriations have fluctuated since then, but currently fifteen are active. These centers combine patient care, research and education in one organizational unit. Several of their educational programs have been described above, but many others are being persued. They fall into the following general areas:

- Improvement and evaluation of rheumatology training for medical students and resident in family practice and internal medicine.
- Development of self-study guides and computer and videotape assisted modes of instruction.
- Development of integrated arthritis oriented curricula for general physicians and allied health workers.
- Improvement of arthritis education of nurses and nurses-aides.
- Improvement of sexual rehabilitation counseling by allied health professionals.
- Improvement of arthritis education of patients and their families by allied health professionals.

These various educational programs are for the most part interdisciplinary and include methods for evaluation of effectiveness.

Turning to health professionals other than physicians, they follow a quite different educational track. Physical therapists, occupational therapists, and health educators typically study in undergraduate institutions that are generically termed "Schools of Allied Health." There are many such schools in the U.S. and they vary considerably in structure and curriculum. Typically such schools are of the 2+2 variety. Students are admitted after the first two years of college and enroll in the professional program of their choice, which is offered in the upper two years (junior and senior). Graduates then receive a B.S. degree in their specialty. In some schools, graduate work is offered leading to the M.S. degree. Most physical therapists, occupational therapists and health educators are now trained in such schools.

Most schools of allied health are divisions of general colleges or universities. Additionally, they establish affiliations agreements with hospitals to offer clinical experience to their students. More often than not they are not affiliated with medical schools even where such medical schools are to be found in the overall university complex. Historically nursing education as well as allied health education began as non-degree training programs based in hospitals. After World War II, both educational tracks separated from hospitals and from medical schools, and from each other. They developed their own faculties and became accredited to offer degrees to their graduates. Today, most allied health programs are also accredited by their appropriate professional organization.

The separation of education in medicine, allied health and nursing has identifiable historical reasons. Nevertheless, this situation does not advance the collaborative efforts that are needed in today's health care. It is to be hoped that educators in these fields will find ways to reduce separation and fragmentation.

Perhaps the numerically largest non-physician health profession participating in rheumatic disease health care is that of physical therapy. This profession had its origins in the need for rehabilitation workers to treat victims maimed in World War I. The profession expanded after World War II and today in the U.S., the number of practicing physical therapists exceeds 50,000. Their work is concerned with a variety of medical rehabilitation situations; i.e., stroke, amputation, accidents and rheumatic diseases. It is difficult to be exact, but perhaps half of physical therapy time is devoted to the patients in the latter category. Physical therapists function in hospitals, as assistants to orthopedists, and increasingly in independent private practice.

Physical therapy (PT) is a very popular undergraduate major. Nearly 140 institutions offer programs and more than 4,000 students are graduated each year. Entry is usually quite competitive. Minimum entry requirements are completion of the first two college years with good grades in chemistry, biology and physics. Increasingly, candidates for PT programs are offering more than the minimum requirements.

Most PT programs graduate students with a B.S. degree. However, educators in the field are concerned with the increasing difficulty of completing the professional curriculum in two years. The trend appears to be to increase the professional component to three years, and to offer the M.S. degree as the entry level to the profession. Discussions have been held regarding the desirability of offering programs leading to the degree, Doctor of Physical Therapy. At least two institutions are doing so.

Current education in this field includes extensive clinical training offered at affiliated hospitals. Graduates take Board exams given by the American Physical Therapy Association. Additionally, state licensure requirements must also be satisfied.

The increased demand for PT care and the shortage of qualified PT practitioners have stimulated the development of Physical Therapy Assistant programs. These are typically two years long and do not require extensive science prerequisites for admission. Such programs are generally offered at community colleges or allied health schools. The student on completion, receives an Associate Degree and/or a Certificate of Completion. The PT profession describes them as "technical" programs in contrast to the longer and more difficult four–five years "professional" programs. Currently, some sixty-nine PT assistant programs are active nationwide.

Occupational Therapy (OT) constitutes a numerically somewhat smaller but nonetheless significant health profession in rheumatic disease care.

Here, too, OT's work in a variety of health care settings, hospitals, rehabilitation institutes, home-care programs and increasingly in private practice. OT education is offered in some sixty-five college-based programs, which lead to the B.S. degree. As with PT, typical curricula are of the 2+2 variety with professional courses given in the upper two years of study. Following completion of the didactic courses, OT students participate in a six-month clinical clerkship which may include advanced elective training. Students become qualified to practice by passing a registry exam of the American Occupational Therapy Association (AOTA) as well as state licensure examinations.

The number of practicing OT's today approaches 45,000. It is estimated that there are about 2,000 new graduates of OT programs each year, a figure which is perhaps 50% of what is needed to fill currently available jobs. In an attempt to increase the number of graduates, some institutions now offer professional OT Master-level programs directed to college graduates currently in other fields. Masters degree programs for qualified OT's in specialty areas, i.e., physical disability, are also available, and one institution offers the Ph.D. degree in OT.

The field of health education is extraordinarily diverse and a number of major divisions are recognized:

- Community or public health education
- School health education
- Sex education
- Patient and family education

Little data exists on the number and distribution of health educators; many, in fact, come from social work or nursing, and are not formally trained. Formal health education is offered in some eighty academic programs nationwide that lead to the bachelor's or master's degree. Some fifteen of these programs are accredited by The Council on Education in Public Health, and additional ones registered by the American Association of Health Educators. Sex education is considered a subspecialty, and sex therapists may be individually credentialed by the American Association of Sex Counselors and Educators.

Doctoral level education is offered in some forty graduate level programs which offer the D.Ph. in Public Health, the D.Ed. in School Health, or the Ph.D. in Health Education.

Another educational track is followed by social workers. These professionals typically prepare at schools of social work, where they obtain the Master's degree after a two-year program. The clinical psychologist usually majors in psychology at the undergraduate level, and then does graduate work leading to the Master's or Ph.D. degree. Nurses are now for the most part educated in separate schools of nursing, or in departments of nursing that are part of allied health schools. In any case, education is general and rheumatologic expertise is usually gained on-the-job. In recent years a group at the Darmouth Hitchcock

Arthritis Center in Hanover, New Hampshire has been studying the activities of nurses working in rheumatologic office practices. They are interested in defining the "rheumatologic office nurse" as a subset of nursing practice. This group has also given seminars and workshops directed to the rheumatologic nurse. Another more defined and recognized specialty, that of rehabilitation nurse, enlists some 5,000 practitioners. However, they are primarily concerned with stroke and trauma problems rather than rheumatology.

It is clear that the different health professionals who participate in the care of patients afflicted with the various rheumatic diseases come from diverse fields of study. There is regrettably little cross-over among students during their period of preparation in medical schools, nursing schools, allied health schools, social work schools as well as all the other departments and programs that offer health education. The real question, however, is how do trained health professionals concerned with arthritis care improve their knowledge and stay current with new research and new treatment.

The answer to this question seems to be primarily institutional. The Arthritis Centers, as we have pointed out, are beginning to grapple with the need for cross-field rheumatologic education that includes residents, fellows and concerned allied health practitioners. Institutions other than Arthritis Centers have done pioneering work in this area. One example is the Arthritis Unit at Johns Hopkins where, under the leadership of Dr. Mary Betty Stevens, important work in the development of team approach to patient care in rheumatology has been done. This approach has of necessity involved multi-disciplinary education in a variety of ways.

Another important educational resource is the Arthritis Health Professions Association (AHPA). This organization now more than twenty years old, currently numbers about 1,350 members, mainly PT's, OT's and nurses. It is the only national forum where both MD and non-MD arthritis health professionals meet on a common ground of interest. The Association sponsors a wide variety of continuing education courses and programs. It also sponsors an annual meeting that is held in conjunction with the annual meeting of the American Rheumatism Association. This meeting offers an opportunity to arthritis professionals to present and to hear research papers on a wide variety of subjects. There are exhibits of teaching materials as well as teaching sessions with senior experienced individuals. Professional groups and topical study groups are also able to meet during this annual meeting. The AHPA plays a useful educational role and it is to be hoped that their membership and outreach can be extended.

Implicit in the philosophy of this chapter and this book is that quality health care for patients with rheumatic diseases requires the team approach and that to develop mature health care teams in rheumatology much more needs to be done in the way of cross professional education. In this endeavor, organized rheumatology must take on more responsibility than it has in the past. Organized rheumatology must improve modes of teaching of non-MD health workers. Equally important is that organized rheumatology must learn from non-MD health workers by recognizing that the accumulated professional experience of PT's, OT's and all the others, is of significant value in advancing the field of rheumatology in the quest for better and more effective patient care.

SOURCES OF INFORMATION

American Medical Association
Committee on Allied Health Education and Accreditation (CAHEA)
645 N. Dearborn Street
Chicago, IL 60610
(312) 645-4660

American Occupational Therapy Association
1383 Piccard Drive
Rockville, MD 20850
(301) 948-9626

American Physical Therapy Association
1111 North Fairfax Street
Alexandria, VA 22314
(703) 684-2782

American Society of Allied Health Professions
1101 Connecticut Ave. NW, Suite 700
Washington, DC 20036
(202) 857-1150

Arthritis Health Professions Association
17 Executive Park Drive NE, Suite 480
Atlanta, GA 30329
(404) 872-7100

American Association of Sex Educators, Counselors and Therapists
600 Maryland Ave. SW
Washington, DC
(202) 462-1171

Association of American Medical Colleges
One Dupont Circle NW, Suite 200
Washington, DC 20336
(202) 828-0400

Council on Education for Public Health
1015 15th Street NW
Washington, DC 20005
(202) 789-1050

Multipurpose Arthritis Centers
National Institute of Arthritis
Diabetes, Digestive and Kidney Diseases
National Institute of Health
Bethesda, MD 20206
(301) 496-7495

V AFTERWORD

"And my bones shall cry out"
35th Psalm

AFTERWORD

Harry Spiera, M.D.
Irwin Oreskes, Ph.D.

With all that has been said in these pages, it is nevertheless a fact that most individuals with musculoskeletal complaints do not seek medical attention. Most people are subject to occasional minor aches or pain and these events do not result in a trip to the doctor. It is only when pain or discomfort is persistent or when loss of function is clearly evident that help is sought.

To whom do they go? Certainly the vast majority of those with such complaints are seen by general practitioners, family practice doctors, or internal medicine specialists. In most cases these professionals are perfectly competent to diagnose and treat. Indeed far less than 10% of these patients have potentially life-threatening disease such as lupus, scleroderma, dermatomyositis or polyarteritis. Of the remaining 90+% with rheumatoid arthritis or osteoarthritis, no more than a small percentage of these can be expected to go on to crippling disease.

Given these considerations, the primary care provider must, on the one hand avoid over-diagnosis and over-treatment but on the other hand recognize when the expertise of a specialist is required. Thus in perhaps 20% of cases a rheumatologist or orthopedist will be required to establish or confirm a diagnosis and administer therapy.

It is clear that effective utilization of our health care resources depends on the ability and willingness of primary care providers to make the above distinction. For rheumatologists or orthopedists to take on primary care responsibility is not only wasteful but in fact is not possible. There just aren't enough of them! However, if primary care physicians are to be effective in dealing with rheumatic disease then their rheumatologic education needs to be improved first in medical school and later during their career by periodic refresher and updating experiences.

The HMO movement certainly includes the above approach but observers are concerned that in the zeal for cost containment HMOs may hinder the proper flow of patients from primary doctors to specialists. Both the medical profession and concerned lay groups must pay close attention to this issue.

In a related issue of cost containment the Federal Government has imposed tighter Medicare restriction on reimbursement of physicians who treat elderly persons. Such a policy if continued may well adversely affect the availability of specialty care to rheumatic disease patients.

Given the chronic nature of most rheumatic diseases the specialist will often turn to one or another ancillary health care providers to give specific exercise, splinting, psychological or social therapies. In developing *any* therapeutic approach for patients with chronic illness utmost individualization is essential. In the absence of specific cures the patient must be educated to understand both the goals and possibilities of the prescribed therapy. To do otherwise is to skirt quackery.

Probably the largest group providing care to rheumatic patients are the physical therapists. These providers work in hospitals, as employees of physicians and in independent practice. Patients are accepted by physician referral and prescription. The main job of the physical therapist is to administer and teach exercise modalities to the rheumatic patients. Their goal is to maintain or improve function and to encourage independence to the maximum possible extent. Thus the ideal physical therapist not only treats but teaches. Moreover, the physical therapist must communicate effectively with the referring physician, giving information on patient progress and making suggestions regarding diagnosis or further therapy.

How many rheumatic patients need or use the services of a physical therapist? This question is difficult to answer. Some physicians refer less than 5% of their patients to physical therapists. Their general attitude seems to be that most patients can be directly educated in the matter of exercise and function. On the other hand, orthopedists (especially those with physical therapists in their employ) may refer 80% or more of their patients to a physical therapist. Given that these patients are for the most part post-surgical, this difference is understandable. Again the criterion of judgement must be individuation with clear goals and reasonable expectations.

A related area of therapy is that delivered by occupational therapists. In general they are concerned with problems of daily living and their job is to help patients overcome limitations in the doing of every day tasks. This may be accomplished by using physical devices (splints, prostheses) or by functional retraining. Here too, individualization with a realistic goal, is essential. In some respects the work of the occupational therapist may overlap that of the physical therapist. Nevertheless the expertise of the occupational therapist is distinctive and vitally important to appropriate patients.

The stress of chronic disease and its effects on everyday life of patients may require help from one or another mental health worker, e.g., psychiatrists or psychologists. The former deal with clear concurrent mental disease and may prescribe drugs. The latter are more concerned with behavioral issues and family stresses related to the effects of disease. The social worker deals directly with the problems of daily living, family adjustments, mechanics of health provision and the like. There appears to be considerable overlap among these three professions. In their work in a defined environment their different roles do tend to get sorted out.

Again we may ask how many rheumatic patients actually need the aid of one or another of these professionals. In the context of private practice this figure for some physicians is perhaps no more than 1%. By contrast among those hospitalized because of their illness, the figure may approach or exceed 20%. For patients who need such help the work of the psychologist or social worker is essential to successful progress. Again clear goals and reasonable prospects must be part of such therapy. In this area there seems to be little limit to the amount of therapeutic time professionals believe that patients can profitably use. Still, issues of cost-effectiveness are real and referring physicians must scrutinize mental health therapy or social work support as they would (or should) scrutinize physical or occupational therapy.

Numerous other health workers are involved at one time or another in the care of the rheumatic disease patients, dieticians, nurses, orthodists, physiatrists, etc. Indeed this book is devoted to detailing their work and interrelationships. If indeed there is a message here, it is that the effective treatment of the rheumatic diseases requires not merely the activities of a variety of health professionals but also their close cooperation. This is a distinctive feature of chronic disease care.

It is appropriate to restate that we know very little about the etiology or pathogenesis of most of the various rheumatic diseases. We do not know what causes rheumatoid arthritis, systemic lupus erythematosus, scleroderma and most of the other entities listed in the Appendix. Answers to a variety of questions continue to elude us.

Among these questions are:

1. What is the etiologic role of viruses, bacteria, environmental agents or diet?
2. What is the role of the immune system in these diseases?
3. How do biologic mediators or antagonists relate to the process of inflammation?
4. What is the mechanism of collagen breakdown. Can it be stopped or reversed by chemicals, exercise or diet?
5. How does genetic make-up predispose to disease and can we modify such susceptibility?

In spite of these unanswered questions we can nevertheless point to many practical therapeutic successes.

1. Arthritis of clearly infectious origin is readily treatable with antibiotics.

2. Gout is well understood and easily treated. Renal complications and joint destruction formerly common, are now quite rare.
3. Joint replacement is now standard, successful and common.
4. Systemic lupus although its etiology remains unknown, is far more successfully treated with steroids and other drugs. Twenty years ago 90% of patients did not survive five years after diagnosis; today this figure is only 10%.
5. Availability of newer non-steroidal anti-inflammatory drugs (NSAIDS) though they do not stop disease, in many instances offer significantly improved symptomatic relief.
6. Other drugs which are disease-altering, are finding their place in the management of severe RA.
7. Research on prosthetic devices and joint surgical techniques promise more effective therapy for damaged ankles, elbows and shoulders.
8. Total joint replacement by means of transplants is in sight in the not too distant future.

The successes that have been achieved are a direct consequence of both basic and applied (clinical) research. A generation of M.D. and Ph.D. investigators have tackled many scientific questions arising from the rheumatic diseases and new theoretical knowledge has been translated in practical therapy. Our expectations for more and better therapeutic answers will only be realized if the tempo (and the funding) for both basic and applied research is maintained. Practical encouragement for young researchers to concern themselves with problems pertinent to rheumatic diseases is vital. Research, it must be emphasized, is not only molecular but must also be concerned with epidemiological and social questions. Finally the participation of new types of health professionals in the research process must be nurtured and encouraged.

An old saw in epidemiology is that 100% of all subjects die—the question is when and how. In the last 40 years we have seen remarkable decreases in the death rate due to infections, heart disease and stroke and therefore, increases in longevity. As our population ages the incidence of osteoarthritis, osteoporosis and associated other rheumatoid disabilities will inevitably increase. In an ironic way we have become victims of our own successes in medicine and public health. The potential market for rheumatic disease care, especially rehabilitation will continue to increase and surely, so will costs. Ultimately the question is, how much is enough? This is not so much a medical question as it is a public policy question. It is necessarily related to, how much we can afford? In other words it is the public through its legislators and in other ways who must decide on the appropriate level of rheumatic disease care for our population. America could use a national policy on levels of health funding and apportionment of that funding. Is cancer more important than arthritis? Do the old have priority over the young? Health care or military funding—or sewer repair? Health care professionals have considerable responsibility in helping formulate the terms of this debate.

It is true to say that we are doing the best we can for our patients but we must also recognize that this effort is not yet good enough. This is so because we don't know it all! It behooves us individually and collectively in our professions to encourage the acquisition of new knowledge, to educate each other by sharing experiences and information, and to educate our patients so that they are active participators in their own therapy.

GLOSSARY

Acromioclavicular Joint: Where the collar bone joins the shoulder.
Alopecia: Hair loss.
Amenorrhea: Absence of the menses.
Amphiarthrosis: A form of articulation permitting little motion.
Amyloid: An abnormal protein which sometimes deposit excessively in tissues causing disease (Amyloidosis).
Anaphylaxis: An unusual or exaggerated allergic reaction of an organism to foreign protein or other substances.
Androgens: Male hormones.
Anergy: Diminished immune reactivity to specific antigen(s).
Angiotensin: A polypeptide hormone involved in blood pressure control.
Ankylosis: Immobility of the joint.
Antibody: An immunoglobulin protein produced in lymphoid tissue in response to antigen. Antibody reacts with specific antigen by virtue of its specific amino acid sequence.
Antigens: Any substance which is capable, under appropriate conditions, of inducing the formation of antibodies.
Antinuclear Antibodies: Antibodies that react with constituents of cell nuclei, i.e., centromers, DNA, etc.
Anxiolytic Agents: Tranquilizers.
Arachidonic Acid: A fatty acid metabolic precursor of prostaglandins.
Arthralgia: Pain in the joint.
Arthrocentesis: Puncture and aspiration of a joint.
Arthroplasty: Plastic surgery of a joint.
Ataxia: Failure or irregularity of muscular coordination.
Atlanto-Axial Joint: Joint between first two neck (cervical) vertebra.
Auto-Antibodies: An antibody (immunoglobulin) that reacts with one of the individual's own body constituents.
Auto-Immune Response: An immune response directed against the body's own tissue.
Axial Joints: Central joints, i.e., shoulder, spine, hip.
Azotemia: An excess of urea or other nitrogenous compounds in the blood. Often seen in kidney failure.
Balance: Where dietary intake and metabolic synthesis equal excretion. Typically applied to toal nitrogen and particular components, e.g., uric acid. If intake plus synthesis exceed excretion, then accumulation in the blood results.

Basement Membrane: The delicate layer of extra-cellular condensation of mucopolysaccharides and protein underlying the epithelium of mucous membranes and secreting glands.

Birefringent: The quality of transmitting light unequally in different directions.

Blast Cells: An immature blood cell.

Blood Dyscrasia: Any abnormal or pathological condition of the blood.

Bradykinin: A blood peptide with inflammatory and other physiological properties.

Calculi: Kidney or bladder stones.

Carpal Tunnel Syndrome: A clinical condition resulting from irritation of the median nerve at the wrist.

Chemotaxis: The movement of a cell, such as a leukocyte, in response to a chemical stimuli.

Chondrocytes: A cartilage cell.

Collagen: The principal structural protein of connective tissue.

Collagenase: An enzyme that breaks down collagen and gelatin.

Complement: A complex series of enzymatic proteins found in normal serum that interact with antigen-antibody complex.

Corticosteroids: Any of the steroid hormones produced by the adrenal cortex, including cortisol, cortisone and aldosterone. Also their synthetic equivalents.

Dactylitis: Inflammation of finger or toe.

Diathesis: A predisposition to a disease.

Dysmenorrhea: Painful menstruation.

Dyspnea: Difficult or labored breathing.

Enteritis: Inflammation of the intestine, especially the small intestine.

Eosinophiles: White blood cell containing granules, stainable within easin dye. Increased numbers often seen in allergic reactions.

Erythrocyte: Red blood cell.

Erythema: Redness of the skin produced by congestion of the capillaries.

Estrogens: Female sex hormones.

Fibroblast: A connective tissue cell.

Free Radicals: Short-lived highly reactive chemical substances with one extra electron.

Gelling Phenomena: Joint and muscle stiffness after inactivity.

Glomerulus: One of the filtering units of the kidney.

Glossitis: Inflammation of the tongue.

Glycoprotein: Any of a class of proteins chemically bound to a carbohydrate group.

Glycosoaminoglycans: A class of complex polysaccharides widely distributed in connective tissue.

Gonococcus: The micro-organism which causes gonorrhoea.

Gram Stain: Procedure devised by Gram in which microorganisms are stained with crystal violet dye. Those that retain the crystal violet stain are gram positive and those that lose the crystal violet stain by decolorization, but stain with a counterstain (usually safranin) are gram negative.

Hemarthrosis: Bleeding or leakage of blood into a joint or synovial cavity.

Histamine: A chemical mediator involved in certain allergic and inflammatory processes.

Histocompatibility Complex: A series of white blood cell antigens associated with autoimmunity, disease susceptibility and transplant rejection.

Hyaluronic Acid: A polysaccharide present in synovial fluid that determines its viscosity. It is composed of glucosamine and glucuronic acid.

Hyperkeratosis: Hypertrophy of the corneous layer of the skin.

Hyperuricemia: Excess of uric acid in the blood.

Hyperuricosuria: Excess of uric acid in the urine.

Hypoglycemic: An agent that acts to lower the level of glucose in the blood.

Iatrogenic: Resulting from the activity of physicians. Any adverse condition occurring as the result of treatment by a physician or surgeon.

Ileum: The distal portion of the small intestine, extending from the jejunum to the cecum.

Immune Complexes: A soluble complex of antigen and antibody circulating in the blood. Also, antigen-antibody complex.

Immunoelectrophoresis: A method combining electrophoresis and immune double diffusion for distinguishing between proteins and other materials by means of differences in their electrophoretic mobility and antigenic specificity.

Immunodeficiency: An absence or reduction in immune response.

Immunoglobulins: Plasma proteins endowed with antibody activity.

Immunosuppressive Agents: Chemical or biological substances that diminish or prevent the immune response.

Interphalangeal Joints: Finger and toe joints between phalanges.

Juxtaarticular: Situated near a joint or in the region of a joint.

LE Cell: A mature neutrophilic polymorphonuclear leukocyte, which has phagocytized a spherical, homogenous-appearing inclusion, itself derived from another neutrophil; a cell characteristic of lupus erythematosus.

Leukopenia: Reduction of the number of leukocytes in the blood.

Leukotrienes: Chemical mediators of inflammation.

Lymphocyte: A white blood cell also termed a mononuclear leukocyte. It is chiefly a product of lymphoid tissue and participates in both humoral (B cell) and cell-mediated (T cell) immunity.

Lysosomes: Intracellular structures found in many types of cells containing various hydrolytic enzymes. Injury to a lysosome is followed by release into the cell of enzymes, which may damage the cell.

Macrophage: Any of the large phagocytic cells. They are components of the reticuloendothelial system and are usually immobile, but when stimulated by inflammation become actively mobile.

Megakaryocyte: The giant cell of bone marrow from which mature blood platelets originate.

Metacarpophalangeal: Referring to joints connecting metacarpals and the phalanges.

Monocyte: A mononuclear phagocytic leukocyte.

Muscle Enzymes: Normally found in heart or skeletal muscle. Following muscle damage they may leak into the blood. Blood levels are measured to assess muscle damage.

Mycobacteria: A microorganism, one type of which is responsible for tuberculosis.

Myeloproliferative Disorders: A group of disease characterized by excessive proliferation of bone marrow elements, e.g., leukemia.

Myocarditis: Inflammation of the muscular walls of the heart.

Neutrophil: A type of polymorphonuclear leukocyte.

Olecranon: The proximal bony projection of the ulna at the elbow.

Osteomyelitis: Infection of bone.

Pannus: An inflammatory exudate originating from the joint synovial membrane characteristic of rheumatoid arthritis.

Pericarditis: Inflammation of the membrane surrounding the heart.

Pericardiocentesis: Removal of fluid by aspiration from the sac enclosing the heart.

Periosteum: A specialized connective tissue, covering all bone of the body and possessing bone-forming potentialities.

Phlogistic: Inflammatory.

Plasmapheresis: Removal of blood, separation of plasma by centrifugation and reinjection of the packed cells. Used in the treatment of certain pathological conditions.

Platelet: A disk-shaped cell found in the blood of all mammals and chiefly known for its role in blood coagulation.

Pleuritis: Inflammation of the pleura, the membrane investing the lungs and lining the thoracic cavity.

Polycythemia: An increase in the total red cell mass of the body.

Polymer: A compound, usually of high molecular weight, formed by the combination of simpler repeating molecules or monomers.

Polymorphonuclear Cells: White blood cells in which the nucleus is deeply lobed. Principal function is phagocytosis.

Prostaglandins: A group of naturally occurring fatty acids with diverse biological activities among which are induction of inflammation.

Proteoglycans: A protein-polysaccharide complex.

Pruritus: Itching.

Purpura: A group of disorders characterized by purplish or brownish red discoloration of the skin caused by hemorrhage.

Purine Bases: Information carrying substances in DNA, e.g., adenine and guanine.

Pyrimidine Bases: Information carrying substances in DNA, e.g., cytosine and thymine. Uracil is found in RNA.

Reticulo-endothelial System: System of organs and tissues involved in immune response and phagocytosis.

Sclera: The tough white outer coat of the eyeball.

Serotonin: A vasoconstrictor found in plasma and many body tissues.

Sterno-clavicular Joint: Where the sternum meets the clavicle.

Steroids: A group of chemicals of similar structure which include various hormones such as: cortisone, estrogens and androgens (see Corticosteroids).

Subchondral Bone: Bone beneath cartilage.

Subluxation: An incomplete or partial dislocation of a joint.

Synarthrosis: A form of articulation in which the bony elements are united by continuous intervening fibrous tissue.

Synovitis: Inflammation of a synovial membrane.

Synovium: Tissue lining of the joint, one of whose function is secretion of synovial fluid.

Tenosynovitis: Inflammation of a tendon sheath.
Thrombocytopenia: Decrease in the number of blood platelets.
Titer: A measure of antibody concentration.
Tophus: A chalky deposit of sodium urate found in the tissues in gout.
Ulna: The inner and larger bone of the forearm.
Uric Acid: One of the normal products of purine metabolism.
Vitreous Humor: Fluid-like substance within the eyeball.

APPENDIX

CLASSIFICATION OF THE RHEUMATIC DISEASES

I. Diffuse connective tissue diseases
   A. Rheumatoid arthritis
   B. Juvenile rheumatoid arthritis
      1. Systemic onset (Still's disease)
      2. Polyarticular onset
      3. Pauciarticular onset
   C. Systemic lupus erythematosus
   D. Systemic sclerosis
   E. Polymyositis/dermatomyositis
   F. Necrotizing vasculitis and other vasculopathies
      1. Polyarteritis nodosa group (includes hepatitis B associated arteritis and Churg–Strauss allergic granulomatosis)
      2. Hypersensitivity vasculitis (includes Henoch–Schönlein purpura, hypocomplementemic cutaneous vasculitis, and others)
      3. Wegener's granulomatosis
      4. Giant cell arteritis
         a. Temporal arteritis
         b. Takayasu's arteritis
      5. Mucocutaneous lymph node syndrome (Kawasaki disease)
      6. Behçet's disease
      7. Cryoglobulinemia
      8. Juvenile dermatomyositis
   G. Sjögren's syndrome
   H. Overlap syndromes (includes undifferentiated and mixed connective tissue disease)
   I. Others (includes polymyalgia rheumatica, panniculitis (Weber-Christian disease), erythema nodosum, relapsing polychondritis, diffuse fasciitis with eosinophilia, adult onset Still's disease)
II. Arthritis associated with spondylitis
   A. Ankylosing spondylitis
   B. Reiter's syndrome
   C. Psoriatic arthritis
   D. Arthritis associated with chronic inflammatory bowel disease
III. Degenerative joint disease (osteoarthritis, osteoarthrosis)
   A. Primary (includes erosive osteoarthritis)
   B. Secondary
IV. Arthritis, tenosynovitis, and bursitis associated with infectious agents
   A. Direct
      1. Bacterial
         a. Gram-positive cocci (staphylococcus and others)
         b. Gram-negative cocci (gonococcus and others)
         c. Gram-negative rods
         d. Mycobacteria
         e. Spirochetes including Lyme disease
         f. Others including leprosy and mycoplasma
      2. Viral including hepatitis
      3. Fungal
      4. Parasitic
      5. Unknown, suspected (Whipple's disease)
   B. Indirect (reactive)
      1. Bacterial (includes acute rheumatic fever, intestinal bypass, postdysenteric—shigella, yersinia, and others)
      2. Viral (hepatitis B)

V. Metabolic and endocrine diseases associated with rheumatic states
   A. Crystal-induced conditions
      1. Monosodium urate (gout)
      2. Calcium pyrophosphate dihydrate (pseudogout, chondrocalcinosis)
      3. Apatite and other basic calcium phosphates
      4. Oxalate
   B. Biochemical abnormalities
      1. Amyloidosis
      2. Vitamin C deficiency (scurvy)
      3. Specific enzyme-deficiency states (includes Fabry's, Farber's, and others)
      4. Hyperlipoproteinemias (types II, IIa, IV, others)
      5. Mucopolysaccharidoses
      6. Hemoglobinopathies (SS disease and others)
      7. True connective tissue disorders (Ehlers-Danlos, Marfan's, osteogenesis imperfecta, pseudoxanthoma elasticum, and others)
      8. Hemochromatosis
      9. Wilson's disease (hepatolenticular degeneration)
      10. Ochronosis (alkaptonuria)
      11. Gaucher's disease
      12. Others
   C. Endocrine diseases
      1. Diabetes mellitus
      2. Acromegaly
      3. Hyperparathyroidism
      4. Thyroid disease (hyperthyroidism, hypothyroidism, thyroiditis)
      5. Others
   D. Immunodeficiency diseases, primary immunodeficiency, acquired immunodeficiency syndrome (AIDS)
   E. Other hereditary disorders
      1. Arthrogryposis multiplex congenita
      2. Hypermobility syndromes
      3. Myositis ossificans progressiva
VI. Neoplasms
   A. Primary (e.g., synovioma, synoviosarcoma)
   B. Metastatic
   C. Multiple myeloma
   D. Leukemia and lymphoma
   E. Villonodular synovitis
   F. Osteochondromatosis
   G. Other
VII. Neuropathic disorders
   A. Charcot joints
   B. Compression neuropathies
      1. Peripheral entrapment (carpal tunnel syndrome and others)
      2. Radiculopathy
      3. Spinal stenosis
   C. Reflex sympathetic dystrophy
   D. Others
VIII. Bone, periosteal, and cartilage disorders associated with articular manifestations
   A. Osteoporosis
      1. Generalized
      2. Localized (regional and transient)
   B. Osteomalacia
   C. Hypertrophic osteoarthropathy
   D. Diffuse idiopathic skeletal hyperostosis (includes ankylosing vertebral hyperostosis—Forestier's disease)
   E. Osteitis
      1. Generalized (osteitis deformans—Paget's disease of bone)
      2. Localized (osteitis condensans ilii; osteitis pubis)
   F. Osteonecrosis
   G. Osteochondritis (osteochondritis dissecans)
   H. Bone and joint dysplasias
   I. Slipped capital femoral epiphysis
   J. Costochondritis (includes Tietze's syndrome)
   K. Osteolysis and chondrolysis
   L. Osteomyelitis
IX. Nonarticular rheumatism
   A. Myofascial pain syndromes
      1. Generalized (fibrositis, fibromyalgia)
      2. Regional
   B. Low back pain and intervertebral disc disorders
   C. Tendinitis (tenosynovitis) and/or bursitis
      1. Subacromial/subdeltoid bursitis
      2. Bicipital tendinitis, tenosynovitis
      3. Olecranon bursitis
      4. Epicondylitis, medial or lateral humeral
      5. DeQuervain's tenosynovitis
      6. Adhesive capsulitis of the shoulder (frozen shoulder)
      7. Trigger finger
      8. Other
   D. Ganglion cysts

E. Fasciitis
F. Chronic ligament and muscle strain
G. Vasomotor disorders
    1. Erythromelalgia
    2. Raynaud's disease or phenomenon
H. Miscellaneous pain syndromes (includes weather sensitivity, psychogenic rheumatism)

X. Miscellaneous disorders
A. Disorders frequently associated with arthritis
    1. Trauma (the result of direct trauma)
    2. Internal derangement of joints
    3. Pancreatic disease
    4. Sarcoidosis
    5. Palindromic rheumatism
    6. Intermittent hydrarthrosis
    7. Erythema nodosum
    8. Hemophilia
B. Other conditions
    1. Multicentric reticulohistiocytosis (nodular panniculitis)
    2. Familial Mediterranean fever
    3. Goodpasture's syndrome
    4. Chronic active hepatitis
    5. Drug-induced rheumatic syndromes
    6. Dialysis-associated syndromes
    7. Foreign body synovitis
    8. Acne and hydradenitis suppurativa
    9. Pustulosis palmaris et plantaris
    10. Sweet's syndrome
    11. Other

INDEX

A

B

C

Q

R

T